INTERVENTIONAL RADIOLOGY PROCEDURE MANUAL

INTERVENTIONAL RADIOLOGY PROCEDURE MANUAL

MICHAEL A. BRAUN, M.D.

Chairman, Department of Medical Imaging
St. Mary's Hospital
Milwaukee, Wisconsin
Former Assistant Professor, Department of Radiology
Northwestern University Medical School
Former Associate, Section of Vascular and Interventional Radiology
Department of Radiology, Northwestern Memorial Hospital
Chicago, Illinois

ALBERT A. NEMCEK, JR., M.D.

Associate Professor, Department of Radiology
Northwestern University Medical School
Chief, Section of Ultrasonography
Associate, Section of Vascular and Interventional Radiology
Department of Radiology, Northwestern Memorial Hospital
Chicago, Illinois

ROBERT L. VOGELZANG, M.D.

Professor, Department of Radiology
Northwestern University Medical School
Chief, Section of Vascular and Interventional Radiology
Department of Radiology, Northwestern Memorial Hospital
Chicago, Illinois

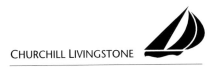

CHURCHILL LIVINGSTONE

New York, Edinburgh, London, Madrid, Melbourne, San Francisco, Tokyo

Library of Congress Cataloging-in-Publication Data

Braun, Michael A. (Michael Andrew). 1959-
    Interventional radiology procedure manual / Michael A. Braun,
Albert A. Nemcek, Jr., Robert L. Vogelzang.
        p.   cm.
    Includes bibliographical references and index.
    ISBN 0-443-07921-8 (alk. paper)
    1. Interventional radiology.   I. Nemcek, Albert A.
II. Vogelzang, Robert L.   III. Title.
    [DNLM: 1. Radiography, Interventional—methods. WN 200 B825i
1997]
RD33.55.B73   1997
617′.05—dc21
DNLM/DLC
for Library of Congress   96-53121
                                                            CIP

© **Churchill Livingstone Inc. 1997**

Distributed in the United Kingdom by Churchill Livingstone, Robert Stevenson House, 1–3 Baxter's Place, Leith Walk, Edinburgh EH1 3AF, and by associated companies, branches, and representatives throughout the world.

Medical knowledge is constantly changing. As new information becomes available, changes in treatment, procedures, equipment and the use of drugs become necessary. The editors/authors/contributors and the publishers have, as far as it is possible, taken care to ensure that the information given in this text is accurate and up to date. However, readers are strongly advised to confirm that the information, especially with regard to drug usage, complies with the latest legislation and standards of practice.

The Publishers have made every effort to trace the copyright holders for borrowed material. If they have inadvertently overlooked any, they will be pleased to make the necessary arrangements at the first opportunity.

Acquisitions Editor: *Michael J. Houston*
Assistant Editor: *Ann Ruzycka*
Production Editor: *Paul Bernstein*
Production Supervisor: *Laura Mosberg Cohen*
Desktop Coordinator: *Kathy Jo Dunayer*
Cover Design: *Jeannette Jacobs*

Printed in the United States of America

First published in 1997   7   6   5   4   3   2   1

*To our wives and families
for their patience and understanding
while we pursued this work.*

Preface

Over the past several years the radiologic disciplines of angiography and cross-sectional interventional radiology have solidified into the established field of interventional radiology. The popularity of this field has been fueled by widespread acceptance of minimally invasive techniques. The combination of ultrasonography and fluoroscopy expanded radiology into the areas of venous access and pleural drainage. The new technology of hydrophilic coatings and coaxial microcatheters has facilitated superselective catheterizations. These technologic advances, combined with enthusiasm and creativity on the part of radiologists, has led to the development of several new procedures. In particular the introduction of stents has made possible both percutaneous creation of a portosystemic shunt and durable repair of vascular occlusive disease. Such new procedures and rapid technologic changes have made this an exciting time for experienced radiologists to practice. But it has placed a greater demand on residents and fellows to learn not only the fundamental skills of angiography but also these new techniques.

The *Interventional Radiology Procedure Manual* grew out of the Northwestern Memorial Hospital radiology residents procedure manual. It was written both to teach the fundamental skills necessary to practice interventional radiology and assemble information on the newer techniques that were not covered in the classic textbooks on angiography. The newer techniques are discussed in greater detail relative to the traditional angiographic procedures. The book focuses on the indications for a given procedure and details the technical steps necessary to accomplish the indicated goal. It is intended as an introduction to the discipline of interventional radiology and is written in a concise style so that it can be read while on a busy interventional radiology service. Emphasis is placed on covering the wide spectrum of procedures performed, rather than on a detailed discussion of pathophysiology and procedural outcomes. Current references are listed at the end of each chapter to guide further reading. The *Interventional Radiology Procedure Manual* is dedicated to both the novice and the experienced practitioner of interventional radiology.

Michael A. Braun, M.D.
Albert A. Nemcek, Jr., M.D.
Robert L. Vogelzang, M.D.

Acknowledgments

Positive feedback from residents, fellows, and colleagues has inspired us to write this work. We wish to thank Dorothy Woodward for her considerable help in manuscript preparation. The line art is the work of both Sheila Macomber of Northwestern Memorial Hospital Media Services and Robert Fenn of Medical Center Graphics, Inc. We would like to thank the authors and publishers of previously published illustrations for their permission to use the illustrations in this book. We acknowledge that many of the illustrations in this text are modifications of manufacturers' instructional illustrations or modifications of previously published work. We thank these individuals and companies. Robert Beres and Theresa Braun provided proofreading and much helpful advice.

Fundamental Methods

This section discusses the evaluation and preparation of patients before a procedure is performed. It is important to be familiar with the patient's medical problems and past surgical history to tailor the procedure appropriately. Patient acceptance of procedures is dramatically improved when anxiety and pain are relieved. This requires knowledge of the principles of conscious sedation and other drugs commonly used during procedures. Successful performance of procedures requires familiarity with the tools of the trade and the basic skills for using the available devices. The techniques and methods of diagnostic vascular studies with emphasis on newer procedures are detailed in Chapter 5. A thorough understanding of complications is a necessary part of quality assurance and good medical care.

Patient Evaluation MICHAEL A. BRAUN

Clinical Evaluation of Peripheral Vascular Disease

An understanding of the pathophysiology of atherosclerosis helps in the evaluation of patients with peripheral vascular disease. An atheroma is a fibrofatty plaque that can narrow the lumen of a vessel or secondarily thrombose. Atherosclerosis is responsible for both occlusive disease and aneurysmal dilatation. Atherosclerotic plaques and subsequent stenosis occur at bifurcations and areas of fixation where shear forces and turbulent flow cause endothelial injury. Typical locations are the major aortic branch vessel takeoffs, the aortic bifurcation, the common iliac bifurcation, the common femoral artery bifurcation, and the superficial femoral artery at Hunter's canal. The abdominal aorta is more frequently involved by atherosclerotic disease than the thoracic aorta due to the absence of vasa vasorum within the abdominal aorta.

Occlusive atherosclerotic vascular disease follows certain patterns. The arterial supply to the lower extremity can be divided into aortoiliac inflow, femoropopliteal outflow, and tibioperoneal runoff circulations. Isolated aortoiliac disease is typically found in 40- to 60-year-old smokers. Femoropopliteal occlusive disease is most common in 60- to 80-year-old patients. Atherosclerotic disease is accelerated in patients with diabetes and chronic renal failure. Distribution of the disease is in the smaller vessels below the knee, with sparing of the aortoiliac segment. The profunda femoris is the most important collateral vessel to the leg.

The herald symptom of peripheral vascular stenotic disease is claudication. Claudication is reported as a cramping pain in the calves, which is induced by exercise. It is quantified by the amount of distance a patient can walk before encountering symptoms. Claudication is relieved by rest and reflects muscle ischemia that occurs distal to an arterial stenosis that limits blood flow. The significance of the patient's claudication is relative to the patient's activity level and age. Claudication must be life-style inhibiting before an intervention can be contemplated. Conservative treatment includes cessation of smoking and a regimen of walking. Exercise programs can develop enough collaterals to allow the patient an adequate life-style. The location of the claudication is somewhat helpful in determining the level of the lesion. Claudication symptoms generally occur in the muscle group immediately distal to a stenosis. One would expect aortoiliac disease to manifest as pain in the buttocks or thighs, but 75 percent of patients with iliac stenosis have calf claudication. Thus, claudication is not a reliable indicator of the precise level of the patient's stenosis. Impotence can be the result of aortoiliac disease. Leriche's syndrome is intermittent claudication, impotence, and back or buttock pain.

Rest pain is continuous pain on the dorsum of the foot. It is worse when the patient is lying flat at night and is reduced by dangling the leg over the edge of the bed. It can awaken the patient from sleep. Rest pain is a signal that the patient has converted a stenotic lesion into an occlusive lesion. This puts the patient in the category of having a threatened limb.

The clinical signs of severe peripheral vascular disease are ischemic ulcerations or nonhealing wounds occurring on the affected extremity. Ischemic foot ulcers occur on the distal portion (forefoot) of the affected extremity while venous stasis ulcers occur near the malleoli. The presence of a nonhealing foot ulcer implies that the patient has multiple segments of occlusive peripheral vascular disease or has concomitant peripheral vascular disease and diabetes. Other clinical signs of severe vascular insufficiency are absence of hair, dry skin, atrophic skin, muscle atrophy, diminished temperature, and poor capillary refill. Elevatory pallor and dependent rubor indicate severe vascular occlusive disease.

The blue-toe-syndrome consists of palpable femoral and pedal pulses, with tiny purple petechiae present on the distal portions of the toes and feet. The petechial patches are end arterial infarctions caused by microemboli. Bilateral blue-toe-syndrome implies that the source is above the aortic bifurcation.

The signs and symptoms of an acute arterial occlusion are "the five P's": pain, pallor, paresthesias, paralysis, and pulselessness. Acute vascular insufficiency may be due to an embolus or a thrombosis of an underlying atherosclerotic stenosis. Sudden onset and a cardiac history helps differentiate embolic from thrombotic occlusions. Most emboli are cardiac in origin, lodge at bifurcations, and involve the lower extremity 10 times more frequently than the upper extremity. Irreversible injury may occur after 6 hours if left untreated. Urgent intervention is necessary when all these signs and symptoms are present. The mortality rate of acute ischemia is high at 20 to 30 percent due to coexistent cardiopulmonary disease. Thrombolytic therapy is not recommended when paralysis and paresthesias are present.

The natural history of claudication is relatively benign. Only 5 to 10 percent of patients have progressive disease leading to limb loss in 10 years. Conservative treatment of smoking cessation and exercise can stabilize or improve the symptoms in the majority of patients. The major cause of mortality is from coexisting cardiac and cerebrovascular disease. Patients with rest pain and ischemic ulcerations are considered to have threatened limbs and will lose the extremity unless an intervention is performed.

The symptoms of venous insufficiency are aching, swelling, and night cramps. Venous claudication is described as a heaviness or aching discomfort aggravated by a period of standing. The symptoms are relieved by elevation and result from the increased weight of the extremity caused by the increase in blood volume and interstitial fluid. The signs are brawny induration, edema, dermatitis, and ulceration. Brawny induration refers to the brown pigmentation caused by hemosiderin deposition and the woody feeling to the chronically swollen leg. Venous stasis ulcers are found in the lower third of the leg adjacent to the malleoli.

Noninvasive Evaluation of Peripheral Vascular Disease

The clinical symptoms indicate the significance of the disease. Noninvasive studies were developed to provide a reliable and repeatable evaluation of atherosclerotic disease. Noninvasive studies can predict more accurately the level of the vascular disease and provide objective criteria for assessing the outcome of interventional and surgical revascularizations. Single and multilevel disease distribution can be distinguished by noninvasive tests. Noninvasive studies are used to screen symptomatic patients and can be performed postexercise to document the changes brought on by exertion. The noninvasive test complements angiography by determining whether a borderline stenosis is hemodynamically significant and which stenosis is significant when multiple lesions are present.

The ankle-brachial index (ABI) is the ratio between the brachial systolic blood pressure and the systolic calf blood pressure measured by a continuous wave Doppler device. The normal value is usually equal to or greater than 1.0. Ranges between 0.6 and 0.9 imply underlying stenotic lesions and are associated with claudication symptoms. A value above 0.5 implies a single level of an occlusion. An ABI less than 0.5 implies multiple levels of occlusions or a combination of an inflow stenosis and an outflow occlusion. The normal toe systolic pressure should be approximately 80 to 90 percent of the brachial pressure and is useful when the ankle vessels are noncompressible from calcification. A drop to less than 60 mmHg in the ankle pressure following exercise confirms claudication. An ankle pressure less than 40 mmHg and an ABI less than 0.35 correlate with severe rest pain. Diabetic foot ulcers are unlikely to heal if the ankle pressure is less than 80 mmHg and nondiabetic ulcers if the pressure is less than 55 mmHg. Foot ulcers are unlikely to heal if the toe pressure is less than 30 mmHg but likely to heal if the pressure is greater than 30 mmHg.

The segmental blood flow study can determine the relative location of the arterial disease and the individual significance of multiple lesions. The test consists of segmental evaluations of the pressure and Doppler waveform measurements in the extremity. Typically, four cuffs are positioned and inflated in the high thigh, above knee, below knee, and ankle locations. The arterial waveform is measured at the dorsalis pedis or posterior tibialis arteries at the ankle. The normal peripheral arterial waveform is triphasic. The waveform consists of a sharp systolic upsweep, a brief reverse component in early diastole, and a low forward flow in the late diastole (Fig. 1.1). A mild to moderate proximal arterial stenosis will cause an absence of the reversed flow in diastole. A severe stenosis will cause dampening and widening of the systolic waveform. Occlusive disease causes the waveform to be increasingly dampened and monophasic. The waveforms are measurements of upstream arterial disease. In this manner, the level and quantifiable hemodynamic significance of the arterial disease can be estimated. A gradient of 20 to 30 mmHg between segments indicates intervening disease. The opposite leg can be used as a comparison. Claudication can be induced by treadmill exercise or reactive hyperemia to measure and quantify the exertion necessary to provoke the ischemia. Acute and chronic ischemia have been classified into different categories based on the severity of the disease by Rutherford and Becker. The categories are stratified by clinical criteria and noninvasive assessments to provide a uniform definition of vascular disease status (Tables 1.1 and 1.2).

Preprocedure Laboratory and Medical Evaluation

The patient's history and physical examination should be thoroughly reviewed. The patient's vascular history, current pulse status, symptomatology caused by the peripheral vascular disease, and results of noninvasive blood flow testing help tailor the study to the individual patient. Any previous angiographic studies or cross-sectional imaging studies should be reviewed to help plan the access. The symptoms determine the significance and justify the need for the procedure. This formulates the indication for the procedure. The clinical symptoms and noninvasive testing help predict the level and extent of the peripheral vascular disease. Each procedure should be approached as both a diagnostic study and potentially a therapeutic intervention.

The patient's medical, physical, and emotional status need to be evaluated to assess the patient's ability to withstand the procedure and any possible complications. The evaluation should determine whether the

patient would tolerate an operation if a complication arose necessitating surgery. Atherosclerosis is a systemic disease, and multiple organs other than the legs or arms are often affected. Concomitant coronary artery and cerebral vascular diseases are frequent. Patients frequently are smokers and may have emphysema. The patient's renal status should be evaluated before the administration of radiographic contrast material. The patient's allergy history should be ascertained. A review of the identified cardiac risk factors (smoking, age, family history, cholesterol level, male, hypertension, and diabetes) will help organize a pertinent review of systems.

Before the performance of a procedure, there should be direct patient–physician interaction. Patients (and families) will expect some familiarity with their diagnosis, past medical management, and therapeutic plan. This engenders comfortable conversation and builds confidence. Following this introduction, additional questions are asked to assess the patient's medical status and ability to tolerate the procedure. From the patient's perspective, a routine test is an anxiety-provoking experience. The procedure should be explained in a confident and reassuring manner. This will help alleviate any unnecessary apprehension by the patient. During this interaction, the procedure, alternatives, risks, and benefits should be explained to the patient. This approach establishes a positive patient–physician rapport and satisfies the elements of informed consent. Besides obtaining consent for a diagnostic procedure, consent for therapeutic intervention should be obtained. Any patient who is having an angiogram should have consent obtained for a potential angioplasty or thrombolysis. The patient should be informed that different routes of vascular access (femoral, brachial, or transvenous) are routine and may be utilized. Complications and side effects should be explained to the patient so that the patient is informed but not frightened.

Pertinent laboratory results to review before performing any procedure are the patient's prothrombin time (PT), partial thromboplastin time (PTT), platelet count, hemoglobin, blood urea nitrogen (BUN), and creatinine levels. An abnormality of a coagulation value should direct one to determine whether the coagulopathy is reversible or nonreversible. If the elevated coagulation value is due to heparin or coumadin anticoagulation, the coagulopathy should be corrected before an elective diagnostic procedure is performed. If the pro-

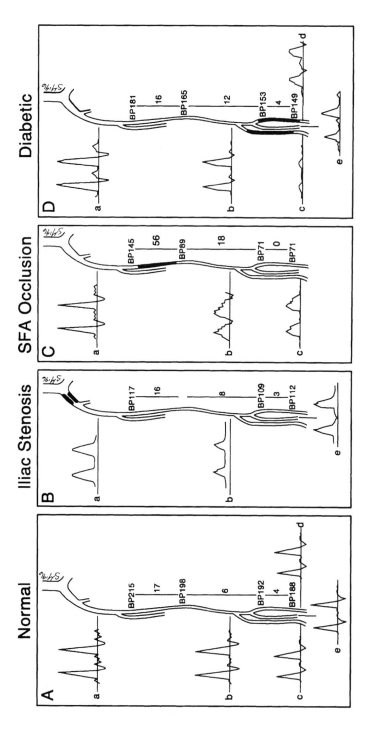

Figure 1.1 *Example of noninvasive blood flow study of the lower extremity.* (**A**) *Normal blood flow examination with triphasic waveforms. The high thigh blood pressure is normally greater than the other pressures due to the relative smaller size of the blood pressure cuff compared with the diameter of the upper thigh.* (**B**) *An aortoiliac stenosis causes loss of reverse flow in early diastole on the waveform and a gradient between the brachial artery and high thigh pressure cuff.* (**C**) *A femoral popliteal occlusion causes a gradient between the high thigh and above knee cuff of > 30 mmHg. The waveform below the occlusion has loss of reverse flow in a diastole and blunting of the systolic peak.* (**D**) *Infrapopliteal occlusive disease is inferred by a combination of abnormal waveforms on the tibial arteries and a pressure gradient. The presence of diabetic-related vascular calcifications can cause a false negative test result. a, femoral; b, popliteal; c, anterior tibialis; d, posterior tibialis; e, dorsalis pedis. (Modified from Gerlock AJ, Giyanani VL, Krebs C: Applications of Noninvasive Vascular Techniques. WB Saunders, Philadelphia, 1988, with permission)*

Table 1.1 *Peripheral vascular disease: clinical categories of acute limb ischemia*

Category	Description	Capillary Return	Muscle Weakness	Sensory Loss	Doppler Signals	
					Arterial	Venous
Viable	Not immediately threatened	Intact	None	None	Audible ankle pressure > 30 mmHg	Audible
Threatened	Salvageable if promptly treated	Intact, slow	Mild, partial	Mild, incomplete	Inaudible	Audible
Irreversible	Major tissue loss, amputation required regardless of treatment	Absent (marbling)	Profound, paralysis (rigor)	Profound, anesthetic	Inaudible	Inaudible

Table 1.2 *Peripheral vascular disease: clinical categories of chronic limb ischemia*

Grade	Category	Clinical Description	Objective Criteria
	0	Asymptomatic, no hemodynamically significant occlusive disease	Normal results of treadmill (5 minutes at 2 mph on a 12° incline)/stress test
I	1	Mild claudication	Treadmill exercise completed, postexercise ankle pressure is > 50 mmHg but > 25 mmHg less than normal
	2	Moderate claudication	Symptoms between those of categories 1 and 3
	3	Severe claudication	Treadmill exercise cannot be completed, postexercise ankle pressure > 50 mmHg
II	4	Ischemic rest pain	Resting ankle pressure >/= 40 mmHg, flat or barely pulsatile ankle or metatarsal plethysmographic tracing, toe pressure < 30 mmHg
III	5	Minor tissue loss, nonhealing ulcer, focal gangrene with diffuse pedal ischemia	Resting ankle pressure < 60 mmHg, ankle or metatarsal plethysmographic tracing flat or barely pulsatile, toe pressure < 40 mmHg
	6	Major tissue loss, extending above transmetatarsal level, functional foot no longer salvageable	Same as for category 5

cedure is needed on an emergency basis, a single wall vessel puncture should be performed by the most experienced operator. Special care will be required when removing the catheter. Minimizing catheter exchanges may help reduce the incidence of bleeding. An option in this situation is to place a sheath within the artery, which can be removed after the coagulopathy is corrected. If a coagulopathy is discovered and there is no obvious reason for it, a hematology consultation should be obtained before performing an elective procedure. If the patient's platelet count is below 75,000, there is a higher risk of a bleeding complication. For an elective procedure the platelet count should be greater than 50,000 and preferably greater than 75,000. If the platelet count is less than 50,000, arrange to have platelets available for transfusion.

Renal insufficiency must be carefully screened for because of the large volumes of contrast utilized in certain angiographic procedures. The only proven prevention of contrast nephropathy is adequate preprocedure hydration with 1 to 1.5 L of 0.45 percent saline. Other proposed treatments for prevention of contrast nephrotoxicity are sublingual nifedipine 10 mg, intravenous dopamine 3 µg/min continuous infusion, and postprocedure mannitol 12.5 g. Mannitol should be given intravenously near the end of the procedure to promote an osmotic diuresis. If the patient has moderate renal insufficiency (creatinine between 2 and 5), it is important to review the patient's history and possibly suggest an alternative test such as a magnetic resonance angiogram, color duplex ultrasound, or CO_2 angiogram. For patients who have chronic renal failure, the contrast load can be removed by hemodialysis. The study should be coordinated with the dialysis laboratory.

A history of an allergic reaction to contrast material requires further investigation. If the patient has had hives, pruritus, or other similar mild contrast reactions, premedication with steroids and Benadryl will usually prevent a second allergic response. The allergy premedication is 50 mg of prednisone given 13, 7, and 1 hour before the procedure. Diphenhydramine, 50 mg, and ephedrine, 25 mg, are given orally or intravenously 1 hour before the procedure. For patients who have had severe anaphylactic reactions, it is best to suggest an alternative procedure that may be utilized to gain the same information without giving intravenous contrast. If no alternatives are suitable, the procedure should be performed during regular working hours following an allergic preparation. It is advisable to have an anesthesiologist monitor the patient who has had a previous episode of bronchospasm.

Patients with insulin-dependent diabetes require special management of their insulin and glucose requirements the day of the procedure. Because preprocedure oral intake is eliminated, a change is required in the patient's insulin administration. Patients with diabetes should be given dextrose intravenously the morning of the angiogram. The standard liter solution of D5W contains approximately 200 calories of energy. The patient's total daily insulin dose is calculated and one-half of the total daily dose is given in NPH insulin in the morning. The remaining one-half total daily dose is given in the early evening before the patient eats dinner. An afternoon fasting blood glucose level is measured.

Suggested Readings

Cohen JR: Vascular Surgery for the House Officer. Williams & Wilkins, Baltimore, 1992

Consigny PM: Pathogenesis of atherosclerosis. AJR 164:553, 1995

Darcy MD: Lower extremity arteriography: current approach and techniques. Radiology 178:615, 1991

Gerlock AJ, Giyanani VL, Krebs C: Applications of Noninvasive Vascular Techniques. WB Saunders, Philadelphia, 1988

Greenberger PA, Patterson R: The prevention of immediate generalized repeated reactions to radiocontrast media in high-risk patients. J Allergy Clin Immunol 87:867, 1991

Kim D, Orron DE: Peripheral Vascular Imaging and Intervention. Mosby-Year Book, St. Louis, 1992

Lasser EC, Berry CC, Talner LB et al: Pretreatment with corticosteroids to alleviate reactions to intravenous contrast material. N Engl J Med 317:845, 1987

Murphy TP, Dorfman GS, Becker GJ: Use of preprocedural tests by interventional radiologists. Radiology 186:213, 1993

Perler BA: Hypercoagulability and the hypercoagulability syndromes. AJR 164:559, 1995

Rutherford RB, Becker GB: Standards for evaluating and reporting the results of surgical and percutaneous therapy for peripheral arterial disease. J Vasc Interv Radiol 2:169, 1991

Silverman SG, Mueller PR, Pfister RC: Hemostatic evaluation before abdominal interventions: an overview and proposal. AJR 154:233, 1990

Solomon R: Effects of saline, mannitol, and furosemide on acute decreases in renal function induced by radiocontrast agents. N Engl J Med 331:1416, 1994

vanSonnenberg E, Barton JB, Wittich GR: Radiology and the law, with an emphasis on interventional radiology. Radiology 187:297, 1993

Zierler RE, Strandness DE Jr: Nonimaging physiologic tests for assessment of extremity arterial disease. p. 201. In Zweibel WJ: Introduction to Vascular Ultrasound. 3rd Ed. WB Saunders, Philadelphia, 1992

Medications MICHAEL A. BRAUN

Interventional procedures are performed with patients under conscious sedation. During all procedures, the patient's electrocardiogram, blood pressure, and pulse oximetry are continuously monitored. It is a standard of care to administer conscious sedation by intravenous access in adults. Drugs given intravenously have a more predictable onset and duration. It is important to maintain concern about the patient and their well-being during performance of the examination. Carefully monitor the patient's comfort level and provide additional sedatives and narcotics when necessary. Careful monitoring of the respiratory and cardiac status of the patient is vital and should be performed by both the physician and nurse monitoring the case.

Analgesics and Sedatives

Conscious sedation is best achieved by a combination of an opiate narcotic and a sedative/hypnotic. It is safest to administer a low dose and titrate upward to manage pain and comfort. Doses should be reduced in elderly patients. The sedation regimen must be tailored to each patient's needs, underlying medical condition, and procedure performed. Conscious sedation is administered and monitored by the nursing staff under the supervision of the physician.

Conscious sedation is not a substitute for good local infiltrative anesthesia. Lidocaine is the most widely used amide-type agent that produces loss of pain sensation by blocking nerve conduction. The maximum subcutaneous dosage is 7 mg/kg or less than 500 mg in a healthy adult. Two percent lidocaine contains 20 mg/ml. The maximum dose in a 70 kg adult is 25 ml of 2 percent lidocaine. The duration of action is 1½ to 2 hours but is prolonged in patients with liver failure. Bupivacaine is an amide-type agent that is four times more potent and three times longer in duration than lidocaine. Bupivacaine is used for regional nerve blocks. Patients with adverse reactions to lidocaine can be given the ester-type agents procaine, pontocaine, or chloroprocaine.

Opiates provide analgesia by blunting the response to painful stimulation, causing drowsiness and clouding mentation. The synthetic opiate fentanyl has a short duration of action (30 to 60 minutes) and is more potent than morphine. Fentanyl has fewer negative cardiac side effects and causes less sphincter of Oddi spasm than morphine. This makes fentanyl the agent of choice for conscious sedation in interventional procedures. Fentanyl is 100 times more potent than morphine (fentanyl 100 µg equals morphine 10 mg or Demerol 75 mg). It is best to titrate the dose of fentanyl by using incremental small doses of 12.5 to 25 µg delivered intravenously. Fentanyl is metabolized in the liver and must be used with care in patients with hepatic insufficiency. It can cause respiratory depression and muscular rigidity in doses as low as 50 to 100 µg. Minor respiratory depression can be readily treated by supplemental oxygen delivery (pulse oxygenation less than 95 percent). Fentanyl can be reversed with Narcan. The dose of naloxone (Narcan) is 0.4 to 0.8 mg IV. If there is no response in 5 minutes, a second dose of 0.2 mg should be given. The half-life of Narcan is short but parallels the half-life of fentanyl.

The benzodiazepine midazolam (Versed) produces sedation by causing amnesia and relieving anxiety. It has anticonvulsant activity, but no analgesic properties. Versed is metabolized in the liver and is twice as potent per milligram as diazepam (Valium). Versed is delivered intravenously in titrated increments of 1 to 3 mg. Side effects are respiratory depression, venoirritation, and paradoxical hyperstimulation. Versed can be reversed using flumazenil (Romazicon). The recommended initial dosage of Romazicon is 0.2 mg IV over 15 seconds. If the desired level of consciousness is not obtained after waiting an additional 45 seconds, a second dose of 0.2 mg can be injected and repeated up to four times at 60 second intervals when necessary.

Vasodilators

Several vasodilators are used in the angiography suite. Nifedipine is a calcium-channel blocking agent that produces relaxation of arterial smooth muscles and is commonly used to prevent prophylactically vascular spasm produced by catheters and guidewires. It is the drug of choice for temporarily reducing high blood pressure. Nifedipine is delivered by placing 10 mg sublingually. The onset of an effect occurs in 10 to 15 minutes.

Papaverine is a direct smooth muscle relaxant. Traditionally, it has been used in infusional therapy for mesenteric ischemia. Papaverine is administered in a 30 mg bolus and then infused at rates of 1 to 3 mg/min.

Nitroglycerin is a direct smooth muscle dilator that may be utilized for preventing catheter- or guidewire-induced vasospasm. Nitroglycerin is injected intravenously or intra-arterially in doses of 50 to 100 μg. It should be diluted in normal saline to provide 100 to 200 μg in 5 to 10 ml of saline. Onset of the vasodilatory effect is rapid and transient. Diagnostic angiography following vasodilatation should be performed within 15 to 30 seconds after injection.

Tolazoline (Priscoline) is a potent vasodilator. The vasodilatory effect is used to improve flow from the arterial to the venous vascular beds for opacification of the portal system. The vasodilatory effect is used to optimally visualize the small vessels within the hand or treat catheter- or guidewire-induced vasospasm. The dose of tolazoline is 25 mg diluted in 10 ml of saline injected slowly over 2 minutes to provide maximum effect. Maximal vasodilatation occurs 5 minutes after injection. Contrast material volumes and rates for diagnostic studies should be increased in response to the vasodilatory effect. Side effects are common including flushing, hypotension, and extreme warmth of the extremity.

Vasoconstrictors

Vasopressin (Pitressin) produces marked splanchnic vasoconstriction and is used in the control of gastrointestinal bleeding, especially for gastric mucosal or colonic diverticular sources. Vasopressin is infused directly into the main trunk of the bleeding visceral artery starting at a rate of 0.2 U/min. The infusion should be titrated to the smallest rate that produces a response angiographically. The maximum infusion rate that can be used is 0.4 U/min. Vasopressin should be used with care in patients who have coronary artery disease. Cardiac arrhythmias, especially bradycardia, may develop. Vasopressin has an antidiuretic effect and may cause electrolyte disturbances and fluid retention.

Anticoagulants

Heparin is used routinely in all angiography flush solutions at a concentration of 5 to 10 U/ml saline. Routine anticoagulation with heparin during angiography is not performed. Heparin should be administered when there is a risk of thrombosis during a vascular procedure and whenever a catheter or guidewire traverses a stenotic vessel and impedes flow. It is routine to give a bolus infusion of 3,000 to 5,000 units before the crossing of a stenotic lesion when performing transluminal angioplasty. The half-life of heparin is approximately 45 to 90 minutes. It varies with the administered dose and is prolonged in patients with renal and hepatic dysfunction. The effects of heparin can be reversed with protamine sulfate; 10 mg of protamine reverses 1,000 units of heparin. At the conclusion of a procedure, an activated clotting time (ACT) can be obtained to quantify the amount of residual anticoagulation. A normal ACT value is 170 seconds or less. If the ACT level is greater than 200 seconds, reversal with protamine should be performed. Protamine is administered slowly for 1 to 2 minutes. Protamine should be used with caution in diabetic patients who have received long-acting insulin preparations (i.e., NPH insulin) because there is a 15 percent chance of an allergic-type reaction. Low molecular weight heparin, which is undergoing clinical investigation, is administered subcutaneously once a day and does not require monitoring of partial thromboplastin time (PTT). It can be given on an outpatient basis and thus eliminates the cost of hospitalization.

Antibiotic Prophylaxis

Prophylactic antibiotics given before a procedure reduce the septic complications of surgery. Antibiotic prophylaxis is designed to provide adequate serum levels of antibiotic to ameliorate the consequences of pro-

Table 2.1 *Antibiotic prophylaxis in interventional radiology procedures*

Procedure	Organism	Recommended Drug	Dosage and Duration
Diagnostic and therapeutic angiography	None	None	—
Diagnostic angiography, angioplasty, vascular stents, IVC filters, thrombolysis, TIPS			
Biliary tract interventions	*E. coli,* *Klebsiella,* *Enterococcus,* *Pseudo- enterobacter*	Cefoperazone or Ceftizoxime	2 g 12 h × 48 h and then 1 h before further drain manipulations 1 gm q8° × 48°
Percutaneous biliary drainage, percutaneous cholecystostomy, biliary endoprothesis			
Genitourinary interventions			
Percutaneous nephrostomy and nephroureteral stents			
Noninfected	None	Cefazolin Bactrim	1 g IV × 1 dose 160 mg IV × 1 dose
Infected, modify according to prior C & S	*Enterococcus,* *E. coli,* *Proteus,* *Enterobacter*	Ampicillin and Gentamicin	2 g IV q6 h 1.5 mg/kg IV q8 h
Abscess	Multiorganism, gram-negative, anaerobes	Gentamicin and Flagyl	1.5 mg/kg IV 500 mg q8 h IV
Arm port	gram-positive, skin flora	Cefazolin	1 g IV 1° before procedure
PICC line	None	None	—
Endocarditis prophylaxis	*Enterococcus*	Ampicillin and Gentamicin (PCN allergic PTS)	2 g IV q8 h × 2 doses 1.5 mg/kg IV × 1 dose
Biliary, GI, GU, interventional procedures only		Vancomycin	1 g IV × 1
Chemoembolization	Bowel flora	Cefoperizone Flagyl then Ofloxacin Flagyl	2 g IV q12 h × 4 doses 500 mg IV q6 h × 8 doses 400 mg po BID × 5 days 500 mg po TID × 5 days
Splenic embolization	Bowel flora	Cefazolin or Ceftizoxime	1 g IV × 1 dose 1 g IV × 1 dose

Abbreviations: GI, gastrointestinal; GU, genitourinary; IVC, inferior vena cava; PAS, periodic acid-Schiff; PCN, penicillin; PICC, peripherally inserted central catheter; TIPS, transjugular intrahepatic portosystemic shunt

cedural-related bacteremia. Distention of abscess cavities and mucosal breaks allow communication of contaminated spaces with the venous, arterial, and lymphatic systems. This causes systemic spread of bacteria and endotoxins. The timing and route of prophylaxis are important. The drug should be given intravenously 30 to 60 minutes before the procedure. The duration of prophylaxis is more controversial and often prescribed arbitrarily. Prophylaxis is usually a single dose of drug. Prophylactic therapy in high-risk patients may require a longer duration of treatment. An example is the 48-hour course of intravenous antibiotics given to chemoembolization patients.

General diagnostic and most therapeutic angiography does not require antibiotic prophylaxis. Antibiotic prophylaxis is given before placing implanted venous access ports but not peripherally inserted central catheter (PICC) lines.

Experience with inferior vena cava (IVC) filters has shown that infection complicating filter placement does not occur. This experience is being extrapolated to intravascular stents. Exceptions are splenic embolizations and hepatic chemoembolization, which both require prophylaxis (Table 2.1).

The infectious complications of biliary interventions are common. Approximately 50 percent of biliary trees are colonized in patients with malignant obstructions and up to 90 percent in patients with common duct stones. The organisms are usually gram-negative enteric bacteria. For prophylaxis of biliary procedures, cefoperazone, 2 g IV every 12 hours, is given for 48 hours and one dose is given before future catheter manipulations. Cefoperazone has only modest antienterococcal activity. It is excreted 75 percent in the liver and 25 percent in the kidney. The biliary excretion is a theoretical advantage to using it in patients with an obstructed biliary system. An alternative choice for biliary intervention prophylaxis is ceftizoxime, 1 g IV every 8 hours. Ceftizoxime has better anaerobic and gram-positive coverage than cefoperazone but no antienterococcal activity. It is not concentrated in the biliary tree.

Genitourinary procedures have fewer infectious complications than biliary procedures. The combination of ampicillin and gentamicin is chosen because of the good enterococcal and gram-negative enteric coverage. In patients with infected urinary tracts, the antibiotic regimen should be culture directed.

Endocarditis prophylaxis is required in patients with rheumatic heart disease or prosthetic valves who are undergoing interventional procedures that may result in iatrogenic bacteremias. Examples are biliary, genitourinary, and gastrointestinal interventions.

Suggested Readings

AMA Drug Evaluations. 5th Ed. American Medical Association, Chicago, 1984

Cragg AH, Smith TP, Berbaum KS, Nakagawa N: Randomized double-blind trial of midazolam/placebo and midazolam/fentanyl for sedation and analgesia in lower extremity angiography. AJR 157:173, 1991

Spies JB, Rosen R, Lebowitz A: Antibiotic prophylaxis in vascular and interventional radiology: a rational approach. Radiology 166:381, 1988

Weinger MB: Principles of conscious sedation. p. 66. The Society of Cardiovascular and Interventional Radiology 19th Annual Meeting Program, March 20–24, 1994, San Diego

Equipment MICHAEL A. BRAUN

A wide variety of equipment is available for performing interventional procedures. A knowledge of the equipment is fundamental for performance of angiographic techniques. One should have a low threshold for using different catheters and guidewires during a problematic catheterization. A slightly different but related catheter shape will often jump into a target vessel that has avoided cannulation with the initially chosen catheter. The time saved is worth the additional cost of the materials. For this reason, it is preferable to stock a wide variety of equipment. Thoughtful management of inventory has taken on increasing importance in this cost-conscious era. Computerized inventory control programs are being developed and tested to aid in inventory control.

The nomenclature for describing needle, catheter, and guidewire size is confusing because each is sized by a different convention of measurement. Needles are sized by gauge, catheters by French size, and guidewires by a thousand fraction of inch diameter. Three French equal 1 mm equal 0.039 inch. The outer diameter of 20 gauge is 0.035 inch. A standard 5 French catheter has a lumen of 0.040 inch and will accept a 3 French catheter or a 0.035 to 0.038 inch guidewire. The tip of catheters are tapered to facilitate insertion through the subcutaneous tissues over a guidewire.

Access Needles

Vascular access needles can be categorized into two sizes. Routinely used 18-gauge needles accept 0.035 to 0.038 inch guidewires; 21-gauge needles are referred to as micropuncture needles and accept 0.018 inch guidewires. The 21-gauge needle takes the smaller diameter mandrel-type wire, which requires an intermediary vascular dilator/sheath to up-size to a 0.035 inch system. Eighteen-gauge needles come with or without stylets. A needle combined with a stylet requires double wall puncture technique. The advantage to double-wall puncture technique is the theoretical reduced rate of causing a dissection or vascular injury. The double-wall technique makes two holes in a vessel and deflects off of heavily calcified vascular walls. Nonstylet needles allow for single-wall puncture and are becoming more popular than stylet needles. The sharpened bevel and hollow lumen easily pass through heavily calcified vessel walls. A single-wall arterial puncture reduces the likelihood of bleeding during thrombolysis.

Guidewires

Guidewires are used to introduce, lead, position, and exchange catheters. A guidewire consists of two basic parts: a mandrel core and a spring guide (Fig. 3.1). The mandrel core is a solid wire that runs the length of the guidewire. The thickness of the mandrel determines the stiffness of the guidewire. The mandrel is tapered at one end, which determines the flexibility of the guidewire. Generally, only the flexible end of the guidewire is placed within the vasculature. The spring guide is a tightly coiled, stainless steel spring. The coils of the spring guide act as a track over which catheters can be advanced. The spring coils are covered with Teflon and heparin to lubricate the surface and reduce the thrombogenicity of the guidewire. The heparin coating lasts for 10 minutes. The J-tip radius may be 1.5, 3, 7.5, and 15 mm in size. A guidewire mandrel can be either fixed or movable within the spring guide. A movable core guidewire tip's flexibility can be varied by moving the inner mandrel core.

Figure 3.1 *Guidewires. (**A**) Fixed core guidewire has a spring coil wound around a central mandrel wire. The distal tip of the mandrel wire may be tapered. (**B**) The flexibility of the tip of a moveable core guidewire can be varied by advancing or withdrawing the core mandrel wire. The length of the taper and the diameter of the taper determine the flexibility of the guidewire tip. (**C**) A 0.018-inch mandrel wire has a solid core body with a spring coil tip for flexibility. (**D**) A tip-deflecting wire can be used to direct catheters across acute bends, reform catheters, or grasp objects. (**E**) The Glidewire has a kink-resistant core of Nitinol covered with a hydrophilic polymer to provide a water-activated slippery surface.*

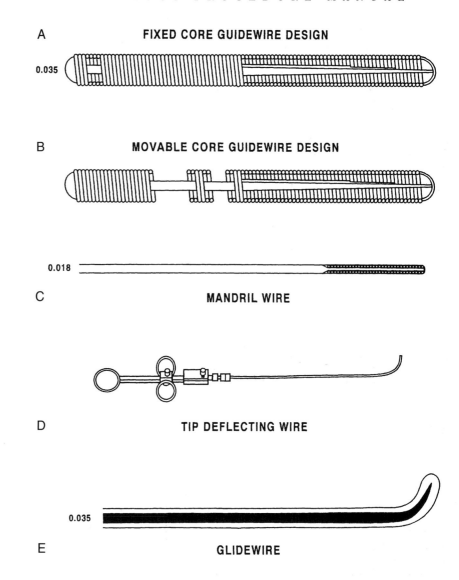

The configuration of the tip helps direct the advancement of a guidewire through a vessel. The J-tipped guidewire is used most often in routine cases. The J-tip helps prevent the guidewire from perforating the intima, causing a dissection. Different tip shapes have evolved to negotiate tortuous, stenotic, or occluded vessels. Angled tip designs are incorporated in guidewires that are used to steer through tortuous vessels or select a desired branch vessel. Angled and straight guidewires have a higher likelihood of causing a dissection and must be carefully advanced under fluoroscopic or roadmap control.

Guidewires are available in lengths of 75, 150, 180, and 260 cm and diameters of 0.018, 0.025, 0.035, and 0.038 inches. In general, the guidewire should be greater than twice the length of the catheter that is being introduced. A 75 cm guidewire is used to introduce short pig-tail drainage catheters. A 150 cm guidewire is used for most vascular procedures in adults because most routine angiographic catheters are 65 to 100 cm long. An example of a routine guidewire is a 0.038 inch diameter, 150 cm long, 3 mm radius safety-J movable core guidewire with heparin coating. A 180 to 260 cm guidewire is used for exchange of long vascular catheters.

The angled-tip Glidewire (Terumo/Medi-Tech, Watertown, MA) has become an invaluable tool for assisting in difficult and superselective catheterizations.

The Glidewire is coated with a hydrophilic material, which is primed by bathing it in saline. The Glidewire must be constantly rewetted to maintain the slippery surface. Its lubricity and torque ability significantly aid in difficult catheterizations. It is very slippery to handle with gloved hands, and special care must be taken when exchanging catheters over this wire. A torque device aids in manipulation and steering of Glidewires. The torque device attaches using a chuck mechanism (Fig. 3.2). Stiff Glidewires have an extra stiff shaft and are unkinkable. They are useful for crossing a steep aortic bifurcation or cannulating a thrombosed vessel.

The Torsional Attenuating Diameter (TAD) wire is used primarily for renal artery angioplasty. The distal end of the wire is tapered from a flexible 0.018 inch diameter tip to a stiff 0.035 inch diameter body. The TAD wire's soft, floppy tip is less likely to elicit spasm within the peripheral renal arteries, and the stiff body of the wire guides angioplasty balloons across the diseased vessel segment. The Wholey wire is 0.035 in diameter and has 1:1 torque ratio with a shapeable tip. It is used for crossing stenotic vessels or selecting a branch vessel. The Bentson wire has a long floppy tip segment that folds readily into a J configuration. It is most useful for traversing tortuous vessels or reversing direction in a vessel (see Fig. 21.5).

The Rosen wire and Amplatz Super Stiff wire have stiff mandrel cores and short segment flexible tips. The Rosen wire is used for catheter exchange and is used during renal angioplasty. The Amplatz Super Stiff was developed for abscess drainage catheter placement and has a stiff, kink-resistant shaft.

A tip-deflecting wire uses a handle attached at the proximal end of the wire to pull on the core mandrel wire, which bends the guidewire distal tip (Fig. 3.1). The amount of tip deflection can be varied from a bend to a coil. The tip can be wrapped around an object for foreign body removal. Other applications are guiding a catheter into an acutely angled vessel takeoff, reforming Simmons catheters, unknotting catheters, and directing a pigtail catheter through a dilated right atrium into the right ventricle.

Small diameter 0.018 inch guidewires are used for small vessel angiography and micropuncture access technique. Micropuncture technique uses a 21-gauge needle to access a vessel and a 0.018 inch guidewire to cannulate the vessel. These wires fit through the smaller lumen of small vessel (sub 4 mm) angioplasty catheters and coaxial microcatheters (Tracker catheters, Target Therapeutics, Fremont, CA).

Catheters

In general, catheters with an outer diameter of 5 French are used for most procedures. These catheters offer the best combination of high flow rate, small outer diameter, and torque control. When additional torque control is necessary, a 6 to 7 French catheter or a braided catheter may be chosen. Braided catheters have a fine wire mesh that reinforces the rigidity of the wall. The increased torquability is achieved at the expense of reduced ability to pass the catheter through tortuous vessels or across an acute bend. A wide variety of catheter tip configurations are available. The exact shape in individual cases will depend on the anticipated anatomy of the vessel to be studied. There are several basic catheter shapes: straight, pigtail, hook, and angled tip catheters.

Straight catheters require little explanation. Straight catheters can have a single end hole or multiple side holes near the distal tip. Straight catheters are used for selective opacification of a vascular tree or for delivery of embolization agents. Flush catheters were developed to inject a high volume of contrast in a tight

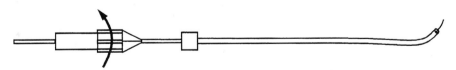

Figure 3.2 *Torque device. The device is attached to a Glidewire 5 to 10 cm from the catheter hub. The torque device increases rotational and directional control of Glidewires. The torque device is useful for pushing a Glidewire through an occluded vessel or selecting the desired branch of vessel bifurcation.*

bolus manner. These catheters prevent the end hole jet effect of a straight catheter, which can injure a vessel. The pigtail catheter is the most common design. Alternative designs are tennis racket and halo catheters (Fig. 3.3). These catheters may be repositioned without a guidewire and can be used to cross the aortic bifurcation or reposition a foreign body.

A hook-shaped catheter is used for selectively catheterizing acutely angled branch vessels such as the branches of the abdominal aorta. These catheters are reformed in the aorta and then pulled into the orifice of the desired vessel. The Neiman visceral catheter (Cook, Bloomington, IN) typifies this design. The Neiman catheter has an approximate 70° bend in its tip (Fig. 3.4). Other examples of these types of catheters are cobra, Simmons, and visceral hook catheters (Fig. 3.5). Cobra catheters have primary and secondary downward-shaped curves and are pulled into the vessel to be selected. They are used routinely in visceral and renal catheterizations. Simmons catheters are shaped like a shepherd's hook. Simmons 1 and 2 catheters are used for both cerebral and visceral selective work. The Simmons catheters have good torque control, but it is sometimes difficult to reform their shape in the aorta. The Rösch inferior mesenteric catheter is an example of a visceral hook catheter. It has a 1 cm radius 180° bend at its tip. This allows for selective catheterization of the inferior mesenteric artery and crossing of the

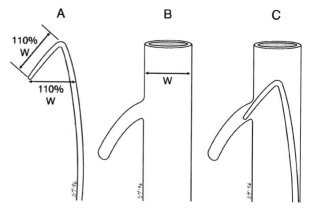

Figure 3.4 *Rule of 110. Pull-type catheters are available in different tip lengths. The primary catheter tip length should be 110 percent of the diameter of the abdominal aorta. The catheter that matches this percentage is the easiest to reform and reposition within the abdominal aorta. The catheter tip that is slightly greater than the width of the aorta will allow the catheter tip to engage the orifice of branched vessels.*

aortic bifurcation. A Mikaelsson catheter is used for selecting the bronchial or intercostal arteries. A spinal angiography catheter can be used for catheterizing vessels that make 90 degree angles with the aorta such as the spinal and intercostal arteries.

Figure 3.3 *Flush-type catheters. These catheters are designed to provide a dense compact bolus of contrast to opacify a large lumen vessel such as the aorta or cava. The multisidehole straight catheter is limited by a jet effect out of the end hole of the catheter. The pigtail, tennis racket, and halo catheters have curled ends that are designed to overcome the end hole jet effect. These catheters can be moved in the aorta or cava without leading over a guidewire.*

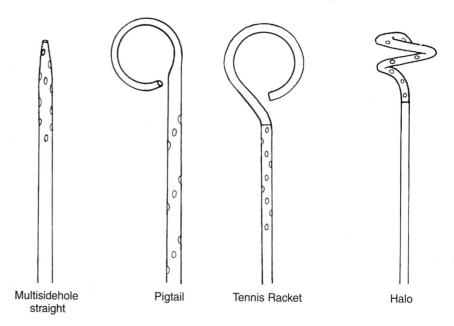

Multisidehole straight   Pigtail   Tennis Racket   Halo

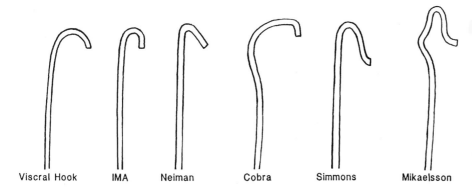

Figure 3.5 *Pull-type catheters. These catheters are reformed in the aorta or cava and pulled into the downward-angled orifice of the desired vessel branch.*

Viscral Hook   IMA   Neiman   Cobra   Simmons   Mikaelsson

An angled-tip catheter is used for selecting an obtuse angle vessel branch or a Y-type bifurcation. These catheters are pulled or pushed into the branch vessel or used to direct a guidewire into the desired branch orifice. All are variations of an angled-tip design. They are primarily used for upward branch vessels such as cerebral and subclavian vessels. The Weinberg catheter has a 30° angled tip and a gentle sweeping secondary curve that directs the primary curve into the vessel orifice. Head hunter catheters have a steeper secondary and tertiary curve than the Weinberg. Berenstein catheters have a 45° angled tip shape with no secondary curve. The JB1 catheter is a modified version of the head hunter catheter (Fig. 3.6).

Coaxial catheter systems facilitate superselective vascular catheterizations. An example is the Tracker catheter system (Target Therapeutics, Fremont, CA). Tracker catheters come in several sizes with several different guidewires available. The Tracker-10 catheter is the most flexible and smallest device available. The Tracker-10 catheter is used for superselective cerebral catheterizations. The Tracker-18 system is used for routine superselective catheterizations. The Tracker-325 system has a larger internal luminal size. It was designed for infusional treatments such as chemoembolization. It is somewhat stiffer than the Tracker-10 and the Tracker-18.

The Tracker-18 is a 3 French outer diameter catheter, which is inserted over a 0.016 inch diameter guidewire. The Tracker-18 fits through the lumen of a 5 French catheter. The 5 French catheter is used to engage the orifice of the vessel and to guide the Tracker catheter into the desired vascular tree. Available guidewires vary from soft and flexible to stiff. The flexible guidewires will negotiate tortuous anatomy, while the stiff guidewires have better torque control to select and direct the catheter across a bend. The Tracker guidewire can be shaped by gently giving its end an angled bend. A torque control device is used to steer the guidewire. The Tracker catheter is advanced over the guidewire. The Tracker catheter's small internal diameter severely limits the flow rate of contrast through it. A 1 ml luerlock tuberculin syringe is necessary when injecting through a Tracker. The small-sized syringe can generate adequate pressures to perform an injection. A Toughy-Bourst valve is used to flush the guiding catheter and Tracker catheter during the procedure.

Vascular Sheaths

Vascular sheaths allow easy exchange and introduction of catheters and guidewires. A hemostatic valve prevents blood reflux and air embolism. Sheaths protect against endothelial and mural vessel wall damage from multiple

Figure 3.6 *Push-type catheters. These catheters are designed to cannulate upward-angled vessel branches or select the desired branch of a Y-shaped bifurcation.*

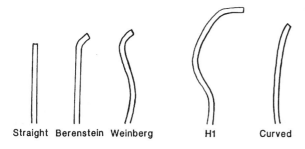

Straight   Berenstein   Weinberg   H1   Curved

catheter exchanges or removal of a foreign body or winged angioplasty balloon. A sheath should be used whenever multiple catheter exchanges are anticipated. Sheaths are always used when performing angioplasty, stenting, and thrombolysis. Sizing of sheaths is based on inner diameter: a 6 French sheath will accept up to a 6 French catheter. A 5 French sheath will accept most diagnostic catheters and 5 French shaft angioplasty balloons (up to 7 mm in diameter balloon). An 8 to 9 French sheath is required when performing angioplasty with balloon sizes 8 to 12 mm in diameter. Peel-away sheaths are used to place drainage catheters and venous access devices. The peel-away sheath is used to percutaneously place a device that cannot be primarily advanced over a guidewire alone. This occurs when the device has a blunt distal end or a permanently connected proximal end. A peel-away sheath helps prevent buckling of a catheter or drain within a long subcutaneous tract. The sheath is peeled apart like a banana skin once the device has been successfully positioned.

Guiding catheters are used to coaxially direct smaller caliber catheters. An 8 French guiding catheter accepts a 5 French angioplasty balloon catheter. Guiding catheters are used for directing balloon catheters and stents into the renal artery. A hook-shaped guiding catheter makes catheterization of the contralateral iliofemoral arteries feasible when there is a steep bifurcation of the aorta or when an aortobifemoral graft is present. An infusion or angioplasty catheter can then be coaxially inserted through the guiding catheter.

Angioplasty Balloons

A wide variety of angioplasty balloon catheters are available from several different manufacturers. Balloon diameters range from 2 to 20 mm and balloon lengths from 2 to 10 cm. The balloon catheter diameter is chosen by comparing to a normal adjacent segment of vessel or other knowledge of the diameter of the native vessel. The balloon diameter is selected to be the same size or slightly larger than the artery being dilated. Common balloon diameters are 8 to 10 mm for common iliac, 6 to 8 mm for external iliac, 4 to 5 mm for superficial femoral, 4 mm for popliteal, and 2.5 to 3.5 mm for infrapopliteal arteries. The length of the balloon is chosen to correspond to the length of the stenosis.

Standard polyethylene balloon catheters have 7 to 9 French shafts with 4 to 20 mm balloon diameter and use low pressure balloon material. Low profile balloon catheters have smaller shaft sizes, which help cross stenotic vessels and reduce puncture site hemorrhagic complications. Meditech Ultrathin balloon catheters have 5 French shafts for balloon sizes ranging from 5 to 8 mm in diameter and 5.8 French shafts for 9 and 10 mm balloons. High pressure balloons have larger catheter shafts and stronger balloon material construction. Meditech's Blue Max balloons can withstand high pressure inflations up to and exceeding 17 atmospheres. These are used to dilate resistant stenoses such as malignant biliary strictures and hemodialysis fistula strictures. Small vessel catheters have 3 to 3.8 French catheter shafts and balloon sizes ranging from 2 to 4 mm in size. The catheters accept 0.018 inch guidewires. These are used for coronary and infrapopliteal artery angioplasty.

The Olbert balloon has a catheter within catheter, which acts as a piston to inflate the balloon. During deflation, the reverse process returns the balloon material to its original profile. This eliminates the excess balloon wings of a deflated conventional angioplasty balloon. The Olbert balloon catheters have 5.8 French shafts for 4 to 8 mm balloons and 7.8 French balloon shafts for 9 to 14 mm balloons. Olbert catheters accept 0.35 inch guidewires and are rated to 10 to 12 atmosphere pressure. The Olbert latex weave balloon material is tacky, which firmly adheres a Palmaz stent to the balloon. The Olbert-Palmaz stent system can be passed through 7 French sheath valves and advanced across a stenosis without previous dilatation.

Stents

Stents are used to buttress open a vessel or parenchymal tract. Intravascular stents were developed to address the angioplasty limitations of elastic recoil and dissection. Stents were also developed to hold open biliary and enteric strictures. The Palmaz stent is a slotted tube that is expanded by balloon inflation (Fig. 3.7). Palmaz stents are approved by the Food and Drug Administration for intravascular use. Palmaz stents do not shorten significantly on dilatation

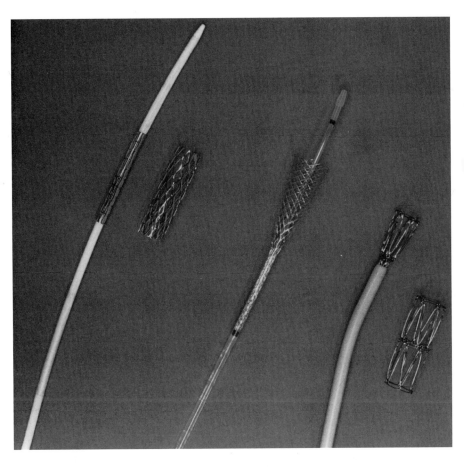

Figure 3.7 *Examples of metallic stents. On the left is a Palmaz stent mounted on an Olbert balloon. In the middle is a self-expanding Wallstent, which is partially deployed by withdrawing the outer protective sheath. On the right is a Gianturco Z stent, which is collapsed and pushed through a deployment sheath.*

and have good hoop strength. They are not flexible and can be pinched by a compressive force. The Wallstent is a tubular braid of stainless steel filaments. It is self-expanding and flexible. The Wallstent shortens longitudinally as it is deployed, making precise positioning of the ends difficult. It is approved for transjugular intrahepatic portosystemic shunt (TIPS), biliary, tracheal, and esophageal stricture treatments. The Wallstent comes in lengths of 20, 48, 60, and 90 mm. The diameter ranges from 2.5 to 30 mm in diameter. The Gianturco Z stent is a self-expanding zigzag pattern cylinder. It is compressed and fed through a catheter to the desired location. Gianturco stents are used for biliary strictures and venous stenosis applications. Fabric- or vein-covered stents are being developed to exclude aneurysms endovascularly. Gianturco Z stents covered with Dacron are used for stent grafting aortic aneurysms.

Thrombolysis Catheters

Successful thrombolysis requires intrathrombus delivery of urokinase into the largest surface area possible within a blood clot. Most thrombolytic infusion catheters have multiple sideholes, which distribute the urokinase into the greatest length of thrombus possible. A variety of multi-side hole infusion catheters and wires are available (Fig. 3.8). Most infusion systems can be used for either continuous infusion or pulse spray technique. The Mewissen infusion catheter is a 5 French catheter with an end hole tapered to fit over an 0.035 or an 0.038 inch guidewire. The catheter fits over a guidewire that has already transversed the thrombosed vessel. A Touhy-Bourst Y adapter is used to infuse urokinase into the catheter around the guidewire and out of the infusion sideholes. The

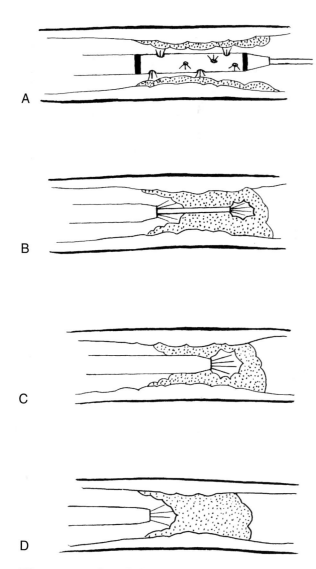

Figure 3.8 *Thrombolytic infusion catheter systems. (A) Mewissen over-the-wire multi-side hole infusion catheter. (B) Example of coaxial infusion via proximal catheter and distal infusion wire. (C) End hole catheter infusion into the thrombus. (D) The least effective method of infusing urokinase is proximal to the thrombus.*

catheter comes in 5, 10, and 15 cm infusion lengths. Coaxial infusion systems combine a proximal infusion catheter with a distal infusion wire to infuse into a long segment occlusion. An example is a Mewissen catheter with a Katzen infusion wire. Katzen infusion wires have infusion lengths of 3 to 12 cm.

Drainage Catheters

Drainage catheters are designed with rigid walls to prevent kinking and buckling and large lumens to maximize drainage of the infected space. Drainage catheters with locking pigtails are preferred because the pigtail helps prevent dislodgement of the catheter. The holes are cut on the inside of the pigtail catheter ring to eliminate plugging of the holes by the walls of the cavity. An 8 French catheter is used for gallbladder drainages. Abdominal fluid collections are drained with 10 to 12 French drains. Thick viscous fluid collections frequently require larger lumen catheters, such as 14 to 18 French pigtails. Pleural space drainage catheters should be 12 French or larger to prevent kinking between the intercostal spaces. Thal-Quick chest tubes measuring 18 to 24 French are available for draining and debriding cavities that contain large chunks of necrotic debris. Sump catheters have two inner channels. The larger channel drains the cavity while the smaller channel provides the sump action. The sump channel vents the cavity and prevents plugging of the drainage holes by the cavity wall tissue. Sump catheters are used for viscous fluid collections, but the majority of abscesses are drained adequately by single lumen catheters of sufficient size.

Table Organization

It is the assistant angiographer's responsibility to keep the angiography table organized and maintained. It is of paramount importance to carefully handle contaminated syringes and sharps. Sharps should be segregated into a corner of the table and placed into a sharps container to minimize any inadvertent needle sticks. Accidental puncture with contaminated syringes and needles does occur. Be extremely careful with sharps. Contaminated flush syringes and contrast injection syringes are emptied and recharged using the closed flush-and-fill system. The flushed syringes should be refilled as they are used with heparinized saline. The saline used during an angiography procedure is heparinized to contain approximately 5 to 10 units of heparin/ml of normal saline. Avoid aerosolizing contaminated blood products and drainage fluid by injecting the syringes into the cups on the table. The table cups are intended for use as reservoirs of sterile saline and contrast. A basin of heparinized saline is used to wet 4 × 4 gauze pads and store coiled wires. The wetted gauze pads are used to wipe catheters and guidewires.

Imaging Equipment

Peripheral catheterization laboratory design trends favor a ceiling mounted C-arm with a pedestal table. The C-arm configuration allows acquisition of complex oblique views or rotational runs, which can provide an optimal view of overlapping structures. The image intensifier should have a large field of view. Reduced radiation dose modes that reduce the dose by pulsing the fluoroscopy are available. The roadmapping feature superimposes an image of opacified vessels on real-time fluoroscopy to aid in selecting the desired branches of an arterial tree. A newer design feature is to give the operator bedside control of many of the operations of the angiography system. This eliminates dependence on an assistant working the system operation in the control room. The study can be rapidly reviewed and subsequent catheterization steps or interventions planned.

Digital angiographic systems have evolved so that they are now the norm in modern angiography suites. Digital subtraction angiography (DSA) has superior contrast resolution compared to cut film technique. This allows for reduction in contrast material concentration and/or volume. Cut film angiography techniques have better linear resolution than DSA and are less affected by motion artifact; however, DSA is now favored because it significantly reduces procedural time by eliminating the significant delay of obtaining scout radiographs and processing film. The rapidity with which images can be acquired, reviewed, and postprocessed is the most significant advantage that DSA offers. The use of digital techniques such as roadmapping, references images, and reduced fluoroscopic patient dosing gives digital units an additional advantage.

The quality of digital subtraction images is significantly degraded by motion. The patient must be carefully coached in breath holding before performing thoracic or abdominal angiography. Care must be taken not to oversedate the patient when performing an abdominal or pulmonary angiogram. The patient should be positioned for optimal visualization of the location to be investigated. In general, maximum coverage of a vascular distribution is desirable. When a specific area of pathology is noted, a more magnified view of this area is often helpful. The area of interest should always be positioned near the center of the film.

Proper collimation and use of filtration are essential to obtain high quality digital radiographs. Good collimation results in reduced patient dose and overall improved film quality. Use of electronic filters smooths out the imaged object's density and results in a more uniform exposure. During pulmonary angiography, a filter should be placed over the lung to equalize the density between the lung and mediastinum. Electrocardiographic leads, intravenous tubing, and contrast-soaked drapes must be compulsively kept out of the field of the angiogram. This maximizes film quality and avoids obscuring diagnostic information. Printing high-quality images is a crucial aspect of the overall angiographic procedure. Subtracted images require careful postprocess editing. Optimal images are obtained when the proper mask image and pixel shifting are done to produce clean images. When filming, be sure to include pictures documenting the arterial, capillary, and venous phases of the angiogram. Print images in both subtracted and nonsubtracted formats. The nonsubtracted images superimpose the bone landmarks for positional reference. Remember the conventional standard is the cut film angiogram in which numerous films are obtained. The films should be labeled appropriate to their anatomic position and side. Be sure to record any pressure gradients, pulmonary artery pressure recordings, or other pertinent clinical information on the films. Avoid labeling films with diagnoses and obvious findings.

Contrast Injectors

Radiographic injectors are designed to inject contrast medium under specifically controlled conditions. Large vessels cannot be opacified adequately by hand injection. Conversely, small vessels must be injected so slowly that an automatic injector is required. In general, the larger the vessel the greater the flow rate.

Contrast injectors contain a syringe, a heating device, and a pressure delivery mechanism. Automatic injectors can be programmed to inject from 1 ml/sec up to 40 ml/sec. Specific flow rates will be discussed within each chapter describing the specific application.

Suggested Readings

Chuang VP: Basic rule in catheter selection for visceral angiography. AJR 136:432, 1981

Frood LR, Smith DC, Pappas JM et al: Use of angiographic needles with or without stylets: pathologic assessment of vessel walls after puncture. J Vasc Interv Radiol 2:269, 1991

Gerlock AJ, Mirfakhraee M: Essentials of Diagnostic and Interventional Techniques. WB Saunders, Philadelphia, 1985

Johnsrude IS, Jackson DC, Dunnick NR: A Practical Approach to Angiography. 2nd Ed., Little, Brown, Boston, 1987

Kadir S: Current Practice of Interventional Radiology. BC Decker, Philadelphia, 1991

Matsumoto AH, Barth KH, Selby JB Jr, Tegtmeyer CJ: Peripheral balloon angioplasty technology. Cardiovasc Intervent Radiol 16:135, 1993

Orron DE, Kim D, Rogaski KJ: Radiographic equipment and angiographic products. p. 61. In Kim D, Orron DE (eds): Peripheral Vascular Imaging and Intervention. Mosby-Year Book, St. Louis, 1992

Schroeder J: Mechanical properties of guidewires. Cardiovasc Intervent Radiol 16:43, 1993

Basic Catheterization Skills

MICHAEL A. BRAUN

Arterial Puncture

The leg opposite the patient's most symptomatic extremity is punctured for the diagnostic portion of the test. This allows the flexibility of doing either a retrograde or antegrade approach to a subsequently identified lesion involving the symptomatic leg. The groin is generously shaved, and antisepsis is obtained by scrubbing the inguinal region three times with povidone–iodine (Betadine) and allowing it to air dry. Dura-prep (3M Healthcare, St. Paul, MN) is a new antiseptic preparation that coats the area with a bacteriocidal film that lasts 24 to 48 hours. The patient is covered generously with drapes, leaving only the puncture site exposed. The importance of proper arterial access cannot be overstated. To provide safe, complication-free access, the artery to be entered should ideally be large, disease free, and easy to compress. Prevention of puncture site complications such as occlusion, pseudoaneurysms, or hematoma demands that the needle (and catheter) be inserted in the common femoral artery. The common femoral artery is best localized by puncturing over the mid portion of the femoral head. In 99 percent of patients, the femoral bifurcation lies well below this point, and the inguinal ligament lies above it. The puncture site is chosen by fluoroscopically localizing the inferior portion of the femoral head (Fig. 4.1). This is more reliable than using the groin crease or palpating the inguinal ligament. Punctures that are too high and enter above the inguinal ligament (in the external iliac artery) risk massive retroperitoneal bleeding. Low punctures (into the superficial femoral or profunda femoris) are associated with a higher incidence of pseudoaneurysms, occlusions, and embolic problems because the punctured artery cannot be compressed against the femoral head. The femoral bifurcation is usually more diseased than the common femoral artery, which can cause a higher incidence of dissections.

Local anesthesia is performed by making a nickel-sized skin weal directly over the puncture site. Deep infiltration of the subcutaneous tissues is done on both sides of the artery. If the pulse is poor, one must be careful when administering anesthetic. Overadministration of local anesthetic may further diminish the already poorly palpable pulse. A 3 mm stab dermatotomy is made with a #11 scalpel. The subcutaneous tissues are generously spread with the tips of a hemostat.

A single wall arterial puncture technique is preferred. An 18-gauge open needle is used. The bevel on this needle cuts through heavily calcified vessel walls rather than deflecting off the vessel. Single wall needles pass more readily through surgical scars and synthetic grafts. The artery to be punctured is palpated with two fingers. The pulse is best felt with the fingertips. The needle is slowly advanced toward the palpated pulse. Pulsations can be felt as they are transmitted through the needle. Sometimes a blood return is not seen as the needle is advanced through the artery. The needle should be slowly withdrawn, watching for a blood return. If a puncture is unsuccessful, the needle should be flushed to remove any subcutaneous debris that may be occluding the lumen. The initial passage of a guidewire is a hazardous point in diagnostic and interventional procedures. It is at this point that subintimal dissections and occlusions frequently occur when the needle tip is not completely intraluminal. To prevent this complication, the operator must observe carefully that there is adequate pulsatile return of blood and that passage of the guidewire is smooth and without resistance. When arterial blood returns, the guidewire (3 mm J) is passed. Resistance to guidewire passage may indicate that the needle is not within the center of the vessel lumen. The guidewire should be gently advanced under fluoroscopic control to determine whether the guidewire is buckling in the vessel or is perivascular. When in doubt, a small injection of contrast through the needle will delineate the relative posi-

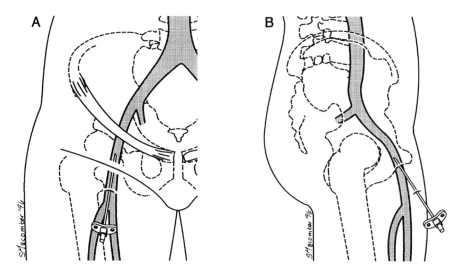

Figure 4.1 *Proper puncture position of the common femoral artery. The femoral head is located fluoroscopically to determine puncture position. The skin dermatotomy is made at the inferior portion of the femoral head. The common femoral artery is punctured over the mid portion of the femoral head. The lateral view demonstrates that the vessel can be effectively compressed against the femoral head when the catheter and needle are removed.*

tion of the needle to the lumen of the vessel. Once this is known, the needle can be redirected and the guidewire advanced under fluoroscopic control. Vessel dilators are reserved for groins that have scars from previous surgeries. Grafts can be punctured that are at least 2 months old. Use of a vascular sheath is recommended when catheterizing a graft to protect the catheters from breakage and to ease the manipulations of catheter movement.

Left brachial artery puncture is the alternative to femoral artery catheterization for diagnostic angiography in patients with aortoiliac disease. A brachial approach is used to selectively cannulate a steeply angled visceral or renal vessel. A low brachial approach is favored over the high brachial or axillary approach. The nerve damage from an axillary puncture site hematoma has greater potential consequences than a low brachial puncture. The brachial artery is punctured two to three finger breadths above the elbow crease. The brachial artery is small and readily goes into spasm. A thin-walled, 19-gauge needle with an 0.035 inch Glidewire or a 21-gauge micropuncture technique is best suited for the initial puncture. Preferably 4 French or at most 5 French catheters are used. Sublingual nifedipine, intra-arterial nitroglycerin, and low-dose

bolus (2,000 to 3,000 units) heparin are given to prevent thrombotic complications from spasm or occlusion. A left brachial approach is used to reduce the potential for stroke complications from a right brachial catheterization of the aorta. The guidewire tends to enter the ascending aorta from a left upper extremity approach. The loop of a pigtail catheter or a hook-shaped catheter is used to direct the wire into the descending aorta.

Puncturing the Poorly Palpable Artery

Certain situations dictate that a poorly palpable artery be punctured. For routine diagnostic work, if both femoral arteries are nonpalpable, a brachial approach should be used. However, puncturing the femoral artery to perform an antegrade or retrograde approach to a stenosis is sometimes required. Several methods have evolved to aid in this procedure. The simplest method is to puncture the groin under fluoroscopic control after a roadmap is performed by contrast delivery through an already indwelling catheter. Similarly, a guidewire can be passed from the contralateral artery into the femoral artery to be punctured. The guidewire can then serve as a fluoroscopic target. Vascular calcifications and bone landmarks can be used as a guide.

The Smart Needle (PSG, Mountainview, CA) was developed as an aid to puncturing a nonpalpable artery. The Smart Needle contains a Doppler probe at the needle tip. The device is primed by flushing it with 10 ml of saline. The Doppler probe is connected to the receptor device, which is turned on and increased to three-fourths volume. The artery should not be palpated as the Smart Needle is advanced. The Smart Needle is moved toward the anticipated location of the nonpalpable artery. An arterial Doppler sound is used to guide the needle to the target vessel. The intensity of the arterial Doppler sound increases as the needle is negotiated closer to the artery. The Smart Needle can be used for performing problematic brachial artery punctures in addition to nonpalpable femoral artery punctures.

Real-time ultrasound guidance of arterial punctures is a useful technique. A 7 MHz transducer is protected by placing a sterile condom over it. The groin is prepared in the usual manner, and the ultrasound probe is held perpendicular and transverse to the course of the femoral artery over the spot where the artery is intended to be punctured. The level of the femoral head should be fluoroscopically marked in addition to using ultrasound guidance. Under direct ultrasound guidance, the needle is directed toward the artery. The tip of the needle is often difficult to visualize. Passage of the needle creates a wave within the tissue, which is more readily seen under ultrasound. This deflection of tissues can be used to infer the position and direction that the needle is passing. Ultrasound guidance is the most reliable means of successful vascular puncture.

Venous Puncture

The common femoral vein is the most frequently used access for diagnostic venography and placement of vena cava filters. The preparation routine is similar to puncture of the femoral artery. The arterial pulse is palpated, and the dermatotomy is made 1 cm medial to the pulse over the femoral head. The pulse is palpated with the fingers of one hand while the other hand is used to advance the needle. A 10 ml syringe or exten-

sion tubing connected to a syringe are used to create negative pressure. The needle is inserted while gentle negative pressure is applied. Often the needle is inserted to the joint space without a venous blood return. The patient is asked to perform a Valsalva maneuver while the needle is withdrawn, watching for blood return. When blood is aspirated, the needle or tubing is disconnected and a guidewire is inserted.

An internal jugular vein puncture is used for transjugular intrahepatic portosystemic shunt (TIPS), liver biopsy, and filter placement. The jugular vein puncture site is halfway between the angle of the mandible and the clavicle. The vein is lateral to the common carotid artery, and the pulse can be used to guide the location of the venipuncture. We use ultrasound guidance on all jugular punctures, preferring the one-stick convenience of imaging guidance. The platysma muscle and fascia resist passage of catheters, necessitating the use of a dilator.

Basic Catheter Skills

The guidewire is advanced into the vessel after vascular puncture. The guidewire should pass easily. If there is any resistance, the guidewire should be observed fluoroscopically for buckling from a stenosis or subintimal passage. A contrast injection through the needle will best evaluate the situation. The guidewire is inserted until the stiff body of the wire is well within the vascular system. If the wire is not inserted far enough, the flexible distal end of the wire will buckle in the subcutaneous tissues when a catheter is inserted. With the guidewire in place, the needle is removed, and the puncture site is compressed with the middle and ring fingers while the guidewire is grasped between the index finger and thumb. The wire is wiped clean with a wet sponge gauze or Telfa pad. The wire is wiped by the assistant starting in the middle and wiping toward the patient end and then the outside end of the guidewire. This simple technique prevents inadvertent removal of the guidewire.

The catheter is threaded onto the end of the guidewire and advanced to the puncture site. The assistant must have control of the end of the guidewire before the catheter is inserted through the puncture site. Catheter insertion is greatly facilitated by the assistant holding the wire taut while the catheter is advanced through the subcutaneous tissues into the vessel. The guidewire should lead the catheter through the vasculature to the desired location. The guidewire is removed and a flow switch or stopcock placed on the end of the catheter. The catheter is flushed using the double flush technique. The initial flush is an aspiration of any potential debris, air, or thrombus within the catheter. The second flush should fill the catheter lumen with heparinized saline.

Catheters are exchanged over a guidewire using the pin and pull technique (Fig. 4.2), a fundamental and important catheter manipulation skill. The guidewire is inserted through the catheter and positioned safely within the vascular tree. The wire is held stationary (pinned) 10 cm from the end of the catheter. The catheter is withdrawn (pulled) the 10 cm while the wire is held motionless. This process is repeated until the catheter is completely withdrawn from the puncture site. The puncture site is compressed, and the wire is firmly grasped similar to insertion of the catheter. Catheter placement and removal over a Glidewire requires special care. The hydrophilic coating on Glidewires must be wetted to be activated. Otherwise, the coating is tacky when dry and will bind within a catheter. The Glidewire must be wiped before the catheter is removed. The Glidewire must be securely grasped at the puncture site before the catheter is totally withdrawn off the wire. The

Glidewire must be pinned carefully and the catheter end supported when a catheter is inserted over a Glidewire into the vasculature.

Selective catheterizations use either an angled or hook-shaped catheter tip. The catheter shape is reformed in the aorta or cava by engaging the renal artery or vein (Fig. 4.3). The catheter tip is positioned above the anticipated level of the vessel to be selected, and the tip is oriented toward the direction of the branch vessel takeoff. The catheter is pulled in a smooth motion toward the branch vessel location. It is best to simultaneously torque the catheter as it is being moved up and down. The catheter tip is observed fluoroscopically for the typical jump in the tip that occurs when the vessel orifice is engaged. The catheter "jump" can sometimes be felt when the tip hooks a vessel orifice. The vessel is identified by a gentle contrast injection. A larger contrast injection confirms vessel identity, catheter position, and catheter stability. Hook-shaped catheters are usually stable enough for power injections when they are fully pulled and seated within the target vessel.

Superselective catheterization refers to placing a catheter in a second- or third-order vessel branch. This is more difficult than selecting a primary aortic branch. Upward branching vessels are simpler to selectively catheterize. An angled-tip catheter can be used to select both the primary and secondary branches (Fig. 4.4). Glidewires facilitate passing a soft, flexible catheter into superselective position. Several methods can be used to cross the aortic bifurcation (Fig. 4.5). Loop catheter technique was devised for superselective catheterization of downward branching visceral and pelvic vessels. A 6 to 7 French cobra catheter is formed into a 10 to 15 cm loop similar in configuration to a shepherd's crook. This is pulled into the primary trunk vessel and negotiated into the desired branch vessel. Loop technique can be complicated by twists, kinks, or knots. For these reasons, coaxial catheterization has predominantly replaced loop technique. Coaxial technique is placing a 3 French catheter through a 5 French catheter that has engaged the primary branch vessel orifice. The 3 French catheter is directed into the desired second or third order branch often with roadmapping guidance.

A hand injection should precede all power injections to confirm the catheter's position and any potential to recoil or migrate during injection. The special contrast injector syringe should be grasped in the palm of the left hand. The right hand's palm is used to

Figure 4.2 *Pin and pull technique. This is the most fundamental and important technique in catheter exchange. The guidewire is held stationary by one hand approximately 5 to 10 cm from the end of the catheter. The catheter is withdrawn to the pinning hand over the wire. This process is repeated until the catheter is removed from the body. This technique keeps the wire stationary as the catheter is removed, preserving the selective position of the wire within the body.*

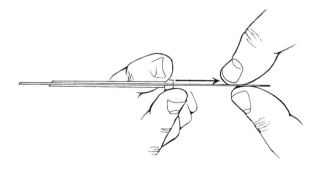

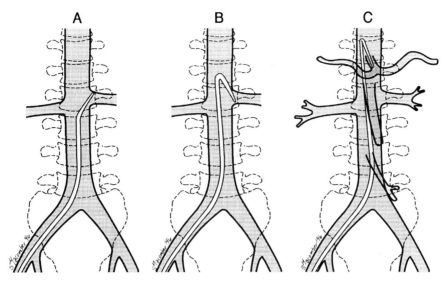

Figure 4.3 *Method for reshaping a visceral hook catheter by engaging the renal artery orifice. The renal artery is usually located at the L2 vertebral body level. (**A**) The catheter tip is directed toward the left renal artery. (**B**) Advancing the catheter with the tip in the orifice of the renal artery reforms the hook shape of the Nieman catheter. (**C**) The catheter is advanced to the L1 vertebral body level and used to select the celiac artery.*

Figure 4.4 *Example of push-type catheter used to select the right subclavian artery. (**A**) The catheter is placed over a guidewire into the ascending aorta and pulled back into the origin of the right brachiocephalic artery. (**B**) The catheter is inserted over a wire into the brachiocephalic artery. The wire is withdrawn, and the catheter is used to direct the wire toward the subclavian artery. (**C**) Once the wire is safely within the subclavian artery the catheter can be advanced over the wire. (Adapted from Gerlock AJ, Mirfakhraee M: Essentials of Diagnostic and Interventional Techniques. WB Saunders, Philadelphia, 1985.)*

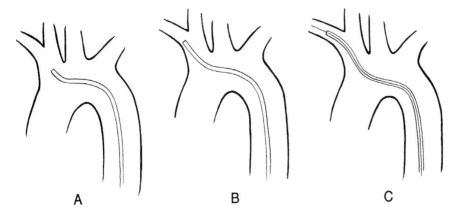

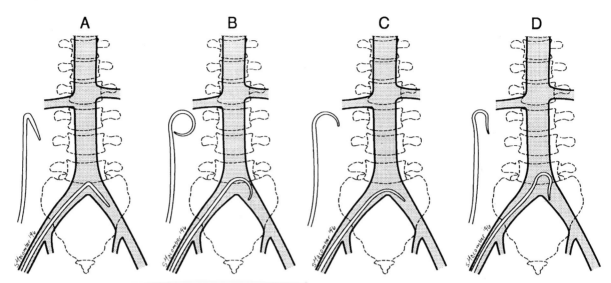

Figure 4.5 *Methods for crossing the aortic bifurcation.* **(A)** *Nieman catheter.* **(B)** *Pigtail catheter.* **(C)** *Rösch inferior mesenteric catheter.* **(D)** *Shepherd's crook-type catheter. The hook-type catheters are reformed in the aorta and pulled down to engage the contralateral iliac artery. The downward-orientated catheters then direct a guidewire into the iliac system. The pigtail catheter uncoils as it is pulled into the iliac artery. This combination of catheter uncoiling and guidewire advancement is used to engage the contralateral iliac artery.*

depress the syringe's plunger. A forceful hand injection is always needed, especially in the aorta. The hand injection is used to help determine the rate of the power injection.

Puncture Site Hemostasis

The study is reviewed and evaluated before catheter removal. A moderate stenosis can be further evaluated with hemodynamic pressure measurements. Additional views to differentiate overlying vessels from an aneurysm are obtained. It is best to preserve access if the diagnostic angiogram becomes a thrombolysis or angioplasty procedure. The catheter is removed after the interventional procedure.

The most frequent complication of diagnostic angiography is hemorrhage from the puncture site. This can be minimized by paying special attention to compressing the vessel once the catheter is removed. Most catheters can be removed primarily from the groin. The exceptions are removing catheters introduced through grafts and removing pigtail catheters from the pulmonary artery. Pigtail catheters must be straightened out over a guidewire before being withdrawn through the heart to avoid valvular injury. The femoral artery puncture should have manual pressure applied using the finger tips for a minimum of 10 minutes. Initially, firm pressure should be applied. After bleeding is controlled, the pressure should be titrated. The pressure must be firm enough to prevent any bleeding but must not occlude the artery. At the end of the holding procedure, there must be no evidence of bleeding. Sandbags are not used and dressings are not applied.

The Femo-Stop (C. R. Bard, Billerica, MA) applies local mechanical compression over femoral artery puncture sites. A Femo-Stop device consists of a belt that slides underneath the patient connected to a plastic pressure arch. Connected to the pressure arch is an inflatable bubble that can be inflated using a standard blood pressure cuff pump (Fig. 4.6). A key to the use of the Femo-Stop is to position the pressure bubble directly over the punctured portion of the artery. This may mean positioning the center of the bubble a few centimeters higher relative to the skin nick. For the first 2 minutes, the bubble is inflated to a suprasystolic

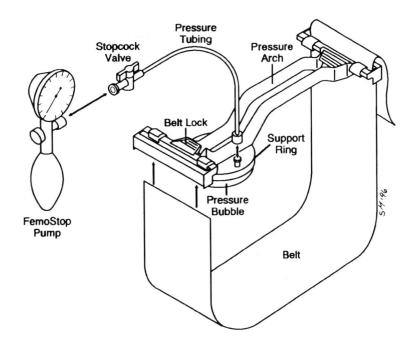

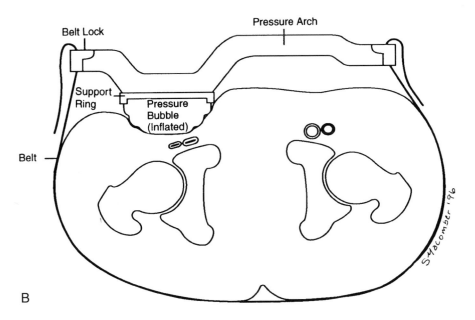

Figure 4.6 *The Femo-Stop system for common femoral artery mechanical compression.* **(A)** *The Femo-Stop consists of an inflatable sterile bubble, which is positioned over the anticipated puncture of the femoral artery. The bubble is attached to a plastic arm, which is fastened around the patient's hips using an adjustable belt. The bubble is inflated by attaching a manual pump with manometer to control the pressure applied.* **(B)** *Proper positioning of the Femo-Stop mechanical compression device effectively compresses the femoral artery compression site against the underlying acetabulum.*

pressure. After 2 minutes, the pressure is lowered at least 40 mmHg or until a palpable pedal pulse is felt. This pressure is maintained for 8 minutes. Following 10 minutes of application of the device, the cuff is deflated and bleeding at the groin carefully checked for. Comparison of the Femo-Stop device with manual compression demonstrated that the Femo-Stop had a lower rate of complications. The device's only disadvantage is the additional cost. The Femo-Stop device helps eliminate operator fatigue when a long period of holding pressure is anticipated. It can be left on the groin for long periods to control minor bleeding.

A formal procedure note is placed in the chart for every procedure performed. The procedure note is modeled after a surgical operative note. This note is a reflection of the consultative role played in the overall care of the patient. A thoroughly documented procedure note improves communication to the referring clinicians, satisfies medical legal requirements, and informs the clinical staff who are caring for the patient. The procedure note format is:

Date; Interventional Radiology Procedure Note
Indication:
Procedure:
Doctor(s):
Results:
Plan:

Routine postangiography orders should document the puncture site. The site should be monitored every 15 minutes × 2, then every 30 minutes × 4, and finally every 1 hour × 4. For an arterial puncture, the patient should be placed on strict bed rest for 6 hours. No sandbags should be used. If the patient is an outpatient and the procedure was uneventful, the period of bed rest may be shortened to 4 hours. Depending on the situation, one should consider ordering postprocedural hydration, prophylactic antibiotics, specific monitoring of a recognized complication, and monitoring of tube output depending on the various procedures performed. All patients who have had a brachial puncture should be seen the next day and examined for any potential delayed complications. All patients

who have had an interventional vascular procedure (e.g., angioplasty, embolization) should be seen daily to monitor the outcome. Patients who have had routine diagnostic angiograms from a femoral approach do not need to be followed up unless there is concern about a procedural complication.

Clinical rounds demonstrate to the referring clinicians that the interventional radiology service is actively participating in the management of their patients and fulfilling the role of a consultant. Clinical rounds serve to monitor the outcomes and complications of the interventional procedures. An appropriate visit includes a brief review of the patient's chart for pertinent details such as catheter output, fever, white count, and appropriate chemistry values. The patient should be visited, briefly interviewed, and evaluated. Any drains or indwelling tubes should be examined to determine the quantity of drainage and the drainage fluid characteristics. For an indwelling drain, a tube injection is performed frequently and is ordered by the interventional radiology service depending on the tube's output. A brief note documenting this visit and outlining the plan of care is recorded daily in the patient's chart.

Suggested Readings

Altin RS, Flicker S, Naidech HJ: Pseudoaneurysm and arteriovenous fistula after femoral artery catheterization: association with low femoral punctures. AJR 152:629, 1989

Gerlock AJ, Mirfakhraee M: Essentials of Diagnostic and Interventional Techniques. WB Saunders, Philadelphia, 1985

Kadir S: Basic catheterization techniques. p. 34. In: Diagnostic Arteriography. WB Saunders, Philadelphia, 1986

Kim D, Orron DE: Techniques and complications of angiography. p. 83. In Kim D, Orron DE (eds): Peripheral Vascular Imaging and Intervention. Mosby-Year Book, St. Louis, 1992

Rupp SB, Vogelzang RL, Nemcek AA Jr, Yungbluth MM: Relationship of the inguinal ligament to pelvic radiographic landmarks: anatomic correlation and its role in femoral arteriography. J Vasc Interv Radiat 4:409, 1993

CHAPTER 5

Diagnostic Angiography

MICHAEL A. BRAUN
ALBERT A. NEMCEK, JR.

The fundamental goal of vascular radiology is obtaining high quality diagnostic images in the safest method available. Diagnostic angiography has traditionally relied on opacification of the lumen of the vessels to define the anatomy of the vascular tree and the morphology of the vessel lumen. The cross-sectional imaging techniques of computed tomography (CT) and ultrasound complement angiography by imaging the vessel wall and surrounding structures. This is most important in evaluating aneurysmal disease. Magnetic resonance imaging (MRI), nuclear medicine, and carbon dioxide angiography offer alternative techniques to contrast angiography to image the vascular tree at a reduced risk to the patient. This chapter discusses the different techniques and applications of diagnostic vascular radiology.

Thoracic Aortography

The indications for thoracic aortography are the evaluation of trauma, atherosclerotic occlusive disease, aneurysm, dissection, aortitis, and congenital abnormality. The thoracic aorta is frequently studied before evaluation of the cerebral or upper extremity vessels. The cross-sectional imaging techniques of spiral CT, magnetic resonance angiography, and transesophageal ultrasound have largely replaced thoracic aortography in diagnosis of aneurysms and dissections. However, thoracic aortography is still used in the preoperative evaluation to define the anatomy of aneurysms, pseudoaneurysms, dissections, and coarctations. Thoracic aortography remains the definitive study for trau-

matic injury to the aorta from blunt or penetrating chest trauma. Less frequent indications include evaluation of Takayasu's arteritis, tumors, postoperative anatomy, and malformations (Fig. 5.1).

A thoracic aortogram is performed with a large caliber pigtail catheter that allows sufficient flow rates to opacify the aorta. A 6 to 7 French pigtail catheter is placed within the ascending aorta just superior to the sinuses of Valsalva. A vigorous hand injection confirms the catheter position and estimates the flow rate before a power injection. The injection rate is 25 to 35 ml/sec for a total of 50 to 70 ml. The base of the great vessels and arch of the aorta are placed within the center of the field of view. At least two but preferably three views of the aorta are obtained. The most important view is a 30° to 45° left anterior oblique, which images the aortic arch en face. The other views are a straight anterior and 30° right anterior oblique. Be sure to remove any extraneous leads or other monitoring devices that may cause artifacts. Rapid film rates are necessary for evaluating traumatic injuries because of the fast flow rate. Typical digital angiography film rates are three to four frames per second. Large aneurysms and aortic valve insufficiency may cause slower flow rates best imaged with a longer contrast injection and film acquisition time. Generally, a large field of view, which is collimated side-to-side, is used, or electronic filters are placed over the lung fields to even out the density to gain a uniform exposure.

The findings of traumatic injury include luminal irregularity, contained transection, and pseudoaneurysm formation at the aortic isthmus (Fig. 5.2). Diagnostic dilemmas are caused by the ductus diverticulum and coexistent aneurysmal disease. Extravasation of contrast, delay of contrast washout, and

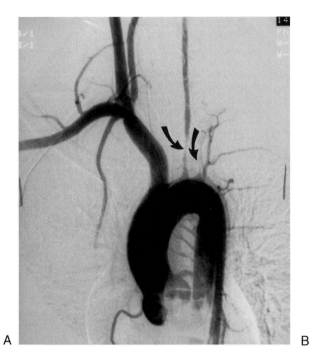
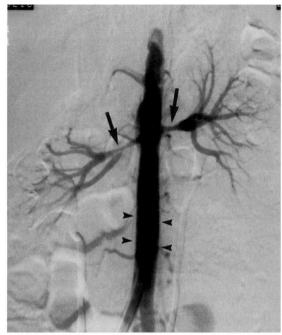

A

B

Figure 5.1 *Takayasu's arteritis. The characteristic arteriographic findings are long segment, tapered stenoses involving the proximal segments of the large aortic branches. **(A)** The left common carotid has a long segment stenosis and the left subclavian has an occlusive stenosis (arrows). **(B)** There are bilateral renal artery stenoses (arrows) and mild dilatation of the infrarenal abdominal aorta (arrowheads).*

luminal irregularity help differentiate traumatic injury from congenital variant. The pigtail catheter is carefully advanced through the aorta when evaluating aortic dissection. A contrast injection is performed when any resistance to catheter or guidewire advancement occurs. The size of the lumen and speed of flow help estimate between the true and false lumen. If it is in the false lumen, the catheter should be redirected into the true lumen. The pigtail is positioned just above the aortic valve, and the power injection and film acquisition rates are adjusted to the estimated flow rate. The demonstration of an intimal flap, the entry and exit site of the intimal tear, involvement of branch vessels, and aortic valve are carefully studied. A reduced power injection into the false lumen can be performed when necessary. Dissections can be described by either the DeBakey or Stanford classification systems (Fig. 5.3).

Upper Extremity Angiography

Indications for upper extremity angiography include trauma, evaluation of thoracic outlet syndrome, and evaluation of ischemic peripheral vascular disease. Other indications include subclavian steal, aneurysmal disease, malformations, preoperative plastic or reconstructive evaluation, and hypothenar hammer syndrome. Upper extremity angiography is commonly performed bilaterally to provide a normal side for comparison, especially for the evaluation of thoracic outlet syndrome.

The examination starts with a thoracic arch angiogram, focusing on the great vessels, which can be performed with a 5 French pigtail placed within the distal ascending thoracic aorta. A 5 French Weinberg catheter is used to select either the right innominate or left subclavian artery (see Fig. 4.4). Other push-type catheters with

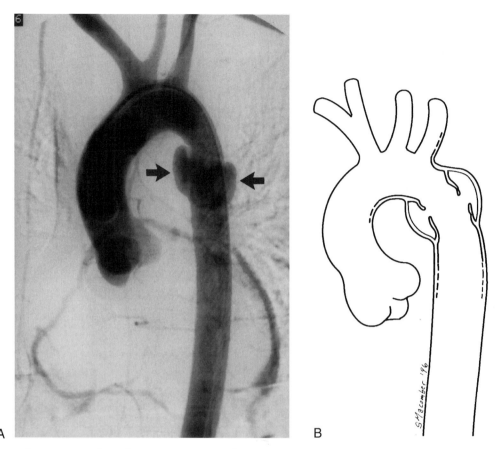

Figure 5.2 *Blunt thoracic trauma results in an aortic transection at the level of the isthmus. (**A**) Thoracic aortogram demonstrating contained traumatic rupture. A contained complete transection has disruption of the intimal and medial planes of the aorta with containment of the pseudoaneurysm by periadventitial tissues (arrows). (**B**) Schematic diagram.*

hockey stick-angled tips may be used. The catheter is positioned within the proximal third of either the right or left subclavian artery. A hand contrast injection assesses the position of the catheter tip and estimates the flow rate. The injection rate is 6 to 8 ml/sec for a total of 20 to 30 ml. In the evaluation of thoracic outlet syndrome, the subclavian artery should be examined in both the neutral and symptomatic positions. The provocative position is the shoulder abducted and the patient's hand placed behind the head (Fig. 5.4).

After examination of the subclavian and axillary artery, the catheter is advanced into the brachial artery and selective injections performed to evaluate the forearm and hand. The forearm or hand is best examined by placing the hand at the patient's side in a pronated position, with the fingers spread slightly apart. Injection rates are approximately 5 to 6 ml/sec for a total of 20 to 30 ml. Magnified views of the hand should be obtained following intra-arterial administration of 25 mg of tolazoline slowly injected over 2 minutes. The radial artery can occasionally have a proximal origin from the brachial artery above the elbow or the axillary artery, which must be kept in mind when selective distal upper extremity arteriography is performed. In general, the radial artery supplies the deep palmar arch, which principally supplies the thumb and index finger. The ulnar artery supplies the superficial palmar arch, which is usually considered the palmar arch

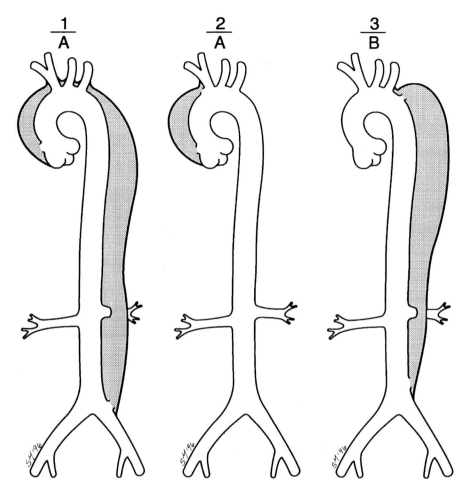

Figure 5.3 *The DeBakey and Stanford classifications of aortic dissections. The DeBakey 1 and Stanford A involve both the ascending and descending aorta (all for one). The DeBakey 2 thoracic aortic dissection involves only the ascending aorta. The DeBakey 3 and Stanford B dissections involve the aorta distal to the left subclavian artery. (Modified from Kadir S: Diagnostic Angiography. WB Saunders, Philadelphia, 1986, with permission.)*

that provides dominant supply to the middle through little fingers (Fig. 5.5). This usual arterial anatomy of the hand is widely variable on angiographic assessment, frequently necessitating comparison with the opposite hand.

The spectrum of disease that involves the upper extremity is different from that of the leg. Upper extremity arterial insufficiency is more commonly from embolism, steal, compression, vasculitis, or repetitive trauma phenomena (Fig. 5.6). The arm has abundant collaterals that readily bypass proximal atherosclerotic occlusive disease.

Abdominal Aortography

The most frequent indication for abdominal aortography is atherosclerotic occlusive disease. Other indications include mesenteric ischemia, preoperative evaluation of an abdominal aortic aneurysm, suspected renal vascular hypertension, and evaluation of a renal transplant donor.

Aortography can be performed from femoral, brachial, or translumbar approaches. The femoral approach is used most often except when there is aor-

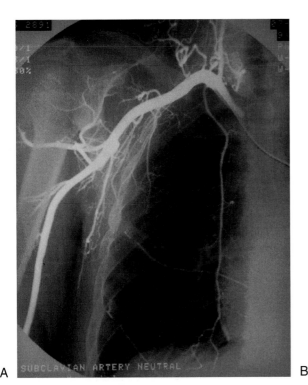

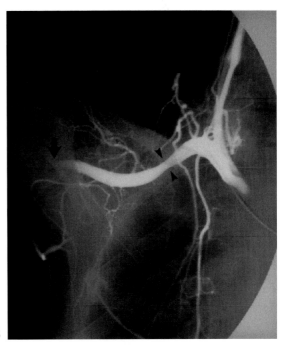

Figure 5.4 *Thoracic outlet syndrome.* **(A)** *Normal right subclavian artery in neutral position.* **(B)** *The right shoulder is externally rotated and abducted into the symptomatic position. The mid subclavian artery is concentrically compressed in the thoracic outlet (arrowheads), and the axillary artery is occluded by compression from the humeral head (arrow).*

toiliac occlusive disease. A 5 French 60 cm pigtail catheter with multiple sideholes is used from the femoral approach and a 4 to 5 French 100 cm pigtail is used from a brachial approach. The pigtail catheter design ensures a localized bolus with less cephalad retrograde flow of contrast. The pigtail catheter tip reduces the jet effect from the catheter end hole. Alternatively, a tennis racket or halo catheter tip configuration can be substituted. Aortography performed as a prelude to a leg runoff evaluates the aorta and renal arteries. The catheter is positioned so that the sideholes below the pigtail catheter bathe the renal arteries, resulting in less filling of the visceral arteries (Fig. 5.7). A forceful power injection may uncoil the pigtail loop, causing the tip to enter an intercostal or lumbar artery. Because the lumbar or intercostal arteries exit the aorta at the level of the vertebral pedicles, the tip of the catheter should be positioned at the level of an intravertebral disk space before the injection.

The injection rate is 20 ml/sec for a total of 40 to 50 ml. The digital images are obtained at three frames per second using a large field of view.

Lateral aortography is obtained in mesenteric ischemia, aortic aneurysm, blue-toe syndrome, penetrating atherosclerotic ulcers, and aortoenteric fistula. The origins of the visceral vessels are evaluated for stenoses or involvement by the aortic aneurysm. The anatomy of the abdominal aorta and the major branches are depicted in Figure 5.8.

Lower Extremity Angiography

Lower extremity arteriography is the most common angiographic study performed in most practices. The most common indications are to evaluate atherosclerotic, stenotic, occlusive, embolic, or aneurysmal disease

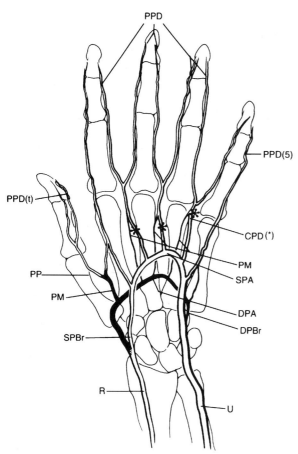

Figure 5.5 *Diagrammatic rendering of the classic arterial anatomy of the hand. Anatomic variation in the hand vasculature is commonplace. R, radial artery; DPA, deep palmar arch; PP, princeps policis artery; PPD(t), proper palmar digital artery (thumb) from deep palmar arch; U, ulnar artery; SPA, superficial palmar arch; CPD, common palmar digital arteries (from superficial arch); PM, palmar metacarpal arteries (from deep arch); PPD, proper palmar digital arteries; PPD(5), proper palmar digital artery (fifth finger) from superficial arch; SPBr, superficial palmar branch (from ulnar artery); DPBr, deep palmar branch (from radial artery). (From Dyer R: Handbook of Basic Vascular and Interventional Radiology. Churchill Livingstone, New York, 1993, with permission).*

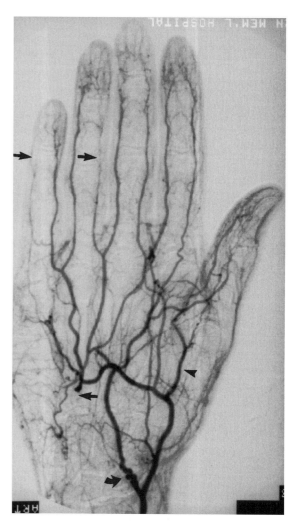

Figure 5.6 *Hypothenar hammer syndrome. Brick glazer who pounded bricks into place with his palm. There are occlusions of the distal ulnar and digital arteries (arrows). The distal radial artery has a focal corkscrew dilatation (curved arrow). The princeps pollicis artery to the thumb is spared (arrowhead).*

(Fig. 5.9). Other indications include trauma, vasculitis, popliteal entrapment, tumors, Buerger's thromboangiitis obliterans, malformations, and popliteal artery cystic adventitial disease. Most patients have been carefully selected for arteriography based on clinical assessment and screening noninvasive tests. Angiography confirms the distribution and extent of disease and is often a prelude to percutaneous or surgical intervention. The diversity of indications and wide variety of angiographic equipment available lead to many different methods and techniques for performing a routine lower extremity angiogram. Regardless of the method, the goals of angiography are to map out precisely the vascular anatomy and to determine the appropriate intervention necessary.

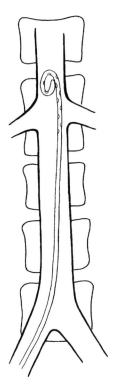

Figure 5.7 *Fluoroscopic bony landmarks are used to position the sideholes of the pigtail catheter. For aortorenal angiography, the sideholes of the pigtail catheter are located at the L2 vertebral body level. For aortovisceral angiography, the sideholes are located at the level of the T12 vertebral body. For bilateral lower extremity runoff, the sideholes of the catheter are located at the L4-L5 vertebral body level to maximally opacify the iliac arteries.*

A lower extremity runoff can be performed from the femoral, brachial, or translumbar approach. The femoral artery with the strongest pulse, preferably opposite the most symptomatic leg, is chosen. Both lower extremities are studied in a runoff because most diseases are systemic. A 5 French pigtail catheter is placed in the abdominal aorta, and the arterial inflow to the legs is evaluated by an aortogram. The pigtail is repositioned at the aortic bifurcation and two 25° to 35° oblique anterior views of the pelvis are taken. The injection rate for the pelvis varies from 8 ml/sec for 24 ml total to 12 ml/sec for 36 ml total, depending on the patient's size and the estimated flow rate. The field of view should encompass the aortic, iliac, and femoral bifurcations, which are common sites for atheroscle-

rotic disease. The hemodynamic significance of a moderate stenosis in the iliac artery is more completely assessed by a pressure measurement. A stress gradient is measured immediately after performing reactive hyperemia or administering an intra-arterial vasodilator in patients with claudication. A resting gradient of 10 mmHg and a stress gradient of 15 mmHg are considered significant.

The runoff examination can be performed by a variety of methods, depending on the equipment available. Image acquisition is by either film screen or digital subtraction techniques. Film screen techniques have the advantage of high spatial resolution and ability to measure vessel size directly from the film. The runoff vessels are imaged by bolus chasing with a stepping table or by imaging the entire leg on a long leg table unit. A long contrast injection at the aortic bifurcation opacifies the vessels of both legs. The injection rate is 7 to 9 ml/sec for 80 to 90 ml. The time from contrast injection in the distal aorta to contrast arrival at the knee estimates the transit time, which is used to match the stepping sequence of the table motion with the progression of contrast flow. A long injection helps compensate for asymmetric flow. A long leg changer images the entire leg at once. The contrast is injected and six films are obtained after a delay to allow opacification of the distal vasculature. Difficulties arise when the blood flow is asymmetric or the estimate of the flow rate does not match the actual flow rate.

Intra-arterial digital subtraction angiography (DSA) has better contrast resolution and allows immediate review of acquired images. The improved contrast resolution improves visualization of the infrapopliteal and pedal vessels. DSA gives a more accurate prediction of the ability to bypass to a given level. Larger image intensifiers allow visualization of both legs with 15 to 16 inch fields of view. The study is performed by contrast injection at the aortic bifurcation, and the legs are sequentially imaged in slightly overlapping stations from the lower pelvis to the pedal arch. Typical injection rates are 8 ml/sec for a total of 36 ml proximally to 60 ml distally. Multiple positions are required, but the images can be obtained and reviewed quickly. Additional projections can be obtained to better define overlapping anatomy, and prolonged acquisition of images can capture late filling vessels. Newer digital angiographic equipment combines bolus chasing technique with real-time image display. This allows the operator to monitor and follow the flow of contrast as the contrast progresses down the legs. A successful bolus chase reduces procedure time and

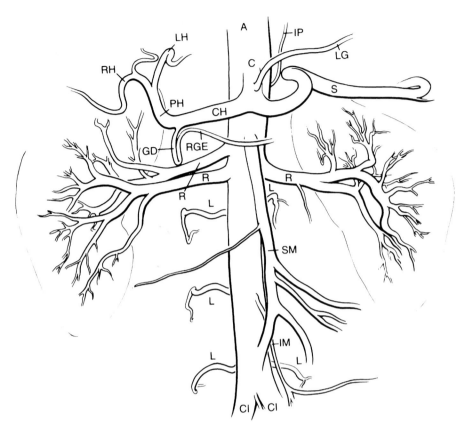

Figure 5.8 *Schematic anatomy of abdominal aorta and branches. A, abdominal aorta; C, celiac artery; LG, left gastric artery; IP, inferior phrenic artery; S, splenic artery; CH, common hepatic artery; GD, gastroduodenal artery; RGE, right gastroepiploic artery; PH, proper hepatic artery; RH, right hepatic artery; LH, left hepatic artery; R, renal arteries; SM, superior mesenteric artery; IM, inferior mesenteric artery; L, lumbar arteries; CI, common iliac arteries. (From Dyer R: Handbook of Basic Vascular and Interventional Radiology. Churchill Livingstone, New York, 1993, with permission).*

contrast load. Real-time monitoring improves visualization of the runoff but does not eliminate the difficulties encountered with asymmetric flow. When there is asymmetric flow, selective leg angiography is used to optimally visualize the patent but late filling vessels.

Small details improve image quality. The patient is instructed to hold the legs still. A center filter is placed between the patient's legs to smooth out the density and reduce shine through. Collimation reduces scatter artifact and improves exposure. A mixture of lidocaine with the contrast makes the injection more comfortable for the patient. The concentration of the lidocaine should not exceed 1 mg/ml of contrast up to a total of

100 mg of lidocaine. Intra-arterial lidocaine is used only in the distal aorta or lower extremities. Nonionic contrast and isosmolar, nonionic contrast are less painful than ionic contrast material.

Distal visualization of the infrapopliteal vessels and pedal arch is necessary for diagnostic and therapeutic planning. Large contrast injections, balloon occlusion angiography, reactive hyperemia, intra-arterial vasodilators, and selective leg angiography can improve opacification of the distal vessels. Selective single leg angiography is probably the easiest strategy to accomplish this goal. Indications for selective leg angiography are the evaluation of trauma, tumors, vas-

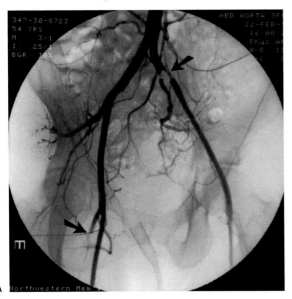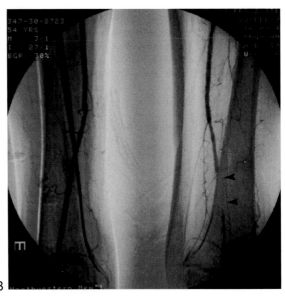

A   B

Figure 5.9 *Acute emboli to the legs from a cardiac source. (A) Filling defects are lodged in the left common iliac bifurcation and the right profunda femoris arteries (arrows). (B) The distal left superficial femoral artery is occluded by emboli (arrowheads). Note the lack of collaterals, which helps differentiate emboli from thrombosis secondary to stenotic disease.*

cular flap grafts, malformations, and severe occlusive disease. A contralateral antegrade study is accomplished by crossing the aortic bifurcation with a pull-type catheter such as a Neiman visceral hook (see Fig. 4.5). Use of a Glidewire or trapping the wire by pressing on the opposite femoral artery facilitates advancing the catheter over the bifurcation. The contrast injection rate varies from 4 to 6 ml/sec for a total of 20 to 40 ml. The ipsilateral leg is studied by a multi-side hole straight catheter positioned in the external iliac artery. The injection rates are similar to the contralateral study. Reactive hyperemia causes transient vasodilatation and is easy to perform by suprasystolic inflation of a cuff on the calf for 5 minutes. Intra-arterial vasodilators reverse spasm associated with trauma and can be safely used in legs with grafts.

Selective contralateral angiography is used to evaluate traumatic injuries with the catheter placed as close as possible to the potential injury. Patients who have proximity injuries to extremity vessels with a normal physical examination can have the angiographic evaluation delayed until normal working hours. Patients with expanding extremity hematomas, pulse deficits, and joint dislocations require urgent angiographic evalua-

tions (Fig. 5.10). Symptomatic young patients should be evaluated for the presence of popliteal artery entrapment, adventitial cystic disease, embolism, and Buerger's thromboangiitis obliterans. The popliteal arteries are examined with the ankle actively plantar flexed or passively dorsiflexed to accentuate the compression on the artery. The majority of cases are due to anomalous course of the artery or anomalous insertion of the medial head of the gastrocnemius muscle, which compresses the artery (Fig. 5.11).

Renal Angiography

Renal angiography is indicated for the evaluation of renovascular hypertension, trauma, tumors, vasculitis, renal transplant donation, and hematuria. Abdominal aortography is performed for renal transplant and renovascular hypertension evaluation. The pigtail artery should be positioned to minimize reflux into the superior mesenteric artery (SMA). The renal arteries usually arise near the L2 vertebral body. Approximately 30

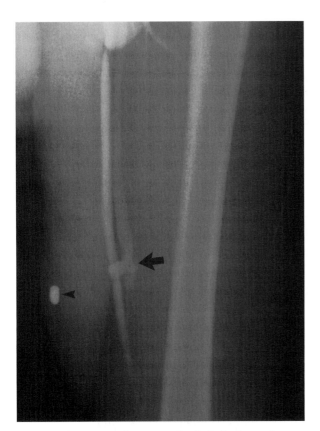

Figure 5.10 *Gunshot wound to left thigh resulting in arteriovenous fistula (arrow). The bullet (arrowhead) is still present in the medial aspect of the thigh.*

to 40 percent of patients have multiple renal arteries. Selective renal angiography is performed to evaluate intrarenal arterial disorders (Fig. 5.12). The renal artery is selected with a 5 French Neiman renal catheter. Other pull-type catheters can be used such as Cobra or Simmons 2 catheters. Selective DSA with mild magnification optimally visualizes the renal vasculature. Two different views are necessary for visualization and evaluation of renal masses. The injection rate is 6 to 8 ml/sec for a total of 14 to 20 ml. The filming rate is acquired at three films per second during the arterial phase and then is reduced to one to two films per second to record the capillary and venous phases.

Renal artery stenosis is usually due to atherosclerotic or fibromuscular disease. Atherosclerotic stenoses involve the main renal artery or aorta, are frequently bilateral, and are smooth concentric or eccentric narrowings. Fibromuscular dysplasia accounts for one-third of reno-

vascular hypertension cases and involves younger individuals than does atherosclerotic disease. Fibromuscular dysplasia lesions are characterized by a string of beads appearance, mural aneurysms, and weblike stenoses (see Fig. 7.3). Fibromuscular dysplasia is classified by the site of involvement in the arterial wall (intima, media, perimedia). Medial dysplasia is the most frequent variant. Multiple intrarenal aneurysms are seen from polyarteritis nodosa, systemic lupus erythematosus, drug vasculitis, trauma, and mycotic etiologies.

Vasogenic Impotence

Impotence can result from psychogenic, hormonal, neurogenic, and vasogenic etiologies. Internal pudendal angiography is reserved for patients who have been carefully screened to exclude the nonvasogenic etiologies of impotence. An absence of nocturnal erections suggests an organic cause for impotence. Screening tests for the arterial supply includes the penile-brachial index and color Doppler interrogation of the cavernosal arteries. The normal penile-brachial index is 0.7 or greater; 0.6 to 0.7 is indeterminate, and less than 0.6 is suggestive. Color Doppler ultrasonography of the cavernosal arteries is performed both before and after intracavernosal injection of papaverine. Arterial insufficiency is suggested when peak systolic flow is less than 30 to 35 ml/sec.

Arteriogenic impotence is studied angiographically to determine the site and morphology of the obstruction. Adequate conscious sedation is necessary to relieve anxiety. Initially, a pelvic arteriogram is performed to study the proximal iliac arteries to exclude inflow stenoses. Bilateral selective internal pudendal arteriography is necessary to define the arterial lesions and select patients for revascularization surgery. The internal pudendal artery arises from the anterior division of the internal iliac artery. The internal pudendal continues as the penile artery. The three main branches of the penile artery are the dorsal penile, bulbar, and cavernosal arteries (Fig. 5.13). The cavernosal artery is the functionally most important erectile artery and is recognized by the helicine arteries. Anatomic variation and collateral circulation are the norm rather than the exception.

Selective internal pudendal arteriography must optimally visualize the intrapenile arteries. Intracaver-

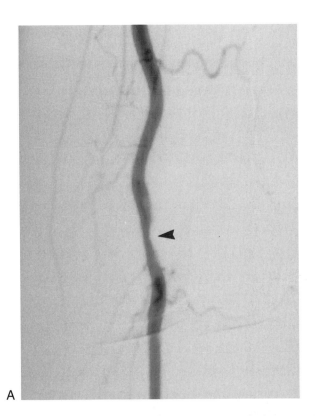

A

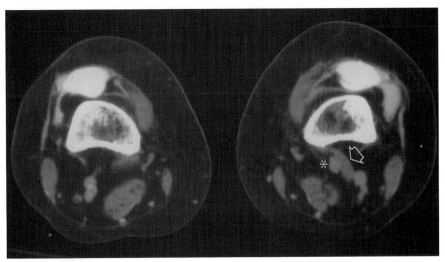

B

Figure 5.11 *Popliteal entrapment syndrome.*
(A) Left popliteal angiogram demonstrates eccentric narrowing of the popliteal artery at the level of the femoral condyle (arrowhead). (B) A CT scan shows that the popliteal artery (*) is deviated medially around the medial head of the gastrocnemius muscle. The muscle courses between the artery and vein (arrow).

Figure 5.12 *von Hippel-Lindau disease. (A) Selected magnified renal arteriogram showing numerous hypervascular masses (arrows). Multiple avascular filling defects are present from renal cysts (arrowheads). (B) CT scan showing multiple renal cysts and solid masses involving both kidneys. Note involvement of head of pancreas with cyst (arrows).*

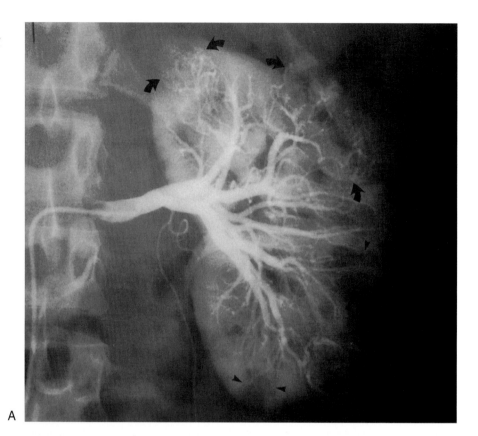

A

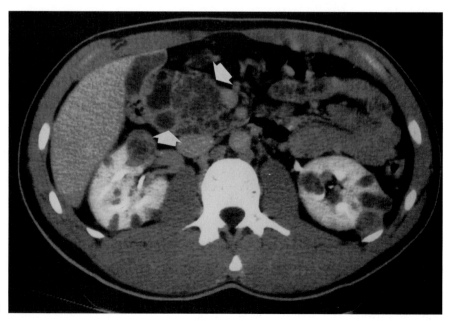

B

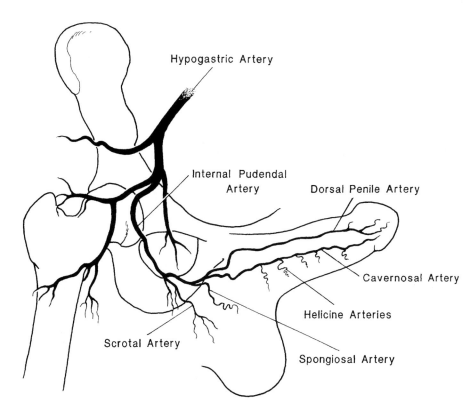

Figure 5.13 *Schematic illustration of the right internal pudendal arterial supply to the penis.*

Labels in figure:
Hypogastric Artery
Internal Pudendal Artery
Dorsal Penile Artery
Cavernosal Artery
Helicine Arteries
Scrotal Artery
Spongiosal Artery

nosal papaverine, 30 to 60 mg, or tolazoline, 25 mg, minimizes venous outflow and maximizes arterial inflow. The contralateral internal pudendal artery is studied first. A Neiman catheter or similar pull-type catheter is used to cross the aortic bifurcation and select the internal iliac artery. The anterior division and internal pudendal arteries are outlined by roadmapping. A Glidewire and angled-tip glide catheter are directed into the internal pudendal artery. Catheter induced vasospasm is treated with intra-arterial vasodilators. The left internal pudendal artery is imaged in the left anterior oblique position, with the penis taped to the right thigh. The injection rate is 3 to 6 ml/sec for a total of 15 to 36 ml. Films are acquired at two to three images per second for the duration of arterial contrast opacification as monitored on real time image review. The ipsilateral internal pudendal artery is imaged in a similar manner. The Neiman or Simmons catheter is used to select the ipsilateral internal iliac artery. Under roadmapping guidance, a torquable guidewire and angled-tip catheter are directed into the anterior division and internal pudendal arteries. A Waltman loop or coaxial technique can be used when the easier methods fail. The penis is taped to the oppo-

site thigh and the films are acquired in the ipsilateral anterior oblique projection.

The arterial anatomy, patency, and distribution of lesions are documented by the study. The anatomy is highly variable, with unilateral origin of the cavernosal arteries, hypoplasia of the dorsal penile, and anomalous origin of the cavernosal arteries being the common variants. There are multiple potential collateral routes. The distribution of lesions tends to be in the base of the penis but is dependent on the age of the patient and the presence of coexistent medical diseases (e.g., diabetes). The arterial lesions must be bilateral to be significant (Fig. 5.14).

Mesenteric Angiography

Mesenteric angiography is the study of the celiac, superior mesenteric, and inferior mesenteric vessels. The use of mesenteric angiography has waned with the advent of endoscopy, cross-sectional imaging, and nuclear medicine techniques but is still useful in certain situations. Current indications are evaluation of

Figure 5.14 *Vasogenic impotence. (**A**) Right internal pudendal arteriogram shows absent right dorsal penile artery and common origin of both cavernosal arteries from the right (arrows). Multiple stenoses are present (arrowheads). (**B**) Left internal pudendal arteriogram demonstrates multiple stenoses in the dorsal penile artery (arrows). The left cavernosal artery is replaced to the right.*

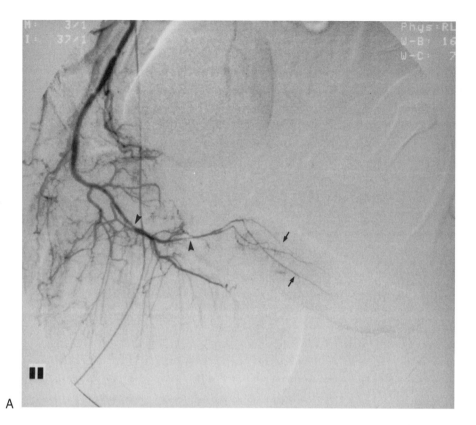

A

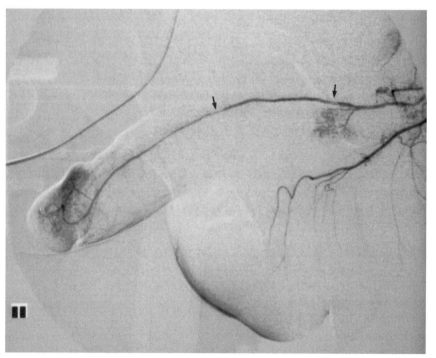

B

gastrointestinal hemorrhage, ischemia, trauma, portal hypertension, vasculitis, aneurysms, and malformations. Mesenteric angiography is used to evaluate mesenteric vascular anatomy before operation, embolization, or CT during arterial portography. Patient preparation includes placing a Foley catheter in patients with gastrointestinal hemorrhage to monitor urine output and to empty the bladder for optimal visualization of the inferior mesenteric artery (IMA).

The femoral approach is used in the majority of cases. The left brachial approach facilitates superselective catheterization when the vessels arise in a steep downgoing course. The Neiman visceral 2 catheter is preferred for catheterization of the celiac or superior mesenteric arteries. This catheter is a simple 70° angled hook shape with a sidehole. The smaller secondary hole helps prevent migration of the catheter out of the vessel during power injections. Alternative catheters are the Cobra or Simmons pull-type catheter designs. The celiac artery arises at the level of the mid T12 to upper L1 vertebral bodies (Fig. 5.15). The SMA is immediately caudal to the celiac. A Rösch inferior mesenteric (RIM) catheter is used for catheterization of the IMA, which arises to the left of midline at the L3 vertebral body level. A lateral aortogram is obtained in patients with ischemia and aortic aneurysms. Otherwise, we directly proceed to selective mesenteric injections without aortography. The order of vessel selection is based on the clinical estimation for the localization of the abnormality. For example, the IMA is examined first when evaluating lower gastrointestinal hemorrhage. It is important to image all the vessels because of the numerous anatomic variants and communications frequently present.

Contrast injection rates for the celiac artery are 6 to 8 ml/sec for a total of 30 to 60 ml. The rate is based on test injections. The injection rate for the SMA is 7 to 8 ml/sec for a total of 40 to 80 ml. An arterial portogram is performed following vasodilatation with 25 mg of tolazoline injected slowly over 2 minutes into the SMA. This promotes rapid arterial-to-venous shunting and optimizes visualization of the portal vein. The injection rate for arterial portography is increased, averaging 8 ml/sec for 80 seconds. Contrast injection rates for the IMA are 3 to 4 ml/sec for a total of 9 to 15 ml. The entire vascular distribution of the IMA cannot be included on a single field of view. Two fields of view should be obtained by positioning over the sigmoid

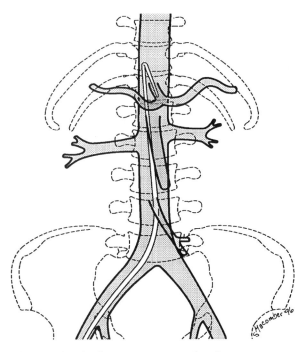

Figure 5.15 *The Neiman visceral catheter is positioned so that its tip is oriented anteriorly and pulled into the orifice of the celiac artery which is located at the level of the T12 vertebral body. Once the celiac angiogram is completed, the catheter is pushed into the body to disengage the celiac artery. The catheter is steered around the celiac artery and pulled into the orifice of the superior mesenteric artery, which is just caudal to the origin of the celiac artery.*

area and the splenic flexure separately. Oblique views of the sigmoid or the splenic flexure may be used to unfold overlapping bowel loops.

Advances in DSA equipment make it our preferred imaging modality despite the decreased spatial resolution and potential for image misregistration from respiratory motion and bowel peristalsis. DSA units with a large (15 to 16 inch) fields of view and 1024 matrix frame size generate diagnostic images with several advantages. There is rapid acquisition of multiple runs, increased contrast resolution, reduced contrast dose, and immediate review of images. A C-arm DSA unit provides superior procedural guidance with roadmapping and rapid image review. The improved postprocessing functions can compensate for image misregistration. Careful coaching of patients on breath holding and inhibition of peristalsis by glucagon improve image quality. If a patient cannot breath hold, we acquire multiple mask images immediately before contrast injection through an entire breath cycle. The mask images are then matched to the contrast images to obtain a clear subtracted image. Filming rates are at a fixed rate of two to three frames per second. The acquisition is carried out until the venous phase is well visualized by viewing the monitor.

Superselective mesenteric catheterization is sometimes required for embolization or infusional procedures. Superselective catheterization techniques include the coaxial 3 French catheter system, the Waltman loop technique, and hydrophilic coated, torque control wires and catheters. The 3 French microcatheter and 0.018 inch guidewire are passed coaxially through a 5 French catheter placed in the orifice of the main vessel trunk. The 3 French catheter can be negotiated deeply into the vascular tree to reach a bleeding site for embolization. The Waltman loop technique is used for selection of second- and third-order mesenteric vessel branches. A 5 to 7 French Cobra catheter is formed into a 10 to 12 cm loop in the iliac, superior mesenteric, or celiac artery. The loop is pulled into the desired mesenteric artery, and the tip is directed into the target branch. Loop technique is more cumbersome than coaxial technique, but it allows larger contrast injections and catheterization of cranially angulated branches of the mesenteric vessels. Hydrophilic coated wires and catheters have lower coefficients of friction, which allow them to pass around bends and through curves easier than conventional devices. The left gastric artery arises superiorly off the downward directed celiac trunk, which can make selective left gastric cannulation problematic. The Rösch left gastric catheter is preshaped to select this branch. The celiac trunk is selected with a visceral catheter and is removed over a long exchange guidewire. The Rösch left gastric catheter tip is advanced beyond the origin of the left

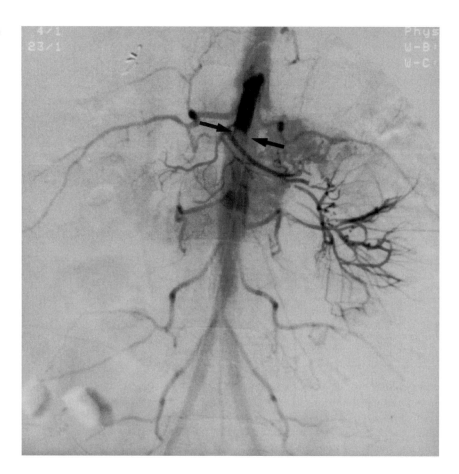

Figure 5.16 *An acute embolic occlusion of the proximal superior mesenteric artery. A meniscus sign is present (arrows).*

gastric over the wire. The catheter's preformed shape directs the tip into the artery as the catheter is carefully withdrawn while injecting small amounts of contrast to identify the left gastric artery.

Most cases of mesenteric ischemia involve the SMA supply. The major causes are arterial embolization or thrombosis, venous thrombosis, and nonocclusive ischemia (Figs. 5.16 and 5.17). Nonocclusive mesenteric ischemia occurs in the elderly who have cardiac disease, hypotension, or sepsis. It is associated with a high mortality rate and is characterized angiographically by arterial vasospasm and diminished venous outflow (Fig. 5.18). Reversal of the spasm confirms the diagnosis and is a therapeutic option. The most commonly used vasodilator is papaverine at 30 to 60 mg/hr. Patients are monitored for hypotension and cardiac arrhythmias during the infusion. Select cases of mesenteric arterial and venous thrombosis can potentially be treated with urokinase thrombolysis. Thrombolysis has a limited role because the duration of a successful infusion may result in the conversion of ischemic bowel to infarcted bowel. Thus, the presence of peritoneal signs is a contraindication to thrombolysis.

During the last decade, angiography has lost its primary role in the diagnosis of acute gastrointestinal hemorrhage to advances in endoscopy and nuclear medicine. Most gastrointestinal bleeding stops spontaneously without treatment or bleeds intermittently. A tagged red blood cell study is now accepted as the most sensitive study for detecting active hemorrhage. Angiography is indicated to localize lower gastrointestinal hemorrhage (Fig. 5.19) and potentially treat massive upper gastrointestinal hemorrhage that has failed endoscopic therapy. The critical rate of bleeding is 0.5 ml/min for detection by angiography. The left gastric artery accounts for 85 percent of gastric hemorrhage. Embolization is the treatment for upper gastrointestinal sources because of the rich anastomotic vascular supply prevents ischemia. Embolotherapy is reserved for carefully selected patients with point sources of bleeding in the lower gastrointestinal tract. A temporary agent such as Gelfoam is used and is placed as selectively as possible to the point source of bleeding but not into the vasa recta. Vasopressin therapy is used for small vessel bleeding, diffuse bleeding, or bleeding from a vessel supplied by one artery. The protocol for vasopressin therapy is to

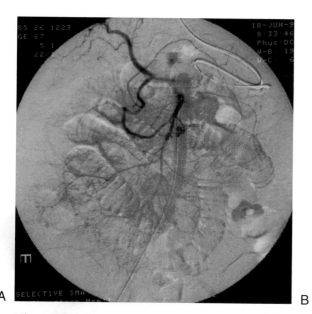
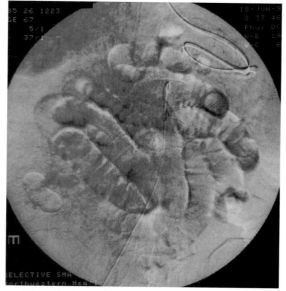

A   B

Figure 5.17 *Superior mesenteric venous thrombosis.* **(A)** *The selective superior mesenteric injection shows spasm involving peripheral arteries with reflux opacification of the hepatic artery via the gastroduodenal artery.* **(B)** *The venous phase of the arterial injection shows an absence of mesenteric veins. The small bowel is dilated from the venous thrombosis.*

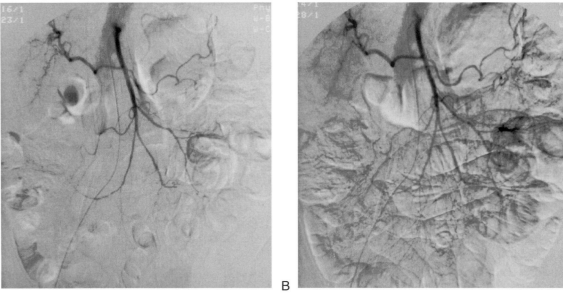

Figure 5.18 *Nonocclusive mesenteric ischemia. (A) Selective superior mesenteric arteriogram showing pruning of the vascular tree and diffuse arterial spasm. (B) Superior mesenteric arteriogram following intra-arterial administration of papaverine, 30 mg. Note significant reversal of the diffuse spasm and filling of the distal arterial tree. The mesenteric vein was opacified following intra-arterial vasodilatation. The patient was treated with a 12-hour infusion of papaverine to treat the ischemia.*

Figure 5.19 *Gastrointestinal hemorrhage. (A) There is extravasation of contrast from the right colic artery (arrow). (B) The puddling of contrast (arrow) that lasts into the venous phase confirms the presence of gastrointestinal hemorrhage and differentiates contrast extravasation from subtraction motion artifact.*

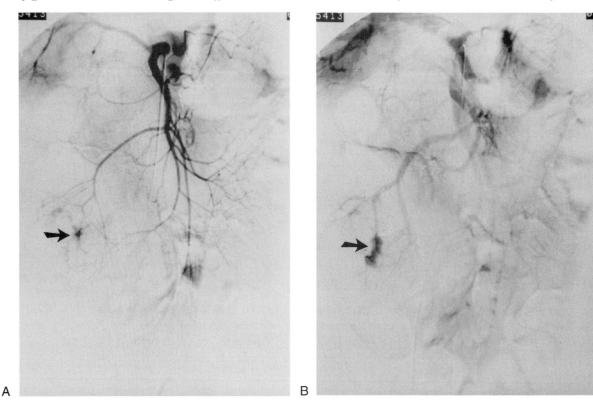

selectively catheterize the bleeding artery. The infusion is started at 0.2 U/min. The arteriogram is repeated in 30 minutes. If the bleeding is stopped, the infusion is continued for 12 to 24 hours, with the patient monitored in an intensive care unit. If the bleeding continues, the rate is increased to 0.3 to 0.4 U/min. If the bleeding stops, the infusion is slowly tapered by 0.1 U every 6 hours and finally replaced with a saline infusion while carefully monitoring for recurrent bleeding with the catheter kept in place. The catheter is removed only after a 6-hour observation period for recurrent bleeding.

Computed Tomography Arterial Portography

Computed tomography during arterial portography (CTAP) is an important technique for evaluating the liver before hepatic tumor resection. The normal liver parenchyma is predominantly supplied by the portal vein, while liver tumors are supplied by the hepatic artery. CT scanning during the portal phase of contrast circulation will depict hepatic tumors as low in attenuation relative to the densely enhancing normal hepatic parenchyma. The hepatic vasculature is well opacified, and the relationship of lesions to the vasculature is optimally localized. CTAP is the most sensitive imaging technique for the detection of hepatic lesions but lacks specificity because the perfusion defects detected with CTAP are not always tumor. Combining CTAP and MRI increases the sensitivity and specificity of evaluating focal liver lesions to a reported rate of 96 percent. MRI has inherent high tissue contrast resolution and is useful for characterizing the lesions discovered on CTAP. MRI alone is hampered by respiratory motion and lower spatial resolution, which limits the detection of lesions smaller than 2 cm.

Indications for performing CTAP are the detection and localization of hepatic metastases and the evaluation of primary hepatic neoplasms. The CTAP technique requires the combination of selected visceral angiography combined with CT of the liver during intra-arterial contrast administration into either the superior mesenteric or splenic artery. The study is started in the angiography suite where a Neiman visceral or similar pull-type catheter is used to select both the celiac and superior mesenteric arteries. Small test boluses (5 to 10 ml) of contrast are injected into each artery to determine the arterial supply to the liver. A replaced right hepatic artery to the SMA occurs in 20 percent of the population. If the patient has a replaced right hepatic artery, the catheter is either advanced distally into the SMA or placed within the splenic artery. The volume of contrast material administered during the initial angiographic portion of the procedure should be minimal to improve the quality of the CT study of the liver.

The patient is subsequently transferred to the CT scanner, and the arterial catheter is connected to the mechanical power injector. A scout scan of the abdomen is obtained to map out the liver size and position. A dynamic or spiral CT scan protocol is programmed to image the liver in 5 to 8 mm table increments. A biphasic injection is programmed at the initial rate of 2 ml/sec for 20 seconds followed by the rate of 1 ml/sec for the remainder of the 150 ml capacity of the power injector. The liver is rapidly scanned with thin sections during the portal phase of contrast circulation. The delay time is 20 to 30 seconds for nonspiral CT scanners and 30 to 60 seconds for spiral scanners. A second CT scan pass through the liver is performed during the systemic phase of contrast enhancement after a 3 to 5 minute delay.

After the CT portion of the test, the patient is returned to the angiography suite where selected visceral angiography is performed. The visceral angiogram maps out the vascular supply for operative planning and depicts hypervascular hepatic lesions. A selective SMA angiogram should be performed at 6 to 8 ml/sec for a total of 40 to 60 ml. Intra-arterial tolazoline administration may be used to optimize visualization of the portal vein. The celiac angiogram uses an injection rate of 6 to 7 ml/sec for a total of 35 to 50 ml. Selective angiography of the hepatic artery with a small field of view covering the liver will improve the specificity in detection of hepatic neoplasms.

Interpretation of CTAP is based on detection of perfusion defects. The shape, attenuation value, and location of the perfusion abnormalities help discriminate malignant from benign lesions. Malignant lesions typically appear as round perfusion defects ranging from 3 mm to 10 cm in diameter. Round perfusion defects with calcifications and perfusion defects with vascular invasion are highly suspicious for being caused by malignant neoplasms (Fig. 5.20). Round perfusion defects, however, can also be caused by cysts, hemangiomas, cirrhotic nodules, focal nodular hyperplasia, and focal fatty change. Small, wedge-shaped perfusion

Figure 5.20 CTAP. *(A) The catheter is infusing into the splenic artery, and the liver is scanned during the portal phase of contrast circulation. (Figure continues.)*

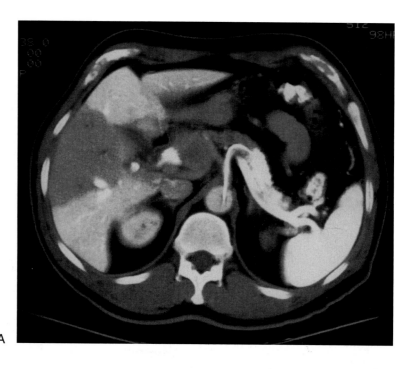

A

defects that are peripherally located are usually benign. Flat perfusion defects in two locations are common pseudolesions. These are perfusion defects adjacent to the falciform ligament and immediately anterior to the porta hepatis in segment 4 (Fig. 5.21). High attenuation lesions are almost always malignant and are due to an aberrant hepatic artery or late scanning during the systemic circulation of contrast material. The location of lesions is described based on Couinard's segmental anatomy (Fig. 5.22).

Spiral CT Angiography

Computed tomography angiography (CTA) is made possible by the speed of spiral CT and the computer programs that can render three-dimensional images. The technique is best suited to imaging the aorta, especially in the evaluation of aneurysmal disease. CTA images both the vascular lumen outlined by contrast and the vessel wall and surrounding structures. CTA can be used to image the carotid and renal arteries for stenosis, the pulmonary tree for emboli, the mesenteric vessels for patency, and the thoracic outlet for compression (Fig. 5.23). Patients sustaining decelerating or blunt chest trauma can be effectively screened with

spiral CT of the thoracic aorta to exclude an injury. This is particularly useful when the patient will be taken to the CT scanner to have a cerebral or abdominal CT study. The CT screening of low to moderate probability aortic injury patients reduces the need for thoracic angiography and expedites the care of trauma patients. If there is a very high index of suspicion for a thoracic aortic injury or a highly suspicious chest radiograph, then a thoracic angiogram should be performed. Three to five pre-contrast scans should be taken of the mediastinal to look for hemorrhage. Findings suggesting aortic injury include pseudoaneurysm formation, intimal flap, luminal irregularity, and mediastinal hemorrhage.

Careful attention to technique is required. The patient is instructed about the importance of breath holding. The length of the scan is 20 to 30 seconds, preferably during a single breath hold to eliminate respiratory misregistration. No oral contrast is given. Contrast delivery is accurately timed to obtain scans during the arterial phase of contrast circulation, which minimizes venous and organ parenchymal opacification. Typical injection rates are 2 to 4 ml/sec for a total of 100 to 150 ml, depending on the area covered. The scan delay time is 10 to 25 seconds. Maximum resolution is with thin collimation (2 to 3 mm) and a pitch of 1. This is important for imaging small vessels. Larger vessels covering a longer length can be satisfactorily imaged with larger collimation (3 to 7 mm) and a

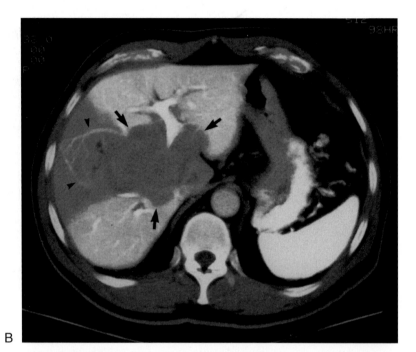

B

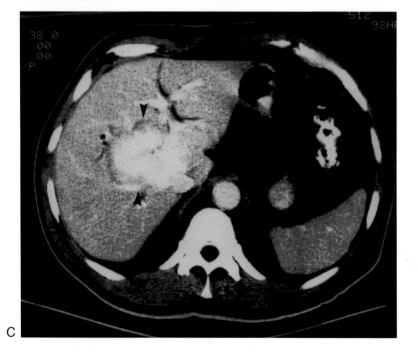

C

Figure 5.20 *(Continued)* **(B)** *The metastasis in the right lobe of the liver is low in attenuation during the portal phase (arrows). The CTAP clearly depicts the compression on the main left portal vein and occlusion of the right anterior segmental portal vein. There are intraportal collaterals (arrowheads).* **(C)** *The metastasis in the right lobe of the liver is hypervascular during the systemic recirculation of contrast (arrowheads).*

Figure 5.21 *CT portogram demonstrating round 4 cm mass in right lobe of liver with vascular compression (arrowheads). The liver is cirrhotic with a nodular border and multiple small round filling defects. These defects were secondary to cirrhotic regenerating nodules. Note the filling defect anterior to the right portal vein, which is a typical pseudolesion location (arrow). Numerous coronary varices are present (curved arrow).*

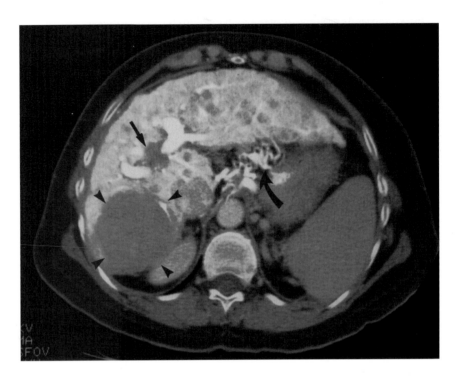

Figure 5.22 *Frontal view segmental anatomy of liver according to Couinaud. The eight hepatic segments are based on portal distribution. The segments are numbered in a clockwise manner.*

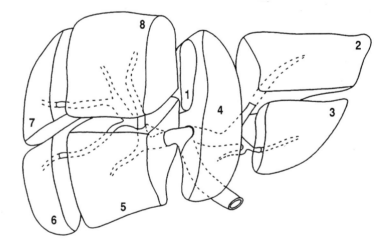

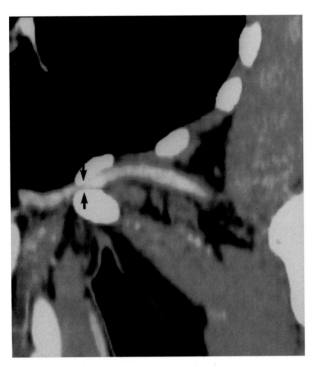

Figure 5.23 *Spiral CT arteriogram of thoracic outlet syndrome. The patient is scanned with the arm abducted in the symptomatic position. Thin axial sections are obtained through thoracic inlet during the arterial phase of contrast injection. The data was reformatted in a curved linear plane. The right subclavian artery is compressed between the clavicle and first rib (arrows).*

slightly longer pitch. Imaging a large volume reduces the spatial resolution. The data are reconstructed with a 33 to 50 percent overlap to diminish partial volume averaging and improve the smoothness of the three-dimensional renderings.

Three-dimensional rendering techniques include maximum intensity projections (MIPs) and shaded surface displays (SSDs). Newer work stations and software have reduced the time and labor necessary to render three-dimensional images. The editing program is used to remove unwanted overlapping structures such as bone and soft tissue and focuses on the vessels. Three-dimensional image rendering starts with choosing a two-dimensional area of interest on the axial image centering on the desired vessel. This is analogous to cropping a picture to isolate the desired interior structures. SSD images are generated by choosing a threshold pixel

value below the density of contrast to eliminate soft tissue density pixels. The image is displayed as a surface illuminated by a light source. SSD images can be rotated to sort out overlapping vessels (Fig. 5.24). An MIP image is generated by casting rays through the volume and encoding the maximum value encountered by each ray. These images are similar in appearance to intravenous digital subtraction angiography (IVDSA). The MIP image always records the brightest pixel encountered along the path of the ray. Thus, MIP images can distinguish calcified plaques in the wall of a vessel from the opacified lumen. However, bone will block the vessels if the bone is either in front of or behind a vessel. The bones must be removed by either cropping the volume or by automated editing. Three-dimensional connectivity editing can remove the bones within the volume of the CTA acquisition. The editor selects a seed point on an axial section on a bony structure. The automatic editing program selects all adjacent voxels that are above the bone density threshold removing unwanted bone within the volume imaged. A third rendering technique displays the volumetric data in coronal, sagittal, or curved planar formats. The image is generated by selecting a straight or curved line to delineate a single voxel thick plane through the volume perpendicular to the view on which the line or curve is drawn. This editing displays the contrast filled lumen of the vessel along with the soft tissue and bone structures within the plane. The postprocessing required to display planar images is easy to perform because cropping and bone removal editing are not required.

Carbon Dioxide Angiography

Carbon dioxide gas can be used as a substitute for iodinated contrast material. The high quality digital subtraction equipment now available can readily detect the minimal differences in density between a carbon dioxide gas filled lumen of an artery and the surrounding soft tissue. The advantage of carbon dioxide angiography is the elimination of iodinated contrast allergic reactions and nephrotoxicity. The indications for carbon dioxide angiography are renal insufficiency, severe contrast allergies, and renal transplant patients. Patients who have renal insufficiency with creatinine values between 2 and 5 are

Figure 5.24 *Rotated SSD renderings of thoracic outlet syndrome. (**A**) Oblique lateral view of right thoracic outlet showing exiting right subclavian artery pinched between clavicle and first rib (arrows). (**B**) Superior view of different patient showing artery being deviated and compressed by right seventh cervical rib (white arrow). The mid right subclavian artery has poststenotic dilatation distal to the cervical rib compression (black arrow).*

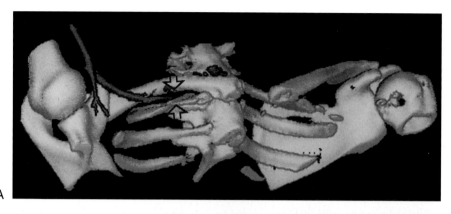

A

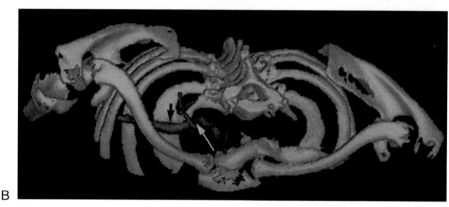

B

ideal candidates. Carbon dioxide angiography best visualizes the larger vessels. It is ideal for doing aortorenal, pelvic, and proximal extremity angiography. Carbon dioxide angiography can provide additional diagnostic information that cannot be attained with iodinated contrast agents: (1) Arterial venous shunting is better demonstrated in malignant tumors, (2) apparently avascular masses become very vascular, (3) carbon dioxide will demonstrate minute amounts of bleeding, and (4) carbon dioxide permits reliable imaging of the portal vein with wedged hepatic venous injections. Carbon dioxide angiography can be used to perform interventional procedures such as angioplasty. Patients with cardiac or renal failure do not need to be prehydrated before undergoing carbon dioxide angiography. Carbon dioxide is inexpensive and is a fraction of the cost of nonionic contrast.

The disadvantages of carbon dioxide angiography are related to the physical properties of the gas, which are compressibility, invisibility, and buoyancy. If there is resistance within the injection system, the gas will compress in volume until an adequate pressure is

developed to overcome the resistance. This results in an explosive-type injection that delivers a large volume of carbon dioxide over a short time. Carbon dioxide is buoyant and preferentially fills nondependent vessels. The target vascular bed must be elevated to adequately visualize it. The carbon dioxide column can fragment as it travels peripherally. Patients frequently have less pain than a contrast angiogram, but some report a tearing sensation with carbon dioxide injections. When this occurs, suspect contamination with air. Carbon dioxide angiography is limited in visualizing small arterial branches, the normally enhancing visceral parenchyma, and veins during arterial injections.

Three important principles must be followed to avoid potentially severe complications: (1) The carbon dioxide should not be contaminated with air, (2) explosive delivery should be avoided, and (3) injection of excess volumes should be avoided. Excess volumes are extrapolated from research. When more than 800 ml of carbon dioxide are injected rapidly in dogs, the heart can fill with the gas and the test animals expire. This occurs with both venous and arterial injections.

The injection of excess volumes can occur when the patient is connected directly to the carbon dioxide tank. Injection of modest volumes of gas is well tolerated because there is an extensive buffering system and capability to eliminate carbon dioxide by the body. Carbon dioxide is 20 times more soluble than oxygen in plasma. The safety of carbon dioxide has been established for injection of modest volumes below the diaphragm both intra-arterially and intravenously. Carbon dioxide angiography is contraindicated for use above the diaphragm within the arterial tree because of the potential neurotoxicity. Carbon dioxide can cause neurotoxicity by capillary blockade resulting in ischemia.

The University of Florida at Gainesville has developed a simple delivery system (Fig. 5.25). This system uses a plastic bag that can hold 1,500 ml of carbon dioxide. Before filling the bag, a 20 ml syringe is used to aspirate the bag creating a vacuum. The bag is filled and purged three times from a disposable cylinder containing medical grade carbon dioxide. The multiple refills reduce the possibility of air contamination. The system has one-way valves to prevent reflux and sealed connections to prevent air leakage. The 60 ml syringe is used for injections and the 10 ml syringe is used to flush the catheter. The key to controlled delivery of carbon dioxide is to clear the catheter of liquid. Because of the low viscosity of gases, carbon dioxide can be injected easily through a catheter that contains only gas. If the catheter contains saline or blood, there is an explosive and uncontrolled delivery of gas.

For abdominal aortography, a 60 ml syringe is filled, and the injection is made over 1 second. A 4 to 5 French halo tip catheter works best at delivering the proper bolus injection. An acquisition is repeated until a diagnostic study is obtained. The renal arteries are imaged in a decubitus position to use the buoyant effect of the gas when standard supine images are inadequate. Pelvic angiography uses an injection of 40 ml of carbon dioxide over 2 seconds. A similar size bolus is used to image the lower extremities. Optimal imaging of the infrapopliteal arteries requires selective placement of the catheter, elevation of the extremity, and intra-arterial vasodilatation (Fig. 5.26). The injection rate is 20 to 40 ml over 2 seconds. A rapid filming sequence of four exposures per second is used. A waiting period of 2 minutes between injections is adequate for complete removal of the injected carbon dioxide.

There is a second technique for performing carbon dioxide angiography, which can be assembled from

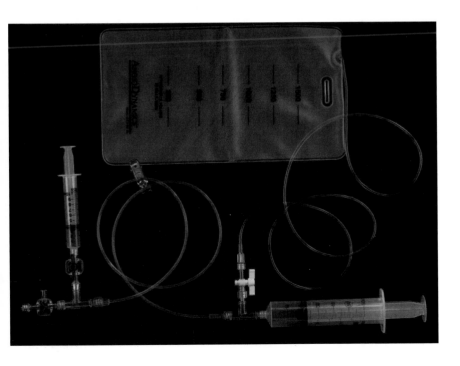

Figure 5.25 The angiodynamic flush bag and connection system modified for use as a carbon dioxide delivery system. The bag is filled with carbon dioxide and is connected to the catheter by a series of tubing and sealed three-way stopcocks containing one-way valves. The 60 ml syringe is the carbon dioxide injector syringe and the 10 ml syringe is the carbon dioxide flush syringe.

Figure 5.26 *Carbon dioxide arteriography. (A) Pelvic arteriogram using carbon dioxide gas injection. Pigtail catheter placed at the aortic bifurcation and carbon dioxide injected at a rate of 40 ml/sec for a total of 60 ml. A renal transplant is anastomosed to the right external iliac artery. (B) Iodinated contrast selective lower extremity arteriogram. (C) Carbon dioxide arteriogram of same extremity. The arteriogram is sufficiently diagnostic for planning surgical or interventional repair. The carbon dioxide arteriogram does not detail as many small vessels compared to the iodinated contrast arteriogram.*

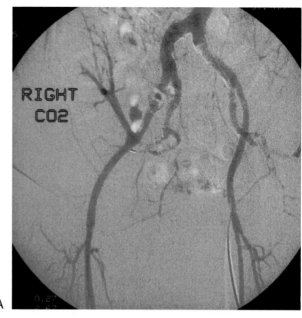

A

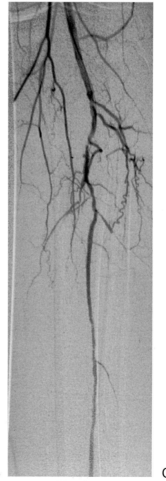

B

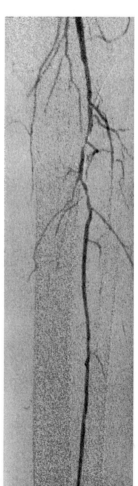

C

materials stocked by most angiography laboratories. The carbon dioxide cylinder is connected to a regulator to control the flow rate of the gas. The regulator is connected through a funnel valve-type connecting tubing to a one-way stopcock device. A series of connective tubing and stopcocks are used to connect the tank to the catheter (Fig. 5.27). The syringes are filled with the regulator set at approximately 5 pounds/square inch. The syringes are filled and evacuated three times to ensure that only carbon dioxide is within the lumen of the syringes. Carbon dioxide is heavier than air and the syringes are purged in an inverted position to preferentially expel the air within them. Once the syringes are filled with carbon dioxide, the 10 ml syringe is used to pre-flush the catheter with carbon dioxide. Immediately following this, the 60 ml syringe is rapidly injected and images acquired of the desired vessel. Larger volumes of carbon dioxide can be delivered using routine injector systems. The injector is filled several times to minimize contamination with air. Injection rates for a runoff range from 60 to 80 ml/sec for a total of 150 to 200 ml. These simple systems have several limitations. A large volume of carbon dioxide can be injected directly into the patient since the carbon dioxide tank is directly connected to the patient. The flush and injection syringes must be filled and purged with carbon dioxide for every injection, which is time consuming.

In general, the decreased density of carbon dioxide is more difficult to image and interpret. Peristalsis, patient motion, and contrast column fragmentation degrade images. Peristalsis is inhibited by injecting 0.5 mg of glucagon. Optimizing the diagnostic studies requires elevation of the injected regions, adequate patient sedation, stacking software, and injection of vasodilators. Selective catheterization improves filling of vessels. One interesting application of carbon dioxide is the reported dramatic ability to demonstrate gastrointestinal bleeding sites. The low viscosity of the gas makes it more easily flow through the arterial rent into the lower extravascular pressure interstitial areas. The gas expands in the interstitial zone and is readily detected.

Lower Extremity Venography

The main indication for lower extremity venography is evaluation for deep venous thrombosis. Less common indications are evaluation of varicose veins, venous insufficiency, and patency of the saphenous vein for bypass grafting. Duplex studies are best for screening for clinically suspected deep venous thrombosis (DVT). Venography is reserved for equivocal noninvasive studies and

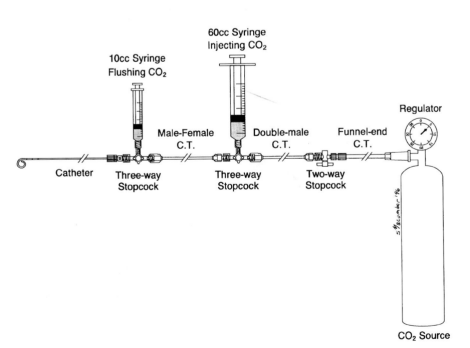

Figure 5.27 *Diagram of carbon dioxide delivery system using direct connection to a carbon dioxide source tank. The tank is connected to the diagnostic angiography catheter and injection syringes via an array of three-way stop cocks and connecting tubes.*

below the knee leg swelling. The etiologic factors for thrombosis are venous stasis, hypercoagulability, and endothelial injury (Virchow's triad). The physiology of venous return is dependent on the calf pump and valves when in the upright position. Compression of the intramuscular sinusoids propels blood upwards towards the heart and the valves prevent reflux. The valves of the calf veins and the sinusoids of the calf are frequently the site of thrombus initiation. The venous anatomy of the lower extremity parallels the arterial anatomy with the exception that the deep calf veins are paired (Fig. 5.28).

The foot of the nonexamined side is placed on a platform so that the examined extremity is non-weight-bearing. The table is tilted in a 20 to 45 degree semiupright position. A 19- or 21-gauge butterfly is introduced into a vein on the dorsum of the foot. This should be done as distal and medial as possible. The veins of the foot tend to be more superficial but readily go into spasm. The veins can be dilated by hot-packing the patient's foot with towels soaked in warm water. To optimally visualize the veins, tourniquets should be used along with tilting the table upright to further engorge the foot veins. If the foot is swollen, a compression dressing or blood pressure cuff can be used to displace the edema.

Tourniquets should be placed both above the ankle and knee to force contrast into the deep venous system. Tourniquets are not used when the superficial venous system is being evaluated. Contrast is slowly injected into the vein under constant visual surveillance. It takes approximately 25 to 35 ml of contrast to fill the deep venous system of the calf. A total of 100 to 150 ml of 43 percent contrast is used in a typical unilateral examination of the lower extremity. Fluoroscopy is used to monitor the filling of the veins and to center the extremity on the overhead film. Anteroposterior and oblique views of the calf, knee, and thigh are obtained. The dump shot is taken once satisfactory visualization of the deep venous system of the leg is obtained. The dump shot centers on the inferior vena cava and iliac vein. Several techniques can be used to maximize visualization of the iliac vein and inferior vena cava. The tourniquets should be released and the patient returned to the horizontal position on the table. The leg is raised and the patient asked to do a Valsalva maneuver while fluoroscopically monitoring the contrast flowing from the leg into the inferior vena cava. Alternatively, the patient is asked to compress the femoral vein and release it as the leg is being raised. The image is obtained during maximum contrast opacification of the veins. The films should be developed

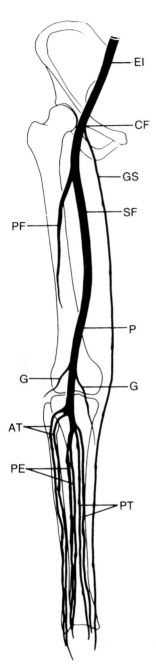

Figure 5.28 *Lower extremity veins. EI, external iliac vein; CF, common femoral vein; GS, greater saphenous vein; PF, profunda femoris (deep femoral) vein; SF, superficial femoral vein; P, popliteal vein; G, gastrocnemius veins; AT, anterior tibial veins; PE, peroneal veins; PT, posterior tibial veins. (From Dyer R: Handbook of Basic Vascular and Interventional Radiology. Churchill Livingstone, New York, 1993, with permission.)*

before the needle is removed from the vein. Saline is infused into the leg to flush the contrast out and reduce the chance of postvenographic syndrome.

A thrombus is identified by a filling defect surrounded by contrast (Fig. 5.29). Nonfilling of veins

Figure 5.29 *Left leg venogram showing extensive thrombus in the deep venous system. The thrombus is outlined as a filling defect surrounded by contrast (arrowheads).*

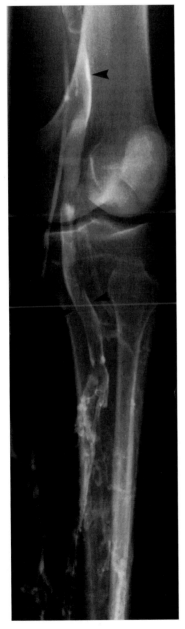

may be due to technique or complete occlusion from thrombus. Chronic DVT findings are linear stranding, absence of valves, and luminal irregularity. Phlegmasia cerulea dolens is extensive DVT that involves the iliac and inferior vena cava segments. It causes severe pain, venous stasis, venous hypertension, and arterial insufficiency. There is a high risk of pulmonary embolism and limb loss. The May-Thurner syndrome is compression of the left iliocaval venous junction between the right common iliac artery and spine (Fig. 5.30). It occurs in young women causing left leg swelling. Paget-Schroetter syndrome or effort thrombosis is axillosubclavian thrombosis resulting from compression at the thoracic outlet. It is associated with a 20 percent rate of pulmonary embolism.

Upper Extremity Venography

The most common indication is to evaluate for an upper extremity deep venous thrombosis, which is usually secondary to an indwelling catheter. Preferably, a 20-gauge or larger intravenous needle is placed within the antecubital vein. Other more distal veins can be used when the antecubital vein is unavailable. Ultrasound-guided puncture of the deep brachial or cephalic vein just above the elbow will gain venous access in patients who have no visible superficial veins. In addition, ultrasound can be used to survey and screen the upper extremity's deep venous system using color flow Doppler. A 30 ml syringe filled with contrast is attached to extension tubing, which is then directly attached to the 20-gauge or larger needle. Digitally acquired films are taken with the subclavian and brachiocephalic vein in the center of the field of view. Patients should be instructed to hold their breath to lessen respiratory motion artifact. It may be necessary to place a 4 or 5 French pigtail catheter to optimally visualize the brachiocephalic and superior vena cava. This may be done from an antecubital approach or a retrograde approach from the femoral vein.

Caval Venography

The inferior vena cava is most frequently examined to rule out a DVT before placing a filter. Other indications include staging of renal cell carcinoma (Fig. 5.31).

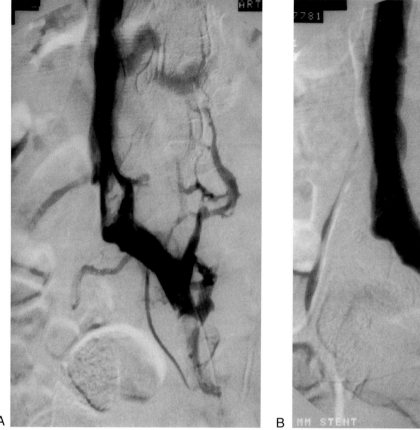
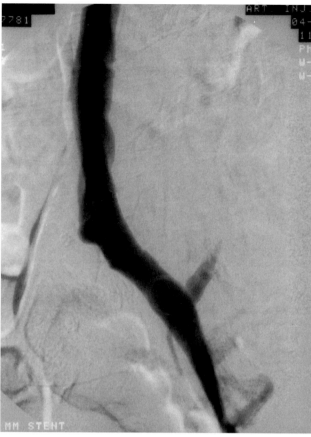

Figure 5.30 *May-Thurner syndrome. **(A)** Complex stenosis of left common iliac vein postulated from compression of right common iliac artery. Note collaterals. Patient had left leg swelling. **(B)** 12 mm Wallstent placed in the complex stenosis eliminated collaterals and the patient's leg swelling.*

The superior vena cava is usually studied to assess for an indwelling catheter related stricture or thrombosis secondary to compression by tumor (superior vena cava syndrome).

The common femoral vein is the preferred route of entry. The femoral head is localized fluoroscopically and the level chosen similar to femoral arterial access. The skin is anesthetized 1 cm medial to the femoral artery pulse. A 10 ml syringe is connected to the needle and suction applied. The femoral pulse is palpated and the needle directed medially to the pulse as the patient performs a Valsalva maneuver. Blood return most frequently occurs as the needle is withdrawn. Alternatively, ultrasound can be used to visualize and guide femoral or jugular venipuncture. Real-time ultrasound guidance greatly simplifies this task. A standard 0.038

guidewire and 5 French pigtail catheter is placed within the venous system. The typical caval injection rate is 15 to 20 ml/sec for a total of 40 to 50 ml. The superior vena cava injection rate is 15 to 20 ml/sec for a total of 30 to 40 ml. A ruler should be placed just to the left side of the lumbar spine to aid in subsequent positioning of caval filters. Films are obtained at the rate of three per second.

Pulmonary Angiography

The common indications are clinical suspicion of pulmonary embolism or evaluation of pulmonary hypertension. Less common indications include evaluation of

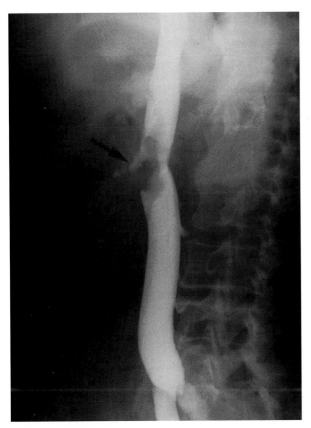

Figure 5.31 *Inferior vena cavogram demonstrating tumor thrombus invading the inferior vena cava from the right renal vein (arrow).*

vasculitis, vascular malformations, stenoses, congenital abnormalities, and tumor encasement. It is important to review the clinical history, chest radiograph, electrocardiogram (ECG), and ventilation/perfusion (V/Q) scan before performing the pulmonary angiogram. It is advisable to recommend that a V/Q scan be performed before obtaining a pulmonary angiogram. A normal or high probability V/Q scan eliminates the need for the pulmonary angiogram. A low probability or indeterminate V/Q scan can be used to tailor the pulmonary angiogram. The perfusion defects visualized on the V/Q scan are used to guide which segments of the lung to examine first. Contraindications to performing pulmonary angiography are a left bundle branch block and severe pulmonary hypertension. Severe pulmonary hypertension is defined as systolic pulmonary artery pressures greater than 70 mmHg or right ventricular end-diastolic pressure greater than 20 mmHg. A left bundle branch block is treated by placing a temporary

transvenous cardiac pacer. In cases of severe pulmonary hypertension, careful selective pulmonary arteriography is done by using small hand injections of contrast.

The study must be done with continuous cardiac ECG monitoring. Pulmonary artery catheters are all slight variations of curved 7 French pigtail catheters. The catheter's shape is re-formed in the right atrium. The secondary curve of the catheter will allow the blood flow to carry the catheter through the tricuspid valve into the right ventricle. Two techniques may be used to advance the catheter from the right ventricle into the pulmonary artery. The Von Aman catheter technique uses a wire to straighten out the pigtail, which directs the wire into the main pulmonary artery. The catheter is quickly advanced over the guidewire and placed within the left or right pulmonary artery (Fig. 5.32). The other technique is to slightly withdraw and rotate the catheter in the right ventricle to orient the tip toward the pulmonary outflow tract. The catheter is advanced when directed toward the pulmonary artery (Fig. 5.33). A Willie catheter (Cordis, Miami, FL) simplifies pulmonary artery catheterization from a jugular approach. The catheter readily forms in the right atrium and is pushed through the right ventricle into the pulmonary artery. The pigtail catheter is straightened out with a guidewire before withdrawal through the right heart valves.

Pulmonary artery pressures are measured before contrast injections. These recordings should be documented on the films and on a paper strip recording. The normal pulmonary artery systolic pressure is 20 to 25 mmHg. The normal diastolic pressure is 8 to 12 mmHg and the mean pressure is 15 mmHg. Right ventricular end diastolic pressure (RVEDP) equals right atrial pressure since the tricuspid valve is open, forming a common chamber. The normal RVEDP is 0 to 5 mmHg. RVEDP greater than 20 mmHg indicates maximal right ventricular afterload. Irreversible right heart failure has been reported following main pulmonary arteriography in these situations. In these cases, segmental vessel injection with reduced volumes should be used cautiously. Pulmonary hypertension is defined as systolic pressures greater than 30 mmHg. There is no strong correlation between pulmonary hypertension and acute pulmonary embolism.

The use of digital versus cut film image acquisition remains controversial. The speed of obtaining multiple views, rapid review of the study, and high contrast resolution make DSA our preferred technique. Selective pulmonary artery injections should be done using a rate

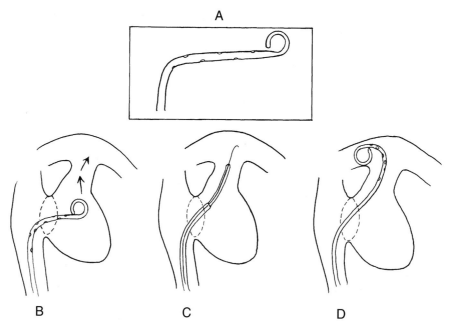

Figure 5.32 *Pulmonary artery catheterization using Von Aman or reversed Grollman catheters. (**A**) The catheter has a 90° bend with the pigtail oriented superiorly. (**B**) The catheter is re-formed in the right atrium and directed across the tricuspid valve into the right ventricle. (**C**) A guidewire is advanced through the catheter. Guidewire advancement unravels the pigtail, which directs the guidewire upward into the pulmonary artery. (**D**) The catheter is advanced over the guidewire and positioned in the pulmonary artery.*

Figure 5.33 *Pulmonary artery catheterization using Grollman catheter. (**A**) The secondary 90° bend proximal to the pigtail is re-formed in the right atrium and used to direct the catheter across the tricuspid valve into the right ventricle. (**B**) The guidewire is advanced across the 90° bend of the catheter. This straightens the bend and orients the catheter in a more superior direction. (**C**) A combination of slightly withdrawing while rotating the catheter orients the pigtail superior toward the right ventricular outflow tract. When the catheter is oriented appropriately, it is advanced forward into the pulmonary artery.*

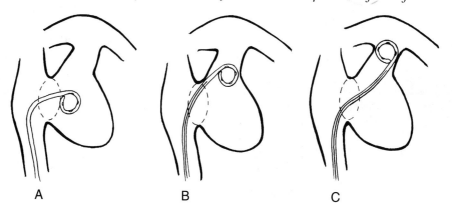

of 20 ml/sec for a total of 50 ml. Two to three views of each lung should be obtained. Breath holding is critical to reducing digital subtraction misregistration. The study is obtained at four frames per second with a filter placed across the lung fields. The electronic filter lessens the abrupt density gradient present between the mediastinum and lungs. The field of view is collimated to bracket one lung field. If the digitally acquired pulmonary angiogram is equivocal, a cut film magnified pulmonary angiogram should be performed using a small focal spot to maximize resolution. The injection rate is the same. The cut film should be centered to include the lower portions of the lung fields. Alternatively, balloon occlusion technique can be used to optimally visualize the small branches and may demonstrate smaller size emboli compared to conventional technique.

The diagnosis of pulmonary embolism is made by demonstrating vessel cutoff, usually with a convex proximal margin, or an intraluminal filling defect surrounded by contrast (Fig. 5.34). Secondary but nonspecific findings are wedge-shaped peripheral parenchymal defects and poor venous outflow. Atelectasis is recognized by crowding of the vessels and a dense parenchymal stain. Most emboli take at least 1 to 3 weeks to naturally lyse, allowing the delay of most studies until working hours. If a positive diagnosis of pulmonary embolus is made, the clinician should be contacted before the venous access is removed and the need for an inferior vena cava filter determined.

Lymphography

Lymphography has been largely replaced by CT for the evaluation of lymphadenopathy. It still plays a limited

Figure 5.34 *(A) Selective magnified left pulmonary angiogram on cut film. Arrows denote filling defect in left lower lobe artery. (B) Selective right pulmonary arteriogram on digital technique. Arrows outline multiple emboli in right lower lobe.*

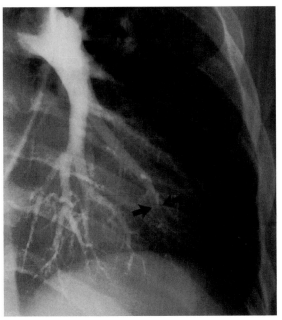

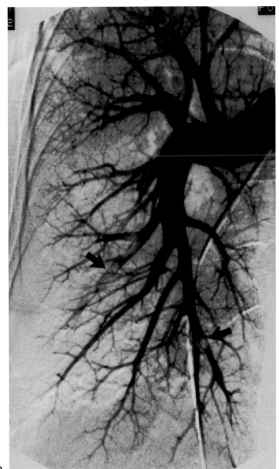

A

B

role in the evaluation of patients with negative CT examinations. The advantage of lymphography over CT is that it permits assessment of the internal architecture of lymph nodes and potentially detects cancer in small lymph nodes. The abnormally visualized lymph nodes can be biopsied for cytologic confirmation. The lymph nodes are opacified for up to 9 months at a time, allowing for simple follow-up examination via abdominal plain films. Radiation portals can be accurately targeted on the opacified lymph nodes. Patients with lymphedema are best evaluated with venography and nuclear scintigraphy. The main indications for performing lymphography are staging cervical cancer, lymphoma, and evaluation of traumatic injury to the lymphatic system. Stage II lymphoma involving lymph node chains above the diaphragm is staged with either a combination of CT scanning and lymphography or CT scanning and surgical exploration. Stage II cervical carcinoma is evaluated using lymphography to determine whether there is evidence of micrometastatic disease to the local lymph node chains.

The patient's feet are prepped and draped according to sterile procedure. A 10 ml mixture of lidocaine and methylene blue dye is injected in the interdigital spaces of both feet. The lymph channels are visualized through the skin as blue streaks. Lymphatic filling can be enhanced by massaging the area of the toes injected with blue dye. The largest visualized lymphatic channel over the dorsum of the midfoot is chosen. Smaller lymphatic channels over the metatarsal area can be used but are more difficult to cannulate.

Lidocaine is used to anesthetize the skin and subcutaneous tissues surrounding the visualized duct. A 3 cm longitudinal incision is made over the lymphatic channel. The incision is made in a single stroke of the scalpel through all the layers of the skin. The subcutaneous tissues are then spread with a hemostat to expose the vessel. The lymph vessel is identified and a narrow piece of wax paper from a Steri-strip is used to elevate and isolate the lymph vessel (Fig. 5.35). Three 4-0 silk sutures are placed around the exposed lymphatic vessel. The proximal ligature is held tight by placing a Steri-strip to occlude the outflow of the lymph vessel. A pair of fine forceps is used to carefully remove the perilymphatic tissues. Massaging the forefoot maximally distends the lymphatic channel. This facilitates successful cannulation of the lymphatic duct.

Figure 5.35 *Lymphangiography technique.* *(A)* *A 3 cm longitudinal incision is made over the blue dye opacified lymphatic in the mid foot region.* *(B)* *The lymphatic vessel is carefully dissected free of adjacent connecting tissue. The lymphatic is isolated by placing a small piece of paper underneath the vessel. Proximal and distal ligatures of 4-0 silk are placed underneath the isolated lymphatic vessel. The proximal ligature is used as a tourniquet to restrict outflow of lymph through the duct.* *(C)* *A 27 or 30 gauge Tegtmeyer needle is used to cannulate the lymphatic vein. The middle ligature is tied around the needle and duct to stabilize the system.*

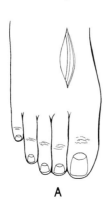
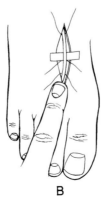
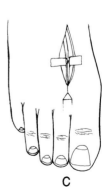

A   B   C

A slight tension is placed on the distal ligature to stabilize the isolated lymph channel. A 27- or 30-gauge Tegtmeyer needle is connected to a syringe containing lidocaine. The needle is carefully advanced into the lymphatic. For successful cannulation, the needle is held almost parallel to the lymph vessel to perform single wall puncture. Once the needle is in the duct, it is secured in place by tying the middle ligature around the duct and needle tip. Steri-strips are used to further stabilize the needle position. The proximal ligature is released, and lidocaine is injected to ensure successful cannulation of the lymph duct.

The contrast medium used for lymphography is ethiodol. Ninety percent of ethiodol is retained in the lymph nodes, and the remainder embolizes the pulmonary vascular bed. In most individuals, this goes unnoticed. In some patients, this may cause temporary dyspnea and transient fevers. A maximum of 10 ml is injected in each leg. The contrast agent is preheated to 40°C and is infused slowly over 30 to 90 minutes. Films of the pelvis are obtained to ensure that there is an adequate amount of contrast injected into the lymphatic system. Adequate opacification of the lymphatic system may occur even with obvious leakage from the injected lymph duct. When leakage occurs, fluoroscopic examination can be used to assess the amount of contrast entering the lymphatic channels. After successful contrast infusion, the wound is cleansed and closed with a subcuticular 4-0 Vicryl suture.

The channel phase films are obtained after the contrast is injected. The channel phase films demonstrate the patency and distribution of lymphatic channels. These are used in conjunction with the nodal phase films to determine whether a filling defect is due to the hilum of the lymph node or is a true filling defect. The nodal phase films are taken after a 24-hour delay.

The size and number of lymph nodes vary in individuals. In general, the fewer the lymph nodes the larger the size. The largest lymph nodes are usually the more peripheral ones such as the inguinal. The accuracy of lymphography for detection of lymphoma is approximately 95 percent. The findings consist of enlarged lymph nodes with a foamy, lacy architecture. The outer margins are usually preserved. Metastatic disease causes small areas of nonopacification of the lymph nodes. Obstructed lymph channels may be visualized. Lymphography does not opacify the internal iliac lymph nodes.

Suggested Readings

Bookstein JJ, Lang EV: Penile magnification pharmacoarteriography: details of intrapenile arterial anatomy. AJR 148:883, 1987

Cohen MI, Vogelzang RL: A comparison of techniques for improved visualization of the arteries of the distal lower extremity. AJR 147:1021, 1986

Darcy MD: Lower-extremity arteriography: current approach and techniques. Radiology 178:615, 1991

Dyer R: Handbook of Basic Vascular and Interventional Radiology. Churchill Livingstone, New York, 1993

Fischer RG, Chasen MH, Lamki N: Diagnosis of injuries of the aorta and brachiocephalic arteries caused by blunt chest trauma: CT vs. aortography. AJR 162:1047, 1994

Friedman SG, Moccio CG: A prospective comparison of intra-arterial digital subtraction and conventional angiography prior to lower extremity revascularization. J Cardiovasc Surg 30:462, 1989

Hawkins IF, Caridi JG, Kerns SR: Plastic bag delivery system for hand injection of carbon dioxide. AJR 165:1487, 1995

Hawkins IF, Kerns SR: Carbon dioxide digital subtraction angiography. p.11.1. In Cope C (ed): Current Techniques in Interventional Radiology. Current Medicine, Philadelphia, 1994

Heiken JP, Weyman PJ, Lee JKT et al: Detection of focal hepatic masses: prospective evaluation with CT, delayed CT, CT during arterial portography, and MR imaging. Radiology 171:47, 1989

Kadir S: Diagnostic Angiography. WB Saunders, Philadelphia, 1986

McDermont VG, Lawrance JAL, Paulson EK et al: CT during arterial portography: comparison of injection into the splenic versus superior mesenteric artery. Radiology 199:627, 1996

Mills SR, Jackson DC, Older RA et al: The incidence, etiologies, and avoidance of complications of pulmonary angiography in a large series. Radiology 136:295, 1980

Moskovic E, Fernando IN, Blake P, Parsons C: Lymphangiography: current role in oncology. Br J Radiol 64:422, 1991

Napel SA: Principles and techniques of 3D spiral CT angiography. p. 167. In Fishman EK, Jeffrey RB Jr (eds.): Spiral CT: Techniques and Clinical Applications. Raven Press, New York, 1995

Nemcek AA Jr, Vogelzang RL: Introduction to angiography of the hollow viscera. p.140. In Gore RM, Levine MS, Laufer I (eds): Textbook of Gastrointestinal Radiology. Vol. 1. WB Saunders, Philadelphia, 1994

Newman GE: Pulmonary angiography in pulmonary embolic disease. J Thorac Imag 4: 28, 1989

Peterson MS, Baron RL, Dodd GD et al: Hepatic parenchymal perfusion defects detected with CTAP: imaging-pathologic correlation. Radiology 185:149, 1992

The PIOPED Investigators: Value of the ventilation/perfusion scan in acute pulmonary embolism. JAMA 263:2753, 1990

Raptopoulos V, Shieman RG, Phillips DA et al: Traumatic aortic tear: screening with chest CT. Radiology 182:667, 1992

Reid JDS, Redman HC, Weigelt JA et al: Wounds of the extremities in proximity to major arteries: value of angiography in the detection of arterial injury. AJR 151:1035, 1988

Remy JM, Remy J, Wattinne L, Giraud F: Central pulmonary thromboembolism: diagnosis with spiral volumetric CT with the single-breath-hold technique-comparison with pulmonary angiography. Radiology 185:381, 1992

Rosen MP, Schwartz AN, Levine FJ, Greenfield AJ: Radiologic assessment of impotence: angiography, sonography, cavernosography, and scintigraphy. AJR 157:923, 1991

Rubin GD: Three-dimensional helical CT angiography. Radiographics 14:905, 1994

Small WC, Mehard WB, Langmo LS et al: Preoperative determination of the resectability of hepatic tumors: efficacy of CT during arterial portography. AJR 161:319, 1993

Smith TP, Cragg AH, Berbaum KS et al: Techniques for lower-limb angiography: a comparative study. Radiology 174:951, 1990

Standards of Practice Committee of the Society of Cardiovascular and Interventional Radiology: Standard for diagnostic arteriography in adults. J Vasc Interv Radiat 4:385, 1993

Vogelzang RL: Arteriography of the hand and wrist. Hand Clin 7:63, 1991

Complications
MICHAEL A. BRAUN
ALBERT A. NEMCEK, JR.

The quality of care can be improved by periodic review and evaluation of complications. Outcomes are monitored to adjust procedures and protocols to minimize complication rates. The definition of what constitutes a complication is not always straightforward or consistently applied. A working definition based on surgical practice defines a complication as any adverse event that occurs during the procedure or within 30 days that can be related potentially or partially to the procedure. Complications are divided into minor and major categories depending on the impact and significance of the complication. Major complications necessitate surgical intervention, prolong hospitalization, or require specific medical treatment. Examples of major complications are hematomas requiring drainage or infections requiring antibiotics. Minor complications are all other adverse consequences that occur within 30 days. Minor complications resolve with no clinical sequelae or minimal treatment. The distinction is not always black and white. Pseudoaneurysms previously would be classified as major complications, but currently with ultrasound-guided compression may arguably be classified as minor.

The majority of the complications encountered in vascular radiology involve puncture site bleeding, iatrogenic vascular injuries, contrast reactions, and contrast nephrotoxicity. Prompt recognition of a complication allows steps to be taken to circumvent the complication or minimize the deleterious effects. If a complication has occurred that may potentially require surgical intervention or medical management, the surgeon or consultant should be notified as soon as possible so that any necessary corrective steps can be taken. Anticipation of a complication aids in appropriate patient selection and pretreatment. An understanding of the mechanisms causing complications will aid the interventionalist in early recognition or avoidance of complications.

The complications of 3,677 diagnostic arteriograms performed from 1993 to 1996 at Northwestern are compiled in Table 6.1. The arteriograms are all noncerebral diagnostic arteriograms including diagnostic studies combined with therapeutic vascular interventions. Data were collected on routine follow-up on both inpatients and outpatients. The complications of 525 arteriograms combined with immediate interventional vascular procedures is reported in Table 6.2. The major complication rate for diagnostic studies was 2.1 percent and for combined diagnostic and therapeutic procedures was 5.3 percent. The complication rates for combined procedures were two to three times those of diagnostic studies. This reflects the presence of diseased vessels, larger catheters, prolonged procedures, periprocedural heparin, and comorbid disease processes.

Arterial puncture site complications are probably the most frequent complications encountered. The incidence of arterial puncture site complications was 3.5 percent for diagnostic and 8.6 percent for interventional procedures. Meticulous attention must be given to the evaluation of the patient before arterial puncture, during the arterial puncture itself, and the removal of a catheter at the end of the procedure. The patient's coagulation status is evaluated by reviewing the patient's history and the laboratory values of prothrombin time (PT), partial thromboplastin time (PTT), and platelet count. A bleeding time is advisable in renal failure patients and patients taking aspirin. Heparin should be discontinued 3 to 4 hours before the procedure. Heparin effects can be quickly assayed with an activated clotting time and then reversed with protamine. Reduction of hypertension with sublingual nifedipine helps control puncture site bleeding. Multiple puncture attempts or improper technique can increase the likelihood of local hemorrhage. An introducer sheath should be used when multiple catheter exchanges are anticipated. A puncture of the common femoral artery above the inguinal ligament places the patient at a higher risk of retroperitoneal hematoma

Table 6.1 *Complications of 3,677 diagnostic arteriograms*

Complication	Number	Percentage
Mortality	1	0.03
Puncture site hematoma	88	2.4
Pseudoaneurysm	30	0.8
Dissection	21	0.6
Renal failure	15	0.4
Embolization	10	0.3
Puncture site thrombosis	10	0.3
Hematoma remote from puncture site	9	0.3
Thrombosis remote from puncture site	4	0.1
Contrast reaction	2	0.05
Total	190	5.2

Table 6.2 *Complications of 525 diagnostic and interventional arteriograms*

Complication	Number	Percentage
Puncture site hematoma	29	5.5
Pseudoaneurysm	14	2.7
Hematoma remote from puncture site	9	1.7
Dissection	6	1.1
Renal failure	6	1.1
Embolization	5	1.0
Puncture site thrombosis	2	0.4
Thrombosis remote from puncture site	2	0.4
Total	73	13.9

pseudoaneurysm is carefully imaged and studied before performing compression. It is important to identify the rent in the artery and the subsequent tract to the pseudoaneurysm, which often contains swirling blood. The groin is anesthetized with a long-acting analgesic such as bupivacaine. The neck and tract of the pseudoaneurysm are targeted, and firm pressure is applied to occlude the neck (Fig. 6.1). Pressure is applied in 10 to 15 minute intervals. Usually 20 to 30 minutes of compression is required to thrombose the pseudoaneurysm (Fig. 6.2). If the patient is systemically anticoagulated, the anticoagulation should be discontinued before attempting pseudoaneurysm compression. Small pseudoaneurysms (< 3 cm) may spontaneously thrombose once the patient is taken off anticoagulation. The common femoral artery and its major branches are studied to

Figure 6.1 *Pseudoaneurysm compression. The neck of the groin pseudoaneurysm is identified with a linear 5 or 7 MHz transducer. The neck of the pseudoaneurysm is occluded by compression with the ultrasound probe. Continuous color ultrasound is used to confirm absence of flow in the pseudoaneurysm with preservation of flow in the femoral artery. Compression is held in 10- to 20-minute intervals until the pseudoaneurysm fills with thrombus.*

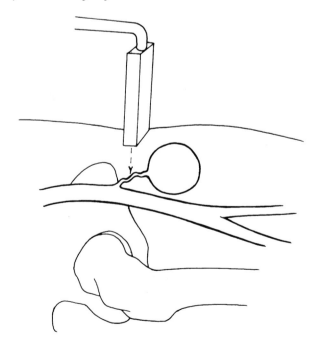

because the artery cannot be effectively compressed against the femoral head.

Pseudoaneurysms occur from low femoral puncture, procedural anticoagulation, or puncture of a branch of the femoral artery. A pseudoaneurysm is suspected when the patient has a painful or pulsatile hematoma. The majority of pseudoaneurysms can be effectively treated with ultrasound-guided compression. The success rate has been reported as high as 90 percent. The study is performed with a 5 to 7.5 MHz linear transducer. The

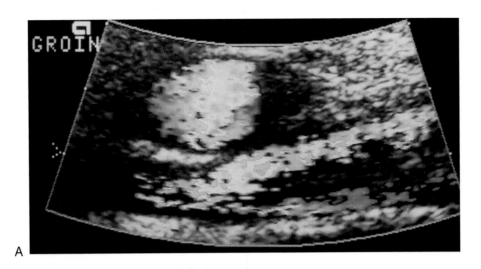

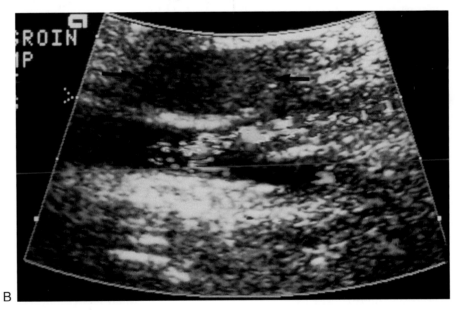

Figure 6.2 *Postcatheterization groin pseudoaneurysm. (**A**) A pseudoaneurysm formed following cardiac catheterization with intraprocedural administration of 10,000 units of heparin. Arrows delineate pseudoaneurysm in subcutaneous tissues superficial to common femoral artery. (**B**) The pseudoaneurysm has completely thrombosed with no flow identified after 20 minutes of ultrasound-guided compression. Arrows indicate thrombosed pseudoaneurysm.*

ensure patency following successful completion of the pseudoaneurysm compression. A follow-up ultrasound is performed 24 hours after compression to ensure complete thrombosis of the pseudoaneurysm.

Puncture complications of brachial artery access occur more frequently compared with femoral artery access. The majority of puncture site thromboses involved the brachial artery. The brachial artery is more difficult to puncture, the catheter to artery ratio is higher, vasospasm occurs more frequently, and the artery is more difficult to compress. Brachial puncture site complications can be minimized by micropuncture technique, ultrasound guidance, smaller 4 French catheters, prophylactic vasodilation, and careful guidewire passage. Extra care must be paid to manual compression of the brachial artery after catheter removal. All patients who have had a brachial puncture should have frequent postprocedure neurovascular checks of the extremity by the nursing staff. The physician performs a 24-hour follow-up check to assess for potential brachial artery injury. The decision between performing low brachial artery puncture (just above the elbow) and high brachial puncture (near the axilla) can be based on potential complication consequences. A hematoma from a high brachial or axillary artery puncture has greater deleterious effects by potentially causing a compressive brachial plexus neuropathy compared to a low brachial puncture site hematoma.

Catheter manipulation complications include dissection, perforation, and embolization. Arterial dissection occurred 0.6 to 1.1 percent of the time. Diffuse atherosclerotic disease is the most important risk factor leading to dissection. Dissections occur from subintimal guidewire or catheter passage at the puncture site or distant to the puncture site. Puncture site dissections result when the bevel of the needle is not completely within the true arterial lumen during initial guidewire passage. This usually happens during difficult punctures. The relationship between the needle tip and the arterial lumen should be assessed by contrast injection when there is resistance to initial guidewire passage. Safety J-tip-shaped and flexible tip guidewires minimize dissections remote to the puncture site by bouncing off rather than tunneling into atheromatous plaques. Arterial perforation is relatively rare and is usually the result of overaggressive manipulation of a stiff guidewire. Embolization may result from a pericatheter thrombosis, introduction of a foreign material, or a disruption of an atheromatous plaque. The incidence of embolization was 0.3 to 1 per-

cent. Embolization is minimized by frequent use of the double flush technique and continuous flushing of guiding catheters and sheaths. Cholesterol embolization is a serious complication and is associated with considerable mortality and morbidity. It is thought to occur from dislodgement of cholesterol crystals from atherosclerotic plaques during catheter manipulations. The cholesterol crystals embolize visceral organs and extremities. Extra care must be taken when traversing a vessel that is heavily involved with ulcerated plaques. Cholesterol embolization should be suspected when postangiography renal failure does not resolve. Diagnosis is suggested by peripheral eosinophilia, leukocytosis, skin petechial markings, and vasculitis-type symptoms. Definitive diagnosis is by biopsy.

Heparin-induced thrombocytopenia occurs in 5 to 15 percent of patients on full-dose heparin therapy and occurs 5 days or more after the start of heparin therapy. White clot syndrome is a rare complication of platelet aggregation mediated by the heparin-dependent antiplatelet antibodies. These antibodies activate platelets causing arterial thromboses that have a high morbidity and mortality. Heparin-coated catheters and heparin flush solutions have induced the syndrome. Recognition of this rare disorder is important and is suggested by thrombocytopenia. One can assay for the heparin-dependent IgG antibody. We have successfully lysed arterial white clot thromboses with catheter-directed urokinase thrombolysis.

Contrast Reactions

Contrast reactions have anaphylactic or allergic-type symptoms. Because circulating IgE antibodies are not consistently recovered in patients with these reactions, they are considered idiosyncratic. Patients who are at risk have a significant atopic medical history or have had a previous contrast reaction. As many as 50 percent of patients who have experienced a prior contrast allergy, however, may not react to a subsequent contrast injection. Fewer contrast reactions are associated with intra-arterial contrast injections compared to intravenous injections. Both allergic-type contrast reactions in the series of 3,677 angiograms occurred during pulmonary angiograms. Contrast reactions are classified as either minor or major. Minor reactions include nausea, vomiting, hives, coughing, and pruritus. These reactions require either no treatment or diphenhydramine, 25 to 50 mg oral, intramuscular, or intravenous, for symptomatic urticaria. Minor reactions are monitored for worsening. Major reactions include facial edema, bronchospasm, cardiac arrest, or hypotension. The majority (reportedly 96 percent) of patients who have a major contrast reaction can recover fully with aggressive treatment. Nonionic contrast significantly reduces the incidence of contrast reactions.

Treatment of anaphylactic reactions includes the basic ABCs (airway, breathing, circulation). Assistance should be sought, the patient assessed, and vital signs taken. Control of the airways is of prime importance. Nasal oxygen should be administered, intravenous access started, and oxygen saturation and electrocardiogram monitored. If the patient is having a bronchoconstrictive episode, it can be reversed by using 0.3 ml subcutaneously of 1 to 1,000 epinephrine. If it is a severe bronchoconstrictive episode associated with hypotension, 3 ml of intravenous 1 to 10,000 epinephrine should be used. Both diphenhydramine, 50 mg, and cimetidine, 300 mg, should be administered intravenously. There have been reports of cimetidine completely reversing anaphylactic reactions. Vasovagal reactions are treated by Trendelenburg position, intravenous fluids, and atropine, 0.3 to 1.0 mg IV, for significant hypotension and bradycardia.

Contrast-induced renal failure is usually nonoliguric, mild, and reversible. Contrast nephrotoxicity is defined as a 25 percent increase from baseline within 48 hours after contrast administration. The serum creatinine elevates usually within 24 hours, peaks by 3 to 5 days, and returns to normal in 1 to 2 weeks. Treatment is usually supportive and consists of monitoring electrolytes and careful hydration. Renal insufficiency and diabetes are the most important risk factors. Other predisposing risk factors are multiple myeloma, congestive heart failure, dehydration, increased volume of contrast, and advanced age. The mechanism of contrast induced renal failure is not understood but thought to be due to a combination of vasoconstriction and direct cytotoxicity of contrast on the renal tubules. The best and only proven way of decreasing the frequency of contrast nephropathy is periprocedural patient hydration. In most patients, this is accomplished by giving 1 to 1½ liters of 0.45 percent saline intravenously in the 8 to 12 hours before the procedure. In patients who have renal insufficiency, the hydration will need to be undertaken more carefully to prevent fluid overload. Nonionic contrast has a lower incidence of nephrotoxi-

city compared with ionic contrast in patients with renal insufficiency. Other treatments include mannitol, renal dose dopamine infusion, theophylline, calcium channel blockers, and atrial natriuretic peptide. None of these agents have a proven effect. Although a beneficial effect is controversial, we give mannitol, 12.5 g intravenously, near the termination of the procedure to any patient who has an increased risk for developing contrast-induced nephropathy. Patients at risk for contrast nephrotoxicity should be prehydrated and monitored after the procedure. The patient's urine output, blood urea nitrogen (BUN), creatinine, and serum electrolytes should be followed for 24 to 48 hours.

The American College of Radiology Standards

The American College of Radiology in conjunction with the Society of Cardiovascular and Interventional Radiology publish standards for the practice of diagnostic arteriography and interventional radiology. The standards were developed to provide a guide to practicing angiographers to ensure that patients undergo arteriography for appropriate reasons, that the methods used in periprocedural care provided are adequate, and that the quality of studies obtained is adequate to answer the clinical questions. These published standards provide a benchmark to which an angiographer's practice can be compared. The 1995 published Thresholds for Complications in Diagnostic Angiography are:

Complication	Threshold
Hematoma	3 percent
Occlusion	0.5 percent
Pseudoaneurysm	0.5 percent
Arterial venous fistula	0.1 percent
Catheter-induced Complications	
Arterial Dissection	2 percent
Subintimal injection	1 percent
Cerebral Arteriography	
All neurologic complications	4 percent
Permanent neurologic complications	1 percent
Contrast Reactions	
All reactions	3 percent
Major reactions	0.5 percent
Contrast-induced renal failure	10 percent

Suggested Readings

Bettman MA: The evaluation of contrast-related renal failure. AJR 157:66, 1991

Cragg AH, Nakagawa N, Smith TP, Berbaum KS: Hematoma formation after diagnostic arteriography: effect of catheter size. J Vasc Interv Radiol 2:231, 1991

Fellmeth BD, Roberts AC, Bookstein JJ et al: Postangiographic femoral artery injuries: nonsurgical repair with US-guided compression. Radiology 178:671, 1991

Harris KG, Smith TP, Cragg AH, Lemke JH: Nephrotoxicity from contrast material in renal insufficiency: ionic versus nonionic agents. Radiology 179:849, 1991

Lautin EM, Freeman NJ, Schoenfeld AH et al: Radiocontrast-associated renal dysfunction: incidence and risk factors. AJR 157:49, 1991

Perler BA: Review of hypercoagulability syndromes: what the interventionalist needs to know. J Vasc Interv Radiol 2:183, 1991

Solomon R, Werner C, Mann D et al: Effects of saline, mannitol, and furosemide on acute decreases in renal function induced by radiocontrast agents. N Engl J Med 331:1416, 1994

Standards for Interventional Radiology p.71. In American College of Radiology Standards, American College of Radiology, Fairfax, VA, 1995

Standards of Practice Committee of the Society of Cardiovascular and Interventional Radiology. Standard for diagnostic arteriography in adults. J Vasc Interv Radiol 4:385, 1993

Waugh JR, Sacharias N: Arteriographic complications in the DSA era. Radiology 182:243, 1992

Interventional Vascular Procedures

This section discusses the variety of percutaneous techniques available for treating both stenotic and occlusive vascular disease. The most well-established endovascular procedure is angioplasty. Percutaneous transluminal angioplasty has proven successful in treating stenotic peripheral vascular disease, especially in large caliber arteries. Balloon angioplasty radially dilates a stenotic lesion within a vessel, which restores the internal luminal caliber of the vessel. The exact mechanism of angioplasty is incompletely understood but is probably a combination of plaque compression, plaque fracture, controlled wall dissection, and vessel remodeling. Despite the widespread success and acceptance of angioplasty, the procedure has limitations. Acute failures result from dissection, spasm, thrombosis, elastic recoil, and rupture. Late failures occur from intimal hyperplasia causing re-stenosis. Atherectomy and stents have been developed and are being used to overcome the shortcomings of angioplasty. Stent grafts are being actively investigated to percutaneously treat aneurysms, arteriovenous fistula, and pseudoaneurysms. Thrombolysis was conceived to dissolve percutaneously both acute and chronic thrombosis, thereby recannulating the occluded vessels. This section describes these interventional vascular procedures and their applications.

CHAPTER 7

Angioplasty MICHAEL A. BRAUN

Angioplasty is the standard among percutaneous interventional vascular procedures. The advantages of percutaneous transluminal angioplasty (PTA) include reduced morbidity, mortality, hospital stay, and recuperative period. The patient's saphenous vein is preserved for potential bypass surgery. The most common indication for angioplasty is life-style-inhibiting claudication caused by stenosis. Angioplasty can be used as an adjunct to a distal revascularization surgery by optimizing inflow or for limb salvage in nonsurgical candidates. Successful PTA can eliminate or reduce the extent of amputation in patients with threatened limbs that are not surgical candidates. It is best performed only when vascular surgery backup is available and after consultation with the referring clinician and patient.

Patient selection for angioplasty or surgery is based on the degree of ischemia, location of the lesion(s), and morphology of the lesion(s). Lesion location is conveniently divided into the suprainguinal ligament and infrainguinal arterial segments. The suprainguinal segment consists of the aorta and iliac arteries. Angioplasty is the procedure of choice for focal aortoiliac stenotic disease, while surgery is indicated for diffuse aortoiliac occlusive disease. Angioplasty, especially when combined with thrombolysis or stents, can be used to treat multiple stenoses or short-segment aortoiliac occlusions. The infrainguinal segment consists of the femoropopliteal and tibioperoneal arteries. Angioplasty is used in focal stenotic or short segment occlusive femoropopliteal disease in patients with life-style-inhibiting claudication. Surgery is indicated in femoropopliteal occlusive disease causing critical ischemia. Infrapopliteal angioplasty is indicated in focal stenotic disease in patients with critical ischemia (limb salvage). The morphology of stenotic lesions can be predictive of success. In general, angioplasty is more effective in concentric versus eccentric stenoses, short rather than long stenoses, nonostial versus ostial stenoses, and stenotic disease versus occlusive.

The technical steps of angioplasty are choosing the approach, estimating the proper balloon size, crossing the lesion, dilating the lesion, and assessing the results. A 5 to 7 French vascular sheath is used in all cases. Iliac lesions can be approached via the contralateral or ipsilateral femoral artery. The ipsilateral approach is the most straightforward but may require puncture of a nonpalpable artery, which can be accomplished using fluoroscopic landmarks, ultrasound-directed puncture, or roadmapping. The contralateral approach requires crossing the aortic bifurcation, which may require a stiff guidewire or a pre-curved guiding sheath. Bilateral common iliac ostial lesions are simultaneously dilated with "kissing balloon" technique. An antegrade femoral approach is preferred when treating lesions in the femoropopliteal and infrapopliteal arteries. A retrograde popliteal puncture in the prone position is an alternative approach to the ipsilateral femoral artery. Choice of approach should take into account the need to measure hemodynamic gradients, which is facilitated by a retrograde approach.

The principle of slight overdilatation of the lesion is recommended. This is accomplished by directly measuring the luminal diameter of the contralateral vessel or unaffected segment near the stenosis on cut film angiography. The slight magnification of the vessels on cut film determines the balloon size. Digital angiography units require calibration estimated from the diagnostic catheter caliber or an external radio-opaque ruler to measure vessel luminal size. The length of the balloon is selected to match the length of the lesion. This avoids injuring the normal, adjacent vessel wall. In general, iliac vessels are dilated with 7 to 10 mm, renal arteries dilated with 4 to 7 mm, femoral arteries with 4 to 6 mm, popliteal arteries with 3 to 4 mm, and tibial arteries with 2.5 to 3.5 mm diameter balloons.

In angioplasty, one is purposefully approaching and attempting to cross a diseased segment of artery, a practice that runs counter to good angiographic principles. Utmost care must be exercised. Stenotic lesions are best crossed by using a steerable angled tip Glidewire or floppy tipped Bentson guidewire. A 5 French angled-tip catheter will additionally steer the guidewire across the stenotic lesion. Digital road-mapping may be used to provide real-time fluoroscopic imaging of the disease segment of artery to guide traversal of the lesion. Heparin should be administered once the diseased segment is crossed. A bolus dose of 3,000 to 5,000 units of heparin is administered intravenously. Vasospasm during angioplasty is reduced by giving sublingual nifedipine 10 mg and/or direct intra-arterial administration of nitroglycerin in 50 to 200 µg boluses. The patient is placed on aspirin, 1 per day, for the rest of their lives following successful angioplasty.

The balloon catheter is positioned across the lesion using either digital roadmapping or anatomic landmarks as a guide (Fig. 7.1). A radio-opaque ruler placed adjacent to the vessel is helpful in localizing the position of the stenotic lesion. The balloon is inflated and monitored under fluoroscopy. The balloon should be inflated to the point of the elimination of the waist caused by the stenosis. There is no standard number for inflation time or number of inflation repetitions. Most operators inflate a balloon between 30 and 60 seconds for a total of one to three inflations. Inflation of a balloon is performed using an inflator device, which has an in-line pressure gauge marked in atmospheres of pressure. Most atherosclerotic lesions can be effectively dilated using approximately 6 atmospheres of pressure. Eccentric and calcified stenoses often require greater pressure inflations. Most balloon angioplasty catheters with 5 French shaft sizes are considered low pressure systems. These angioplasty catheters can be inflated to 10 to 12 atmospheres of pressure before the balloon ruptures. High pressure balloon angioplasty catheters have 6 or 7 French shaft sizes and can be inflated to 18 atmospheres or greater of pressure.

Monitoring of patient pain is a method of determining a successful angioplasty. Transient pain that resolves with deflation results from stretching of the adventitial nerve fibers and is a useful indicator of adequate dilatation. Painless inflation may indicate inadequate dilatation and the need for a larger balloon. Severe pain that persists after deflation is a warning of a possible vessel rupture. The balloon is held stationary during inflation. This prevents converting the intimal fissures and cracks into a flow-limiting dissection.

It is important to preserve access across the dilated stenosis until a satisfactory result is documented by performing either an angiogram or pressure measurement. Angiographic, hemodynamic, intravascular ultrasound, and clinical criteria can be used to ascertain whether the diseased segment is adequately dilated. The dilated segment rarely appears normal on postangioplasty angiograms (Fig. 7.2). The residual stenosis should be no greater than 30 percent. Postangioplasty angiograms may demonstrate small, focal dissections or luminal irregularity. This results from contrast media entering the large fissures between the intima and media that were formed after cracking of the atheroma. An important angiographic finding demonstrating adequate dilatation is elimination of the collateral vessels. Hemodynamic parameters are important in assessing the angioplasty result. In the resting state, any gradient greater than 10 mmHg is considered significant. In patients with claudication, intra-arterial vasodilators are used to simulate exercise-induced claudication. Tolazoline (Priscoline), 25 mg, or nitroglycerin, 100 to 200 µg is administered intra-arterially into the outflow of the diseased artery. Postvasodilatation, any gradient greater than 20 mmHg is considered significant. After angioplasty, the gradient should be eliminated or significantly reduced. Clinical indications of a successful angioplasty are restoration of femoral or distal pulses, improvement in skin color, and relief of any distal pain. The ankle/brachial index should increase by a minimal of 0.15.

Results depend on multiple factors. A short segment concentric stenosis has the most favorable response. Long segment stenoses, occlusions, anastomotic stenoses, and eccentric stenoses generally respond less favorably to angioplasty. Diabetes, smoking, and poor distal runoff diminish the length of patency. The approximate 2-year patency rate is 80 to 90 percent for iliac angioplasty, 60 percent for superficial femoral artery (SFA) angioplasty, and 40 percent for popliteal angioplasty.

Complications of angioplasty include puncture site hematoma, dissection, embolization, thrombosis, and vessel rupture. Abrupt occlusion may be due to spasm, thrombosis, or a dissection. Intravascular stents are excellent at salvaging dissected vessels or inadequate angioplasty results. Thrombolytic therapy can be used for thrombosis at the angioplasty site or distal embolization. Vessel rupture, seen angiographically as a contrast extravasation or pseudoaneurysm formation, is controlled by immediate reinflation of the angioplasty balloon to tamponade the bleeding site. The vascular surgery backup is immediately notified to repair the injury.

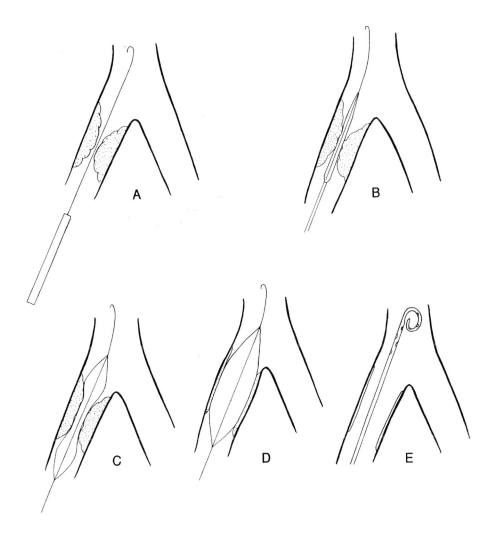

Figure 7.1 *Technique of angioplasty. (**A**) A vascular sheath is placed in common femoral artery for a retrograde approach to a common iliac stenosis. A steerable guidewire is negotiated across the stenosis. (**B**) The angioplasty balloon of appropriate diameter is positioned across the stenosis. The balloon is positioned using bony landmarks, road mapping, or a radio-opaque ruler. (**C**) The balloon is inflated under fluoroscopic monitoring with the waist in the center of the balloon confirming position. (**D**) The balloon is inflated until the waist disappears. (**E**) The result is evaluated by angiography and pressure measurements. Access across the dilated lesion is maintained at all times until a satisfactory result is documented on angiography.*

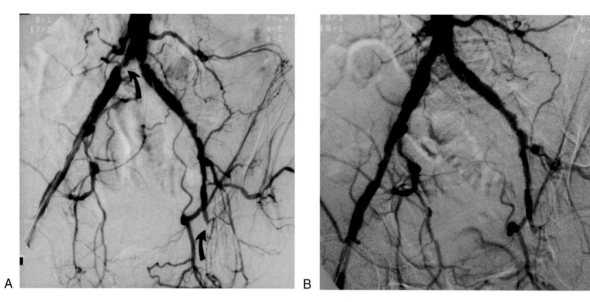

Figure 7.2 *Iliac angioplasty. (**A**) There is an eccentric stenosis in proximal right common iliac artery and an occluded left femoral artery (arrows). (**B**) The post-angioplasty angiogram demonstrates less than 20 percent residual stenosis and a decrease in the size of the collaterals.*

Renal Artery Angioplasty

Indications for renal artery angioplasty include uncontrollable hypertension and renal insufficiency. The multifactorial causes of hypertension and the presence of a concomitant disease process contributing to the patient's renal failure makes patient selection for renal angioplasty problematic. There are many noninvasive studies that can be used for screening for renovascular hypertension. Examples are renal scintigraphy, duplex ultrasound, spiral computed tomography, and magnetic resonance angiography. Each screening study has limitations. Angiographic findings suggestive of a significant renal artery stenosis are a 50 percent or greater stenosis, a gradient of 10 mmHg or greater, and atrophy of the affected kidney. Renal vein renin sampling has been recently discounted because of the inability of renal vein renin levels to positively predict response to revascularization either by surgery or angioplasty. Stenotic lesions caused by fibromuscular dysplasia respond more favorably than atherosclerotic lesions. Renal artery angioplasty of ostial or heavily calcified stenoses have less favorable results. Angioplasty can be used to treat transplant artery stenosis.

Angioplasty of native renal arteries is usually performed from a retrograde femoral artery approach. Antegrade brachial access may be required in the instance of a steep downward-angled renal artery take-off. Angioplasty can be performed either over a guidewire or through a curved-tip guiding sheath (similar to coronary angioplasty). A 7 to 9 French renal curve guiding catheter is used to coaxially guide wires and balloons into the renal artery. The blunt ended guiding catheter is used to engage the orifice of the renal artery. An angioplasty balloon catheter is passed through the lumen of the guiding catheter over a guidewire. This prevents buckling of the balloon catheter as it is passed around a steep bend through a stenosis. The completion angiogram is easily performed through the guiding catheter postdilatation. In the over-the-guidewire technique, a Neiman renal or similar downward-seeking catheter is used to select the diseased renal artery. A torsional attenuating diameter (TAD) wire or steerable wire is used to cross the stenosis. The distal portion of the TAD wire can be gently shaped so that the guidewire conforms to the angle formed by the renal artery origin from the aorta. The TAD wire has a floppy 0.018 inch tip designed to minimize spasm in the distal renal branches. The TAD wire tapers rapidly to a stiff 0.035 inch shaft. The stiffer part of the wire is placed into the renal artery facilitating tracking of the angioplasty balloon around the bend of the renal artery origin. The guidewire should not be placed within the distal renal artery branches because of the frequent incidence of severe renal spasm. Liberal use of intra-arterial nitroglycerin is advised during renal artery angioplasty, and the patient is given heparin when the stenosis is crossed.

Several specialized balloon catheters are commercially available for renal artery angioplasty. The renal angioplasty balloons are short, with a short tip and tapered balloon segment. Preshaped balloons on catheters with downward-seeking curves are available. These pre-curved designs facilitate passage of the balloon catheter across the stenotic vessel segment. Usually, a 5 to 6 mm diameter balloon is used for dilatation. Following dilatation, the access across the dilated segment must be preserved while evaluating the result. The TAD wire is removed and replaced with a 0.018 to 0.025 inch guidewire. The balloon catheter is retracted from the stenosis into the origin of the renal artery. A Touhy-Borst Y adapter is attached over the guidewire to the balloon catheter. A digital angiogram can be performed to assess the angioplasty results (Fig. 7.3). Dilatation is considered successful if the residual stenosis is less than 30 percent and flow is improved. Postangioplasty, there often is fissuring and clefts that give the appearance of an unsatisfactory result. Remodeling will usually correct this appearance. Transient pain indicates an adequate dilatation. Severe, persistent pain is a sign of potential arterial rupture and should not be ignored. Hemodynamic measurements that demonstrate reduction or elimination of the gradient indicate a therapeutic response.

Following renal artery angioplasty, the patient is monitored for blood pressure fluctuations in an inten-

Figure 7.3 *Renal artery angioplasty for fibromuscular dysplasia. (**A**) Preangioplasty left renal arteriogram shows the typical angiographic findings of fibromuscular dysplasia, which are weblike stenoses and a string of beads appearance (arrow). (**B**) Post 6-mm angioplasty arteriogram shows residual luminal irregularities, but the long segment stenosis has been improved in caliber. This is an adequate angioplasty result.*

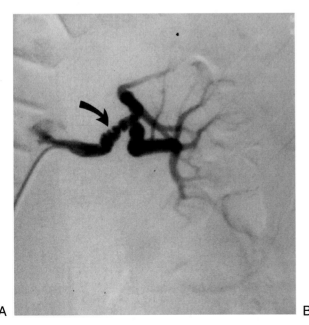 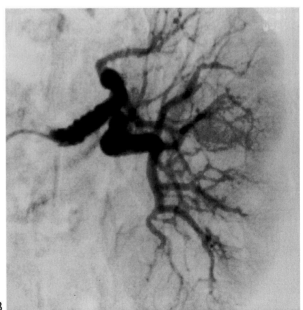

A   B

sive care unit for 24 hours. The patient's blood pressure is carefully monitored and controlled using short-acting antihypertensives such as sublingual nifedipine. Before the performance of the renal artery angioplasty, the patient's long-acting antihypertensive should have been discontinued and replaced by short-acting antihypertensives. Long-term aspirin antiplatelet aggregation therapy is recommended.

The reported clinical benefit of renal PTA ranges from 33 to 90 percent based on review of 13 papers involving 1,000 patients. In patients with fibromuscular disease there is an approximately 40 to 50 percent cure rate of the patient's hypertension and a 30 to 40 percent improvement in hypertension control. In atherosclerotic disease, there is only a 20 percent cure rate and a 40 percent improvement in hypertension control. Improvement in renal function occurs in approximately 40 percent of patients after angioplasty. Renal artery stenoses are prone to recur at an incidence between 5 and 33 percent. For recurrent renal artery stenoses, a second angioplasty is advocated; only when this fails should surgical intervention or stenting be considered.

The Society of Cardiovascular and Interventional Radiology has identified guidelines to provide uniform reporting standards. The reporting categories are cured, improved, or failure. Technical success is less than 20 percent residual stenosis and significant hemodynamic improvement. A cure in angioplasty for renal vascular hypertension is diastolic blood pressure less than 90 mmHg without medication. Improved diastolic blood pressure is less than 90 mmHg or between 90 and 110 mmHg, with a 15 mmHg decrease with similar or reduced medication regimen. Failure is all other cases. The guideline for success in treating renal failure is a decrease in creatinine to normal or by 20 percent.

Complications are spasm, dissection, thrombosis, rupture, hematoma, and renal failure. Renal artery recoil and dissection can be salvaged with stent placement. Rupture is treated by balloon reinflation and tamponade as a temporizing method before surgical repair. Cholesterol embolization can cause renal failure and hypertension by tiny particles of cholesterol occluding the renal arterioles. Widespread cholesterol embolization is associated with a significant mortality rate. Cholesterol embolization can mimic contrast nephrotoxicity or systemic vasculitis causing leukocytosis and eosinophilia.

Atherectomy

Atherectomy is the direct removal of obstructing atheroma. The technique was developed to treat the failures of angioplasty and to expand the role of percutaneous recannulation of femoropopliteal occlusions. Atherectomy requires blind passage of a large caliber, relatively stiff shaft device through heavily diseased vessels. The costs, procedural time, and complications of the currently available devices surpass simple angioplasty, with similar intermediate and long-term results. Hydrophilic guidewires, stents, and thrombolysis have replaced atherectomy devices for recannulation of occluded vessels. Directional atherectomy is a second line treatment modality reserved for failures of simpler techniques. Atherectomy may be considered in focal eccentric, calcified, or anastomotic stenoses after angioplasty has failed. The Simpson atherectomy device (Advanced Cardiovascular Systems, Temecula, CA) is the most widely used. The device combines a side cutting window with an angioplasty balloon. Balloon inflation presses the side cutting window into the atheroma. The plaque is shaved off and collected into a chamber for later analysis by a disposable drive unit. The device is rotated and the procedure repeated until the plaque is removed satisfactorily.

Suggested Readings

Becker GJ, Katzen BT, Dake MD: Noncoronary angioplasty. Radiology 170:921, 1989

Do-dai-DO, Triller J, Walpoth BH: Comparison study of self-expandable stents vs. balloon angioplasty alone in femoropopliteal artery occlusions. Cardiovasc Intervent Radiol 15:306, 1992

Johnstone KW: Femoral and popliteal arteries: reanalysis of results of balloon angioplasty. Radiology 183:767, 1992

Kim D, Gianturco LE, Porter DH et al: Peripheral directional atherectomy: 4-year experience. Radiology 183:773, 1992

Martin LG, Cork RD, Kaufman SL: Long-term results of angioplasty in 110 patients with renal artery stenosis. J Vasc Interv Radiol 3:619, 1992

McLean GK: Percutaneous peripheral atherectomy. J Vasc Interv Radiol 4:465, 1993

Roubidoux MA, Dunnick NR, Klotman PE et al: Renal vein renins: inability to predict response to revascularization in patients with hypertension. Radiology 178:819, 1991

Rutherford RB, Becker GB: Standards for evaluating and reporting the results of surgical and percutaneous therapy for peripheral arterial disease. J Vasc Interv Radiol 2:169, 1991

Tegtmeyer CJ, Sos TA: Technique of renal angioplasty. Radiology 161:577, 1986

Vogelzang RL: Long-term results of angioplasty. J Vasc Interv Radiol Suppl 7:179, 1996

Vascular Stents   MICHAEL A. BRAUN

Stents work by buttressing open the lumen of a diseased vessel. The holes in the stent filaments allow the vascular endothelium to cover the stent, incorporating the stent into the vessel wall. A stented artery has an optimal morphologic result and elimination of the pressure gradient, significant improvements compared with angioplasty alone. The role and indications for intravascular stents are evolving. Stents salvage the angioplasty failures of elastic recoil and dissection. In large vessels, the stented repair appears more durable compared with angioplasty alone. In smaller vessels, the incidence of restenosis equals angioplasty, resulting in similar outcomes.

The Palmaz stent is approved for suboptimal iliac angioplasty results. The initial optimal result and more durable repair have expanded the use of stents in iliac disease. In a 5-year angiographic follow-up comparing iliac stenting versus angioplasty, Richter et al reported a 94 percent patency for stented lesions versus 65 percent for angioplasty alone. These results have led some interventionalists to primarily place stents in iliac stenotic disease instead of angioplasty alone. At Northwestern, a 10-year follow-up study of iliac angioplasty showed a 40 percent patency rate. The 10- to 15-year patency rate for aortoiliac grafting is approximately 75 percent. At Northwestern, almost all iliac stenoses are being repaired with intravascular stents to provide a long-term repair potentially equal to aortoiliac surgery. This increased patency of a stented iliac artery is important when combined with a distal surgical revascularization procedure. Stents provide a means to treat percutaneously long segment iliac stenotic and chronic iliac occlusive disease not previously amenable to angioplasty. Chronic iliac occlusions can be recannulated by stents with or without prior thrombolysis.

Preliminary results for treating vessels smaller than the iliacs with stents have not been superior to results from angioplasty alone. Stent restenosis has limited the durability of the repair of small vessels. Comparison of femoropopliteal stenting with angioplasty has yielded similar patency rates. This does not justify the additional costs of primarily stenting these lesions. Stents remain an important tool for salvage of angioplasty failures in the infrainguinal vessels.

There are several techniques for using intravascular stents. Angioplasty of an iliac stenosis is usually done using a retrograde approach. A long 9 to 10 French vascular sheath is positioned across the lesion. The patient is anticoagulated with heparin. The Palmaz P308 stent (Johnson and Johnson Interventional Systems, Warren, NJ) is mounted on an 8 mm diameter × 3 cm long PEMT balloon (Meditech, Watertown, MA). The metal stent is centered over the balloon and crimped into place using either a rolling motion with the fingers or the crimping tool. The mounted stent on the balloon catheter is advanced through the vascular sheath over a guidewire (Fig. 8.1). A small plastic or metal introducer is used to open the sheath's hemostatic valve so that the stent can be passed safely through the valve. Once the stent is passed through the valve, the introducer is removed from the valve. The stent is advanced through the sheath and positioned across the stenosis. The sheath is withdrawn, exposing the balloon stent combination. A small contrast injection through the sheath will confirm appropriate position of the stent across the lesion. The stent is deployed by inflating the balloon. The inflator device can be filled with saline, which allows better fluoroscopic visualization of the deployment of the stent. The deflated balloon is twisted to free the balloon wings from the stent before withdrawing the balloon. This helps prevent the wings of the deflated balloon from becoming entangled within the stent and possibly causing stent migration. A contrast injection determines the result and the need for additional stents or stent expansion. The stent should be expanded to match the diameter of the adjacent normal vessel (Fig. 8.2). Multiple stents can be nested together to repair a long segment of diseased

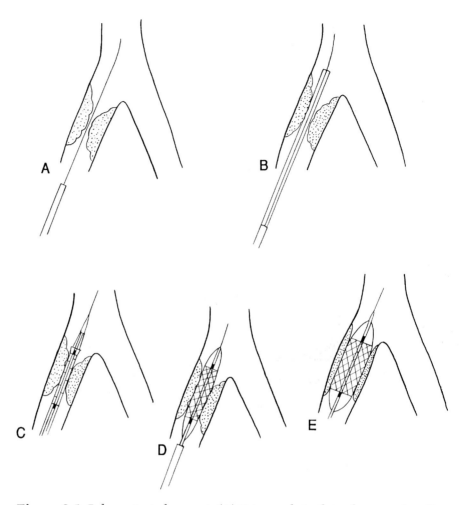

Figure 8.1 *Palmaz stent placement. (A) Retrograde ipsilateral approach to iliac stenosis. The guidewire is passed through the stenosis, and the patient is anticoagulated. A vascular sheath is placed within the common femoral artery. (B) The long vascular sheath and dilator are passed through the lesion. Most lesions have been predilated. (C) The mounted stent and balloon catheter are passed through the sheath across the stenotic lesion. (D) The sheath is withdrawn exposing the stent/balloon. A contrast injection will further confirm position. (E) The stent is dilated by inflating the balloon. Inflating the balloon with saline will aid in visualization of the stent.*

vessel. The stents should be overlapped by several millimeters. Care must be exercised when performing exchanges, especially when removing balloon catheters through deployed stents or passing wires through stents.

An alternative method for placing stents uses a 5.8 French Olbert balloon catheter. Olbert balloons have a low profile and return to their original shape following inflation. There are no excess balloon wings, which can catch and dislodge the stent. The balloon has a tacky surface that binds the stent in place. The stent and balloon can be advanced through the sheaths hemostatic valve without the introducer. The stent balloon combination more readily can be crossed over the aortic bifurcation or pushed through a lesion without dislodg-

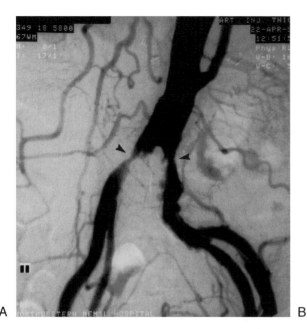
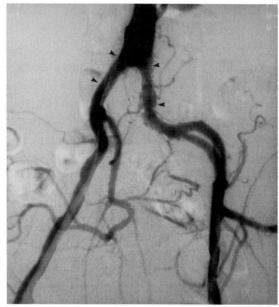

Figure 8.2 *(A) Bilateral common iliac stenoses. Note the presence of large, dilated collaterals. (B) Bilateral common iliac Palmaz stents have been deployed. Note absence of collaterals. The small arrowheads mark the ends of the stents.*

ing the stent. Another advantage to this system is that a smaller 7 French vascular sheath can be used to deploy the stent, reducing the formation of postprocedure groin hematomas. This technique simplifies primary stenting of iliac lesions and is our favored method of deploying stents.

The Wallstent (Schneider, Zurich, Switzerland) differs from the Palmaz stent. It has a low profile and can be deployed through a 7 French vascular sheath. The stent has longitudinal flexibility and is self-expanding. It can be deployed across the aortic bifurcation into a contralateral iliac artery. The stent's flexibility suits it well for tortuous arteries. Wallstents are available in lengths of 20 mm, 42 mm, 68 mm, and 90 mm. A single stent can be used to treat a long-segment occlusion or stenosis. The disadvantage in using a Wallstent is that it shrinks in length as the stent itself expands. A partially released stent can be repositioned but only in the withdrawing direction. Wallstents can be released in a nondilated stenosis followed by angioplasty to dilate the stent to match the adjacent vessel caliber. It can be advanced over a guidewire that has traversed a chronic occlusion. Theoretically, the Wallstent traps the occlusive material

against the vessel wall, preventing embolization. This immediately repairs the occlusion, eliminating the cost and risks of thrombolysis (Fig. 8.3). Chronic iliac occlusions can also be treated by thrombolysis and stenting. Stenting the recannulated and diseased arterial segment is more effective than angioplasty alone (Fig. 8.4). Acute thrombosis is thought best treated with thrombolysis followed by stenting, although this theory has not been validated by clinical studies.

Puncture site complications, thrombosis, embolization, and dissection are increased relative to diagnostic angiography from the large sheaths necessary for deployment of stents. This risk can be reduced by using the smaller deployment systems and eliminating or reducing the use of periprocedure heparin. Acute or subacute thrombosis is increased in hypercoagulable patients. Long-term restenosis is predicted by any post-stent gradient greater than zero. This gradient can occur from underexpansion of the stent, which optimally should be dilated 10 to 15 percent greater than the diameter of the vessel to embed the stent into the vessel wall. Overdilatation should be avoided to prevent vessel rupture or dissection.

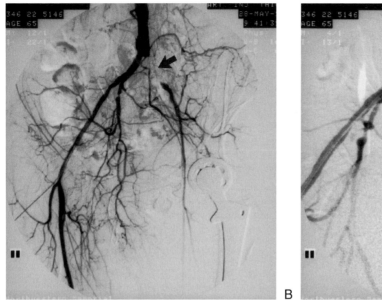
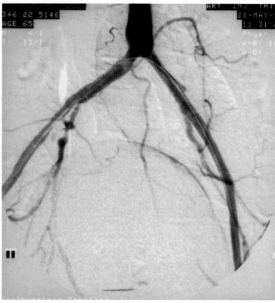

A   B

Figure 8.3 *(A) Chronic left common iliac occlusion (arrow). The occlusion was traversed from an antegrade contralateral approach using a Glidewire. (B) The iliac occlusion was primarily recannulated by contralateral placement of an 8 mm diameter × 68 mm long Wallstent. This is the postangiographic result of a single Wallstent placement. Note absence of collaterals and normal caliber of the left iliac and femoral arteries poststent recannulation.*

Renal Artery Stenting

Renal artery stenting is being used for the treatment of angioplasty failures and atherosclerotic renal ostial stenosis. Stents can salvage the angioplasty technical failures due to elastic recoil or dissection. The treatment of renal ostial lesions with angioplasty is marginal. Ostial stenoses occur from plaques located both within the wall of the aorta and the renal artery. These plaques are displaced rather than dilated by angioplasty. Stents offer a percutaneous repair of ostial lesions that do not respond to angioplasty alone. The role of stents in the treatment of renal artery stenosis is under investigation. Conservative proponents use stents only after angioplasty has failed or resulted in a 30 percent or greater residual stenosis, or for a flow-limiting dissection. Late postangioplasty restenosis is treated with repeat angioplasty, reserving stents for failures of reangioplasty. Others are stenting all ostial lesions and

restenoses. The immediate technical results of stenting are excellent, with elimination of hemodynamic gradients and residual stenosis. Long-term results of cure or improvement in hypertension are reported in approximately 60 to 80 percent of patients based on several investigations. The limiting factor for stents is restenosis in the range of 20 to 32 percent, compared to an estimated 30 percent for angioplasty alone. Other considerations are the cost of stents and the potential interference with renal bypass surgery.

Palmaz and Wallstents have be used for renal artery stenting. The Wallstent's flexibility facilitates placement around the downward-oriented renal artery origin, but it is difficult to visualize fluoroscopically and place precisely because of its longitudinal shrinkage. The Palmaz stent can be placed precisely but is more difficult to negotiate around the renal artery bend and often requires placement through a large diameter guiding catheter. Most renal arteries require a 5 to 7 mm diameter × 15 to 20 mm long stent.

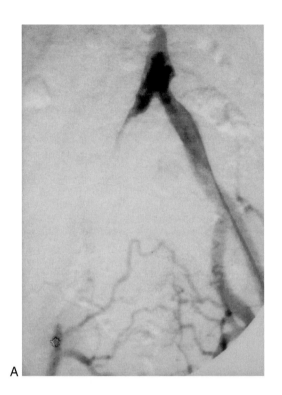

A

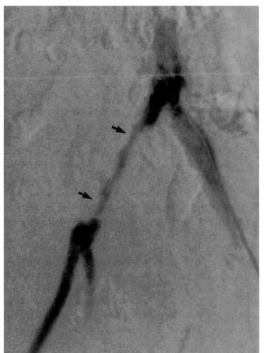

B

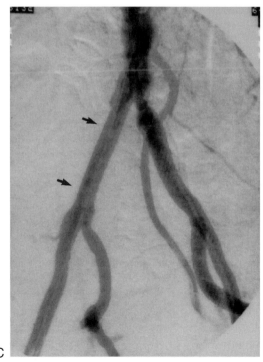

C

Figure 8.4 *Thrombolysis and stenting of chronic right common iliac artery occlusion. (A) The chronic right common iliac artery occlusion is approached from the contralateral left femoral puncture. A guidewire and infusion catheter were placed into the occluded vessel. (B) Right iliac arteriogram following overnight infusion of urokinase. An irregular and narrow lumen has been recannulated through the chronic iliac occlusion (small arrows). (C) The right femoral artery was punctured and Palmaz stents placed across the iliac artery occlusion effectively recannulated the affected vessel segment (small arrows).*

Most renal artery stents are deployed after renal artery angioplasty. Wallstents have been used primarily in Europe. The patient is anticoagulated with a heparin bolus. The appropriate size Wallstent is passed over a guidewire into the renal artery and positioned across the stenosis using fluoroscopic landmarks. The stent is released from the delivery catheter after careful positioning. Poststent deployment balloon dilatation was used only in a minority of cases.

Palmaz renal artery stenting commonly uses a guiding catheter to deliver the protected balloon stent combination around the renal artery bend. Conventional angioplasty is used for the stenosis, and an exchange length guidewire is left in place across the stenosis. Stenting of an ostial lesion requires precise positioning of the stent flush in the origin of the renal artery. The proper oblique view to tangentially image the renal artery origin is necessary. Preliminary oblique aortograms to choose this orientation are performed. An 8 French vascular sheath is placed in the femoral artery approach. A Touhy-Bourst Y adapter is attached to the 8 French guiding catheter for hemostasis and contrast injections. The appropriate diameter balloon catheter is preloaded through an 8 French angled-tip renal guiding catheter. The balloon catheter is passed through guiding catheter to expose the balloon for stent mounting. The stent is crimped on the balloon catheter and the stent is carefully retracted into the distal tip of the guiding catheter. This process saves pushing the stent-mounted balloon through the guiding catheter preventing dislodgement. The tapered tip of the balloon catheter should protrude slightly from the guiding catheter. The Y adapter is tightened for hemostasis.

The stented balloon and guiding catheter assembly are advanced over the wire and positioned across the stenosis (Fig. 8.5). The hemostatic valve is loosened, and the guiding catheter is partially withdrawn to expose the stent. A contrast injection reconfirms position. The guiding catheter is withdrawn to fully expose the stent. The stent is deployed by balloon inflation. The balloon catheter is withdrawn and a completion angiogram performed by contrast injection through the guiding catheter (Fig. 8.6). The stent diameter should match or slightly exceed (not more than 10 percent) the caliber of the native renal artery. Numerous technical variations exist. The stent can be mounted on a small diameter (4.5 French) balloon catheter and passed through a 6 French guiding catheter. An Olbert balloon, with its tacky surface to hold the stent in place, may be used.

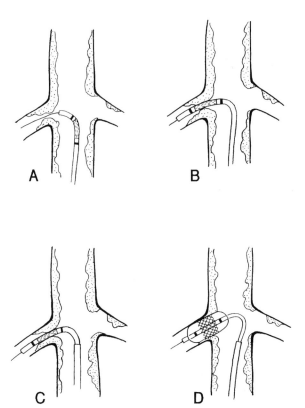

Figure 8.5 *Renal artery stenting. (A) A stiff guidewire is placed across the renal artery orifice stenosis. A 6 mm balloon catheter is passed through a long renal guiding catheter. The stent is mounted on the balloon and then it is pulled back into the sheath. The guiding catheter is placed over the wire through the vascular sheath and into the renal artery. (B) The stent, which is housed within the protective sheath, is positioned across the origin of the renal artery stenosis. The proper obliquity is chosen to image the renal artery origin in profile. This aids precise placement of the stent across the ostial lesion. (C) The outer sheath is slightly withdrawn and contrast injected to further confirm position of the stent. (D) The balloon is inflated, deploying the stent across the stenosis. The stent position is assessed when the balloon is deflated by contrast injection through the sheath.*

Complications are similar to renal angioplasty. Unique complications to stents are dislodgement with migration or malposition. Percutaneous retrieval or repositioning with snares can be judiciously attempted. The contrast load should be tailored or supplemented with carbon dioxide angiography to reduce contrast nephrotoxicity.

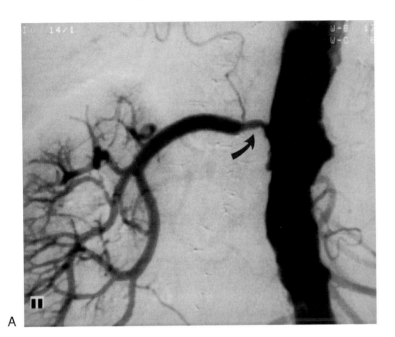

A

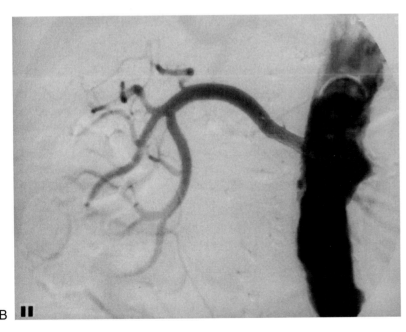

B

Figure 8.6 *Renal artery stent placement in a solitary kidney with an unsatisfactory angioplasty result.* **(A)** *There is a 40 to 50 percent residual stenosis following angioplasty in the right renal artery origin stenosis (arrow).* **(B)** *Poststent deployment arteriogram showing improved luminal caliber compared to the postangioplasty result.(Figure continues.)*

Figure 8.6 *(Continued)* *(C) The position of stent in the origin of the renal artery with protrusion into the aortic lumen is demonstrated on computed tomography. This was necessary to keep the plaque in the aorta from occluding the origin of the renal artery.*

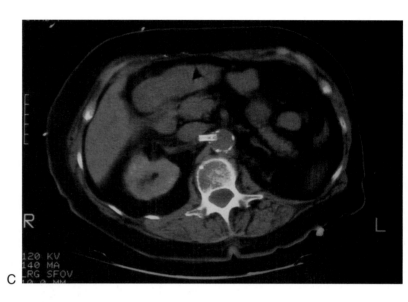

Suggested Readings

Becker GJ: Stent placement for peripheral arterial disease of the lower extremity. J Vasc Interv Radiol Suppl 7:S180, 1996

Bjarnason H, Hunter DW, Ferral H et al: Placement of the Palmaz stent with use of an 8-F introducer sheath and Olbert balloons. J Vasc Interv Radiol 4:435, 1993

Blum U, Gabelmann A, Redecker M et al: Percutaneous recannulization of iliac artery occlusions: results of a prospective study. Radiology 189:536, 1993

Hennequin LM, Joffre FG, Rousseau HP et al: Renal artery stent placement: long-term results with the Wallstent endoprosthesis. Radiology 191:713, 1994

Murphy KD, Encarnacion CE, Le VA, Palmaz JC: Iliac artery stent placement with the Palmaz stent: follow-up study. J Vasc Interv Radiol 6:321, 1995

Palmaz JC, Laborde JC, Rivera FJ et al: Stenting the iliac arteries with the Palmaz stent: experience from a multicenter trial. Cardiovasc Intervent Radiol 15:291, 1992

Raynaud AC, Beyssen BM, Turmel-Rodrigues LE et al: Renal artery stent placement: immediate and midterm technical and clinical results. J Vasc Interv Radiol 5:849, 1994

Rees CR, Palmaz JC, Becker GJ et al: Preliminary report of a multi-center study of the Palmaz stent in atherosclerotic stenoses involving the ostia of the renal arteries. Radiology 181:507, 1991

Rees CR, Palmaz JC, Garcia O et al: Angioplasty and stenting of completely occluded iliac arteries. Radiology 172:953, 1989

Richter GM, Roeren T, Brado M, Noeldege G: Further update on the randomized trial: iliac stent placement versus PTA-morphology, clinical success rates, and failure analysis, abstracted. J Vasc Interv Radiol 4:30, 1993

Saeed M: Aortoiliac and renal stenting. p. 103. In Kandarpa K, Aruny JE (eds): Handbook of Interventional Radiologic Techniques. 2nd Ed. Little, Brown, Boston, 1995

Vorwerk D, Gunther RW, Schurmann K, Wendt G: Primary stent placement for chronic iliac arterial occlusions: follow-up results in 103 patients. Radiology 194:745, 1995

Zollikofer CL, Antonucci F, Pfyffer M et al: Arterial stent placement with use of the Wallstent: midterm results of clinical experience. Radiology 179:449, 1991

Vascular Stent Grafts   MICHAEL A. BRAUN

Metallic stents have revolutionized the treatment of stenotic and occlusive disease. The stents are porous to allow ingrowth of vascular endothelium. Covered stents offer the possibility of endovascularly sealing holes, fistulas, and aneurysms. No approved devices are commercially available, but several designs are being investigated. A home-made stent graft can be fashioned by attaching Dacron fabric, polytetrafluoroethylene (PTFE), or autologous vein to the outside of a stent. The covered stent is positioned across the lesion and expanded to seal the defect from the inside of the vessel. This is in place of suturing the graft from the outside. The bulky nature of these devices frequently requires operative vessel exposure for vascular access or surgical harvesting of the necessary vein. A team approach and close cooperation between intervention radiologists and surgeons are necessary to bring this new technology to fruition.

Palmaz stents covered with PTFE or autogenous vein have been used to repair focal arterial injuries in poor operative risk situations or in difficult to access areas. Impragraft PTFE will radially expand 350 to 400 percent without altering the material's physical and mechanical characteristics. The graft is placed coaxially over the stent and cut to match the length of the stent. The covering is secured to the stent with 6-0 prolene sutures placed at each quadrant of the graft/stent ends and with a circumferential 8-0 prolene suture. Autogenous vein may be substituted for the PTFE prosthetic material (Fig. 9.1). A branch-free segment of 3.0 to 3.5 mm diameter vein is sutured to the stent in the same manner as PTFE. A disadvantage of vein is the possibility of leakage from a tear or unnoticed side branch (Fig. 9.2). The stent graft is delivered through a 12 to 16 French sheath. The tacky balloon surface of an Olbert balloon helps bind the bulky stent graft to the delivery balloon. This facilitates advancing and positioning the bulky device across the target lesion. The balloon length should match the length of the stent.

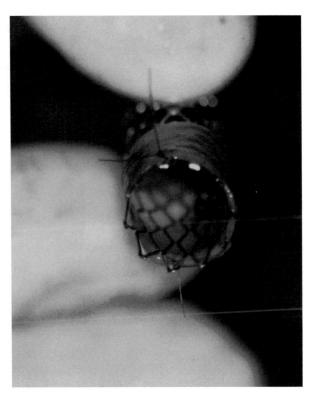

Figure 9.1 *A 3.5 mm diameter segment of saphenous vein was mounted on a Palmaz stent. Sutures were placed at the four quadrants at the edge of the stent and vein. The length of vein mounted on the stent was only half the length of the stent for demonstration purposes.*

Longer length balloons inflate in a dumbbell configuration, which shrinks the length of the stent-covering material. The rest of the procedure is similar to that for deploying a stent.

Large stent graft devices are being investigated in the endovascular repair of abdominal aortic aneurysms or inoperable thoracic aortic aneurysms. Endovascular

Figure 9.2 *(A) Spiral computed tomography angiogram depicting saccular aneurysm of left subclavian artery (arrows). (B) Thoracic arch aortogram demonstrating left subclavian aneurysm (arrows). (Figure continues.)*

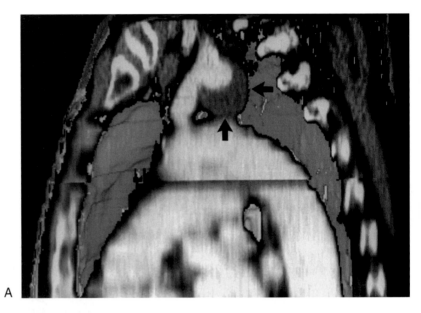

A

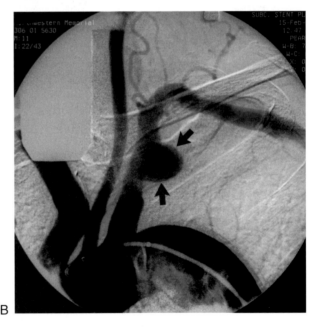

B

repair of aneurysms potentially will reduce the mortality, morbidity, hospital stay, recuperative period, and cost as compared to operative repair. An example is the 23 French Endovascular Technologies (EVT) stent graft, which is placed through a femoral cutdown approach (Fig. 9.3). This device is limited to aortic aneurysms that have 1.5 to 2.0 cm necks above the aortic bifurcation and below the renal arteries. It is placed in the operating room in a team approach between vascular surgeons and interventional radiologists. Each stent graft is custom made to fit the internal dimensions of the patient's aneurysm as measured by computed tomography and angiography. The stents have side hooks, which are used to anchor and seal the connection between the endolumi-

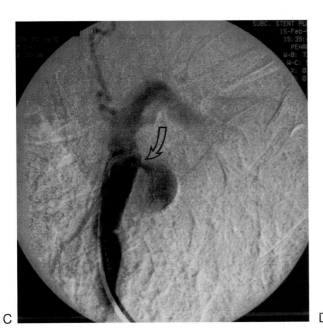

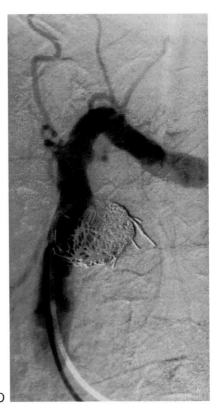

Figure 9.2 *(Continued) **(C)** A vein-covered Palmaz stent was positioned and deployed across the saccular aneurysm. A postdeployment arteriogram demonstrates a small jet of contrast entering the aneurysm from a hole in the vein (arrow). This hole may be from a tear in the vein or a small branch vessel. **(D)** Coils are used to thrombose the lumen of the aneurysm, which successfully excluded the aneurysm.*

nal tube graft and the neck of the aortic aneurysm wall. A tight seal is considered necessary to prevent perigraft leakage and incomplete exclusion of the aneurysm since prevention of rupture is the goal of treatment (Fig. 9.4). The addition of side hooks makes the collapsed EVT deployment device large (23 French). This requires a 7.7 mm diameter iliac artery to accept the device. The EVT tube device is used to repair aneurysms that solely involve the abdominal aorta while the majority of aortic aneurysms extend into the iliac arteries. A bifurcation variant of this original design has been developed to solve the problem of aneurysms that extend into the iliac arteries (Fig. 9.5). Endoluminal stent grafting of thoracic aortic aneurysms is being actively investigated by Dake and

Semba at Stanford. Their design uses a modified Z stent attached to a Dacron tube graft. The radial strength of the self-expanding Z stent has been adequate to anchor the graft in position and prevent leakage (Fig. 9.6).

One of the current limitations of the prototype stent graft designs is their bulky nature. The Corvita endovascular graft offers a low profile (9 French) delivery system to deploy a self-expanding stent covered with polycarbonate urethane fibers. The small diameter and flexibility of this device overcome several of the significant drawbacks of other systems. The device has similar properties and features familiar to the widely used Wallstent. The Corvita graft is not yet approved for use in the United States.

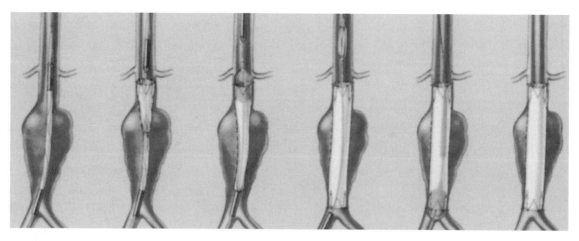

Figure 9.3 *The implantation sequence of the Endovascular Technologies tube stent graft used to exclude abdominal aortic aneurysm. From left to right: tube endograft prosthesis positioned; superior aortic attachment system released; balloon inflated; inferior aortic attachment system released; balloon inflated; implantation completed. (Courtesy of Endovascular Technologies, Menlo Park, CA).*

Figure 9.4 *Abdominal aortogram demonstrating EVT tube stent graft exclusion of an abdominal aortic aneurysm. The aneurysm involved the abdominal aorta only. Metallic markers are distributed along the margins of the Dacron tube graft to delineate the graft radiologically.*

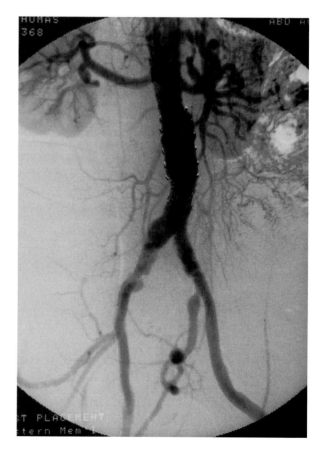

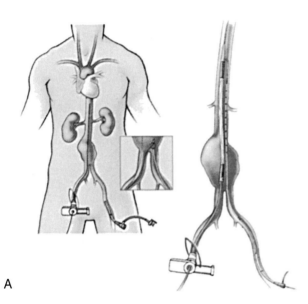

Figure 9.5 *(A) The bifurcated aortic graft requires access from both femoral arteries. The small inset shows the wire controlling deployment of the left graft limb being snared through the left femoral access sheath. The picture at the left depicts initial introduction of the bifurcated stent graft. (B) The implantation sequence of the EVT bifurcated prosthesis. From left to right: bifurcated endograft prosthesis positioned, aortic attachment system released, balloon inflated, contralateral iliac attachment system released; balloon inflated, ipsilateral iliac attachment system released; balloon inflated, implantation completed. (Courtesy of Endovascular Technologies, Menlo Park, CA).*

A

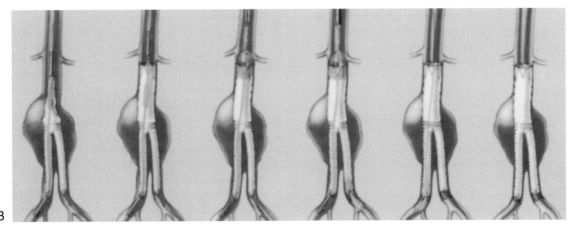

B

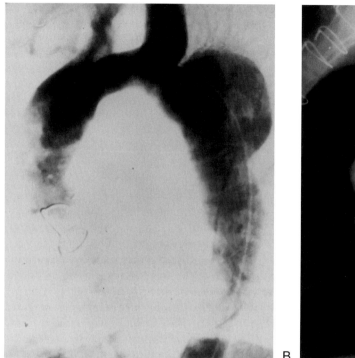
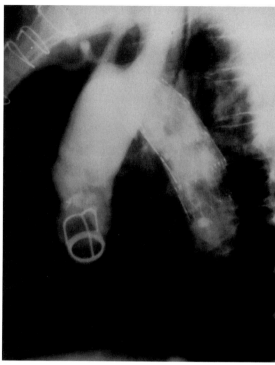

A   B

Figure 9.6 *Endovascular repair of descending thoracic aorta pseudoaneurysm. (A) Lateral thoracic aortogram demonstrating wide-mouth pseudoaneurysm of the descending thoracic aorta. (B) Custom-made stent graft has successfully excluded the thoracic aortic pseudoaneurysm returning the caliber of the aorta to normal. A Star-Edwards aortic valve prosthesis is present. (Courtesy of Michael Dake, Stanford, CA)*

Suggested Readings

Becker GJ, Benenati JF, Zemel G et al: Percutaneous placement of a balloon-expandable intraluminal graft for life-threatening subclavian arterial hemorrhage. J Vasc Interv Radiol 2:225, 1991

Chuter TAM, Donayre CE, White RA: Endoluminal Vascular Prostheses. Little, Brown, Boston, 1995

Laborde JC, Parodi JC, Clem MF et al: Intraluminal bypass of abdominal aortic aneurysm: feasibility study. Radiology 184:185, 1992

Marin ML, Veith FJ, Levine BA: Endovascular Stented Grafts for the Treatment of Vascular Diseases. Springer-Verlag, Heidelberg, 1995

Marin ML, Veith FJ, Panetta TF et al: Percutaneous transfemoral insertion of a stented graft to repair a traumatic femoral arteriovenous fistula. J Vasc Surg 18:298, 1993

May J, White G, Waugh R et al: Transluminal placement of a prosthetic graft-stent device for treatment of subclavian artery aneurysm. J Vasc Surg 18:1056, 1993

Parodi JC, Barone HD: Transfemoral intraluminal graft implantation for abdominal aortic aneurysms. Ann Vasc Surg 5:491, 1991

Thrombolysis MICHAEL A. BRAUN

Urokinase thrombolysis is increasingly being accepted as an alternative form of therapy for embolic occlusions and an important adjuvant to salvage of peripheral graft thrombotic occlusions. Fogarty balloon thrombectomy has been the "gold standard" and is the preferred treatment for embolic occlusions that are readily surgically accessed. Surgical treatment is necessary for the severely ischemic limb that has impending limb loss or the acute postoperative bypass graft thrombosis. The limitations of Fogarty embolectomy are potential damage to the arterial intimal lining and the inability to remove clot in the microvasculature. Infusional thrombolysis can restore patency of the small branch vessels inaccessible to a Fogarty balloon increasing the number of outflow vessels.

Thrombolytic therapy is indicated in any patient who has an acute occlusion within a surgically created bypass graft or a native artery secondary to an embolus or acute thrombosis. Embolic occlusions are signaled by acute onset of the five "P's" and the angiographic findings of a filling defect lodged at a branch point or an occlusion with a meniscus and absence of collaterals. Most emboli are cardiac in origin and can be organized thrombus or mural plaque. Large, accessible emboli are preferably treated with surgical embolectomy. Surgical embolectomy can quickly remove the clot and restore flow reversing critical ischemia. Thrombolysis is used when the emboli are distally located or the patient is a poor operative candidate (Fig. 10.1). Thrombotic occlusion of grafts is the most common indication for thrombolytic therapy, with reported success rates averaging 70 to 80 percent. In general, venous graft thrombosis is best treated urgently to salvage the graft, whereas both acute and chronic occlusions of prosthetic grafts will respond favorably to lysis. Graft occlusion occurring within 30 days of surgery is usually a result of technical failure or patient selection error that is best not treated by thrombolysis.

The patient must be able to tolerate a 24- to 48-hour infusion of urokinase. Patients with neurologic dysfunction or muscle paralysis in the affected extremity should not be considered candidates for urokinase therapy unless no surgical options exist. The general risk of thrombolysis is hemorrhage, which commonly involves the puncture site but can be remote to the treated limb. Contraindications include a recent stroke (3 months), recent surgery or trauma (10 days), active internal bleeding, and a nonviable extremity.

Thrombus is composed of aggregated platelets held together by a fibrin mesh. The fibrin mesh is controlled by the enzyme plasmin, which limits the extent of the clot and removes the clot barrier when it is no longer needed. Three fibrinolytic drugs are available for thrombolysis. Streptokinase is a bacterial protein that indirectly activates plasminogen into plasmin. It is inexpensive but is not used because of its antigenicity and greater bleeding complication rate. Tissue plasminogen activator (TPA) is a direct enzymatic converter of plasminogen to plasmin with affinity for fibrin-bound plasminogen. This affinity was intended to give TPA target specificity for fibrin clots, reducing systemic fibrinolysis. Unfortunately, this has not held up in practice. Recent comparisons of TPA versus urokinase have shown similar efficacy between the two drugs. TPA is more expensive and has a greater bleeding complication rate making urokinase the preferred thrombolytic agent. Urokinase is a direct activator of plasminogen. The half-life of urokinase is approximately 14 to 16 minutes. It is nonantigenic. A side effect of shaking chills can occur and is associated with higher doses used, for example, during pulse spray technique. Prophylactic administration of diphenhydramine, 50 mg, and acetaminophen, 500 to 1,000 mg, can prevent these symptoms or the side effects can be treated with meperidine, 25 to 50 mg, intravenous injection.

The thrombolysis technique starts with a baseline diagnostic arteriogram that assists in planning the ther-

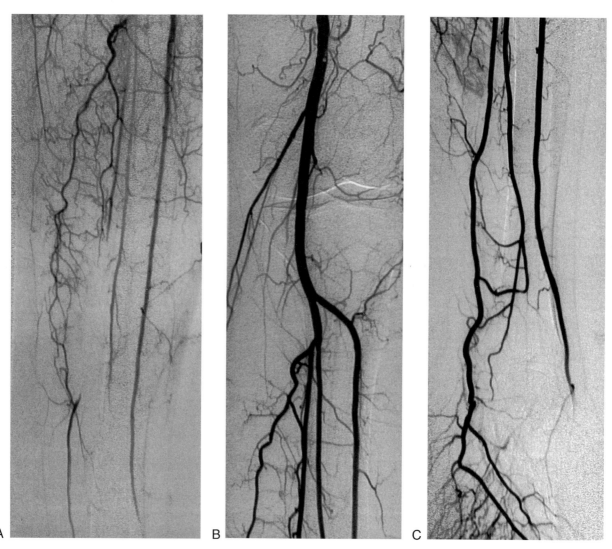

Figure 10.1 **(A)** *The infrapopliteal arteries are acutely occluded from thromboemboli from an upstream pseudoaneurysm causing rest pain.* **(B)** *Left popliteal angiogram after an overnight infusion of urokinase into the popliteal artery.* **(C)** *Left ankle angiogram demonstrates complete lysis of the thrombus in the posterior tibial and peroneal arteries. The dorsalis pedis remained partially occluded.*

apeutic approach and the appraisal of the end result. The thrombolysis treatment option should be considered before performing the angiogram. The contralateral femoral artery is punctured, preferably using single wall technique. A 6 to 7 French vascular sheath is used. The thrombosed vessel or graft stump is identified and carefully probed with an angled-tip catheter and Glidewire (Fig. 10.2). Roadmapping is helpful to guide the probing of the graft stump. The clot often has a rind

that prevents initial penetration by the guidewire. The thrombus rind is optimally crossed by placing the guiding catheter tip in the graft stump, which helps direct the guidewire through the rind into the softer body of the clot. The thrombosed vessel should be traversed with a Glidewire before initiating the urokinase infusion. This helps the lytic agent penetrate the clot more efficiently and mechanically disrupts the clot. Guidewire traversal of the thrombosis predicts a successful out-

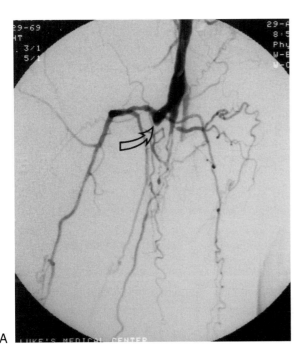
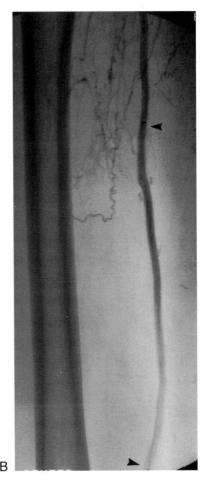

Figure 10.2 *(A) Acute thrombosis of a right femoropopliteal graft. The graft stump is identified by an arrow. The angle tip catheter is used to select the graft stump and direct the Glidewire through the occluded graft. (B) Contrast injection through the proximal infusion catheter shows that the graft is open following 18 hours of urokinase infusion. Note the position of the proximal infusion catheter and distal infusion wire (arrowheads). (Figure continues.)*

come. A 180 to 260 cm stiff Glidewire facilitates catheter placement over steep aortic bifurcations and facilitates exchange of long (100 cm) infusion catheters.

The fibrinolytic agent is delivered directly into the thrombus. Several infusion catheter systems are available for delivery of the urokinase. The fundamental principle of infusion catheter design is even distribution of agent throughout the maximum length of clot possible. Several systems are available with no clinically documented best design delineated. Infusion catheters have the advantage of positional stability over endhole

catheters, which may become dislodged from patient movement. Examples of infusion catheters are the Peripheral Systems EDM, Cook multisideport, Cook McNamara coaxial, Angiodynamics Pro infusion, and Meditech Mewissen. Regardless of the system, it is important to infuse the proximal portion of the thrombus first and then advance the infusion system as necessary. At Northwestern, the most frequently used infusion catheter is a Mewissen. This is a 5 French catheter that has multiple sideholes over a 10 cm length near its distal tip. The distal end of the Mewissen catheter can

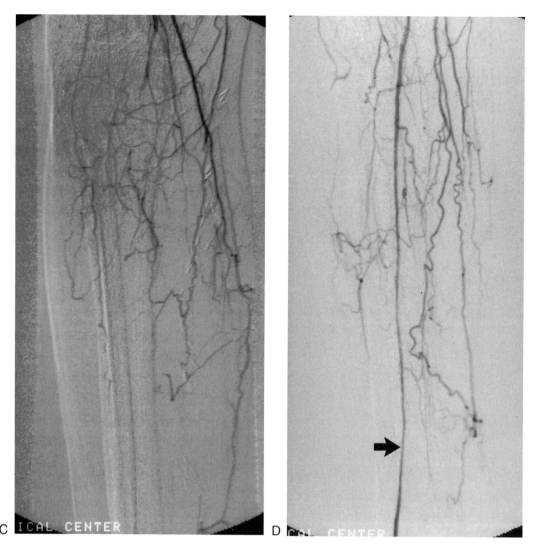

Figure 10.2 *(Continued) (**C**) Prethrombolysis right knee arteriogram showing significant occlusive disease of the popliteal artery and runoff vessels. (**D**) Post-thrombolysis popliteal angiogram showing patency of the popliteal artery with single vessel runoff via the posterior tibial artery (arrow).*

be occluded by placing an appropriate guidewire through it. A Touhy-Bourst Y adapter is connected to the Mewissen catheter. The infusion is given through the sideport of the Touhy-Bourst adapter. This results in intrathrombus infusion via the multiple sideholes along its distal end. Coaxial systems are used to infuse into long segment occlusions. A Mewissen catheter is placed proximally within the clot and a Katzen infusion wire is placed distally within the thrombus (Fig. 10.3).

The urokinase dose is split evenly between the two infusion systems that require two infusion pumps.

The standard urokinase preparation is 1 million units diluted in 250 ml of normal saline. The high-dose urokinase infusion protocol reduces complications and cost by reducing the overall infusion duration. Urokinase is infused initially at a rate of 4,000 U/min for the initial 4 hours and is reduced to 2,000 U/min for the remainder of the infusion. Concomitant

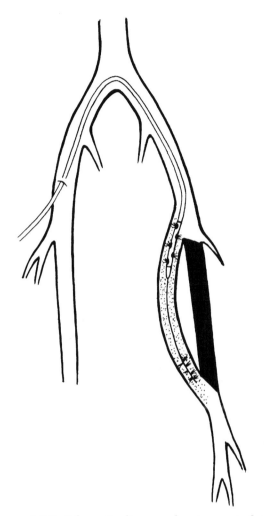

Figure 10.3 *Schematic diagram showing contralateral approach to thrombosed left fem-popliteal bypass graft. A vascular sheath is commonly placed at the puncture site. This facilitates catheter exchanges and blood draws. A coaxial system consisting of a proximal infusion catheter and distal infusion wire maximizes intrathrombus delivery of urokinase.*

administration of low-dose heparin to maintain the partial thromboplastin time (PTT) in a range of 1.25 to 1.5 is performed. This prevents catheter-related thrombus formation and rethrombosis.

The patient should be managed and monitored in the Intensive Care Unit during thrombolytic therapy. The prothrombin time (PT), PTT, fibrinogen level, fibrin split products (FSP), hemoglobin, and platelet count are measured every 4 to 6 hours. No laboratory parameter

accurately predicts the likelihood of systemic bleeding, but a decrease in fibrinogen by 50 percent or to less than 100 mg helps indicate the onset of a systemic thrombolytic state. If this occurs, the urokinase infusion should be decreased by 50 percent and the fibrinogen level remeasured within 2 hours. If the fibrinogen level continues to decrease, the thrombolytic infusion should be discontinued and normal saline infused through the catheter. After a 4-hour interval, the fibrinogen level can be reassessed and thrombolytic therapy restarted at a reduced rate if the fibrinogen level has increased.

Clinical monitoring during infusion includes observation of the infused extremity for evidence of reperfusion or worsening of ischemia. Frequent neurologic and vascular checks should be performed. The puncture site should be carefully observed for bleeding. If bleeding occurs, the urokinase dose can be decreased and direct pressure held to control the bleeding. The patient should be placed on bleeding precautions to prevent any inadvertent induction of bleeding. Perisheath oozing is a frequent occurrence and if it cannot be stopped by pressure, upsizing the sheath by one French size may control the problem.

Follow-up angiography is performed when either logistically feasible or clinically indicated. Angiography is repeated after 18 to 24 hours of infusion. It is not necessary to repeat angiography at a predetermined time, particularly when this involves an after-hours examination, unless there is a pressing clinical reason. Worsening symptoms of ischemia may be due to distal embolization and usually resolves with continued lytic infusion. The follow-up urokinase check is used to assess the amount of clot lysis and reposition the infusion system into the remaining thrombus. Successful thrombolytic infusions generally occur within 24 hours. Most graft thromboses are significantly or completely lysed within 16 to 18 hours. Alternative treatment methods should be considered if complete lysis is not achieved in 48 to 72 hours. Care must be taken when chasing emboli into small distal branches. A catheter placed within a small vessel can lead to local complications such as dissection or vessel injury.

A completion angiogram should search for the underlying etiology that caused the thrombosis. Treatment of the precipitating lesion will prolong patency of the thrombolytic therapy (Fig. 10.4). Causes of prosthetic graft thrombosis are inflow stenosis, progression of distal disease, anastomotic stenosis, hypotensive episode, or hypercoagulability. Venous graft thrombosis is caused by fibrotic valves, clamp

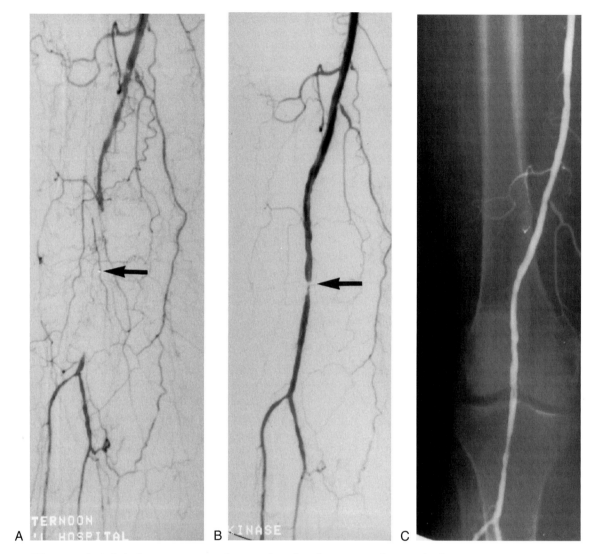

Figure 10.4 **(A)** *Short segment occlusion of popliteal artery resulting in limb ischemia. An infusion catheter has been placed into the chronic occlusion (arrow).* **(B)** *Urokinase thrombolysis dissolved the thrombosis and uncovered the underlying lesion (arrow).* **(C)** *Angioplasty was performed with good result. Angiography of the foot and pedal arch showed no distal embolization.*

injury, ischemia, or strictures from intimal hyperplasia. Identification and treatment of the underlying lesion will increase 1 year patency from 40 percent to 85 percent in successfully lysed grafts.

The most common complication is bleeding. Most bleeding complications are limited to the puncture site and can be controlled as described before. Bleeding complications increase with the duration of the infu-

sion and the use of concomitant heparin. Regional thrombolysis has increased efficacy but has not eliminated systemic hemorrhagic complications. Intracranial hemorrhage is the most feared complication, with an incidence of 1 to 2 percent. Use of concomitant heparinization is not universal, and some centers limit the use to low flow states or when the catheter crosses a stenosis to reach an occlusion. Contrast-induced nephropathy can occur because of the large contrast volume necessary to diagnose and follow the treatment.

The results of thrombolytic therapy are difficult to gauge due to the widely disparate indications. The average technical success rate is approximately 80 to 90 percent using urokinase. Long-term results are more favorable in acute ischemia in native vessel occlusions compared to bypass graft occlusions. Embolic occlusions often require longer infusion times than thrombotic occlusions. Patients with graft thrombosis should be angiographically examined for inflow stenosis, anastomotic stenosis, or progression of distal occlusive disease. These are the common causes of graft failure. Patency results are significantly improved when a focal lesion is identified and treated. Thrombolytic therapy can convert an urgent, major operative procedure to a planned minor correction of a previous limb revascularization. The STILE study compared operative and infusional techniques for acute limb ischemia and found similar patency and limb salvage rates but reduced mortality in the thrombolysis-treated group. The drawback of regional thrombolytic therapy is the prolonged infusion time needed to complete treatment. Pharmacomechanical thrombolysis techniques have recently been tested to accelerate thrombolysis. Pulse-spray infusional techniques are an example of this protocol. When pulse-spray techniques were compared to high-dose infusional techniques, little difference was found between the two treatment regimens. The pulse-spray thrombolysis is more physician time intensive and is not routinely used except for treating thrombosed dialysis access grafts.

Suggested Readings

Comerota AJ, White JV: Overview of catheter-directed thrombolytic therapy for arterial and graft occlusion. p. 225. In Comerota AJ (ed): Thrombolytic Therapy for Peripheral Vascular Disease. JB Lippincott, Philadelphia, 1995

Cragg AH, Smith TP, Corson JD et al: Two urokinase dose regimens in native arterial and graft occlusions: initial results of a prospective, randomized clinical trial. Radiology 178:681, 1991

Flinn WR, McCarthy WJ, Silva MB, Amble S: Thrombolytic therapy in the management of chronic arterial occlusions. p. 269. In Comerota AJ (ed): Thrombolytic Therapy for Peripheral Vascular Disease. JB Lippincott, Philadelphia, 1995

Gardiner GA, Koltun W, Kandarpa K et al: Thrombolysis of occluded femoropopliteal grafts. AJR 147:621, 1986

Graor RA, Olin J, Bartholomew JR, et al: Efficacy and safety of intraarterial local infusion of streptokinase, urokinase, or tissue plasminogen activator for peripheral arterial occlusion: a retrospective review. J Vasc Med Biol 2:310, 1990

Kandarpa K, Chopra PS, Aruny JE et al: Intraarterial thrombolysis of lower extremity occlusions: a prospective, randomized comparison of forced periodic infusion and conventional slow continuous infusion. Radiology 188:861, 1993

Katzen BT: Devices for delivery of thrombolytic agents. p. 291. In Comerota AJ (ed): Thrombolytic Therapy for Peripheral Vascular Disease. JB Lippincott, Philadelphia, 1995

Mewissen MW, Minor PL, Beyer GA et al: Symptomatic native arterial occlusions: early experience with "over-the-wire" thrombolysis. J Vasc Interv Radiol 1:43, 1991

McNamara TO: Thrombolysis as an alternative initial therapy for the acutely ischemic limb. Semin Vasc Surg 5:89, 1992

McNamara TO, Fischer JR: Thrombolysis in peripheral arterial and graft occlusions: improved results using high dose urokinase. AJR 144:764, 1985

Ouriel K, Shortell CK, DeWeese JA et al: A comparison of thrombolytic therapy with operative revascularization in the treatment of acute peripheral arterial ischemia. J Vasc Surg 19:1021, 1994

The STILE Investigators: Results of a prospective randomized trial evaluating surgery versus thrombolysis for ischemia of the lower extremity. Ann Surg 220:251, 1994

Valji K, Roberts AC, Davis GB, Bookstein JJ: Pulsed-spray thrombolysis of arterial and bypass graft occlusions. AJR 156:617, 1991

Embolization
MICHAEL A. BRAUN
ROBERT L. VOGELZANG

Embolization is a core procedure within interventional radiology. The principal advantage of embolization is immediate control of hemorrhage. It is used therapeutically in situations involving trauma, gastrointestinal bleeding, arterial aneurysms and pseudoaneurysms, neoplasms, vascular malformations, varicoceles, pulmonary hemorrhage, and obstetrical hemorrhage. The goals of embolization must be considered before performing the procedure. The vessel or vascular bed must be accessible for selective catheterization to prevent inadvertent blockage of a nontarget vessel. The site of embolization must be anticipated. A proximal occlusion of a distal bleeding artery reduces distal perfusion pressure to allow local hemostasis. Collateral flow will prevent unnecessary tissue infarction. Distal embolization is performed to devascularize tumors to control intraoperative hemorrhage when tissue infarction of the tumor is not a concern.

Embolization agents are best delivered through an endhole catheter. A vascular sheath is always used. A selective angiogram is mandatory before embolization to study the vascular lesion and exclude anomalous anatomy. The catheter must be placed as selectively as possible to avoid reflux of embolic agents into nontarget vessels. The position of the catheter must be secure during coil embolization to prevent migration of the catheter tip when the coil is pushed through the catheter. Embolization materials and catheters should be segregated from diagnostic equipment to prevent inadvertent embolization. Overzealous administration of particulate or liquid agent is unnecessary. Wait 5 to 10 minutes for the induced hemostasis to occur before assessing the results with the postembolization angiogram. Embolization of malformations or large tumors is often performed in stages.

Distal embolization of organs results in the postembolization syndrome from the effects of the tissue infarction. The ischemic pain from embolization is severe and should be anticipated. Prophylactic infusion of injectable lidocaine into the embolization bed can help reduce the pain. Difficult malformation embolizations may require general anesthesia for patient comfort and prolonged immobility. The postembolization syndrome is pain, fever, and leukocytosis. Fever and leukocytosis occur 3 to 7 days after embolization-mimicking sepsis. Prophylactic antibiotics are given before hepatic chemoembolization and splenic embolization.

Embolization materials are classified as either temporary or permanent. The size of the material determines between a proximal or distal occlusion. The classic example of a short-term embolizing material is autologous clot. The drawbacks of an autologous clot is that it is easily fragmented and readily lysed by the patient's own natural thrombolytic system. For this reason, Gelfoam (Upjohn, Kalamazoo, MI) is the temporary embolic agent of choice. Gelfoam is a surgical packing agent that provides contact hemostasis. Because it is absorbable, the occlusion process may result in recannulation after 3 weeks. This is advantageous in situations when short-term embolization is desired such as in traumatic or gastrointestinal hemorrhages. Gelfoam is supplied in different thickness wafers. The wafer can be cut into small pieces to match the caliber of the vessel to be embolized. The Gelfoam torpedo is loaded into the nozzle of a dilute contrast-filled syringe and carefully injected into the target vessel under fluoroscopic guidance (Fig. 11.1). Multiple tiny Gelfoam pledgets or a slurry preparation can be injected to occlude a vascular bed.

Permanent embolic agents include particles, liquids, and mechanical blocking agents. Polyvinyl alcohol (PVA) particles are used to embolize distally the arteriolar bed of a tumor, the small vessel bleeding of the bronchial artery, or the nidus of a vascular malformation. It is commercially available in different sizes, ranging from 150 to 1,000 μ in size. PVA is usually used in the 250 to 500 μ size particles for neoplasm embolization and 500 to 750 μ size for bronchial artery

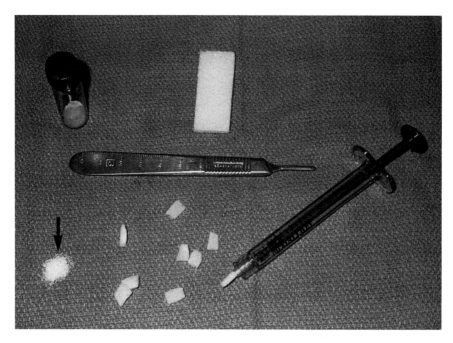

Figure 11.1 *Examples of Gelfoam torpedoes and PVA particles (arrow). The embolization torpedoes are cut from a 3 to 7 mm thickness block of Gelfoam to the necessary size. The Gelfoam pledget is loaded into a nozzle of a 1 ml syringe containing dilute contrast for injection.*

embolization. The particles are suspended in contrast and injected superselectively under fluoroscopic visualization. The particles tend to aggregate and form clumps, which can temporarily occlude microcatheters. The particles cause permanent occlusion by mechanical impaction in the vascular bed.

Alcohol, Sotradecol, 50% glucose, and boiling contrast solutions are examples of liquid embolic agents. Liquid sclerosants are useful in venous embolization since the slower flow rates allow better control of the delivery. Alcohol is a tissue-sclerosing agent that produces occlusion at all levels from the capillary bed to the main artery. Alcohol causes protein precipitation within the vascular bed with clot formation and subsequent infarction. Absolute alcohol is the agent of choice for embolizing peripheral congenital arteriovenous malformations (AVMs). It should be delivered as directly as possible into the nidus of the malformation. Both venous and percutaneous approaches may be used in addition to the traditional intra-arterial administration. Alcohol embolization can cause intoxication and in some instances can lead to transient pulmonary hypotension from pulmonary microembolus or the direct toxicity of alcohol on the pulmonary vasculature. Yates recommends monitoring pulmonary artery pressures during alcohol embolization of large vascular malformations.

Boiling contrast offers the advantage of visualization of the delivery of the agent. Occlusion occurs by heat-induced thrombosis. The poor thermal conductivity of catheter materials prevents heat loss and protects the transited vessels from undesired thrombosis. It has been used successfully in varicocele embolization but is less useful in vascular malformations because the high flow rate dissipates the heat before thrombosis occurs.

Mechanical blocking agents include steel coils, platinum microcoils, balloons, and silk thread. Gianturco coils (Cook Inc., Bloomington, IN) are steel coils with attached Dacron strands that cause permanent thrombosis. Gianturco coil embolization is equivalent to ligating an artery. The coils come in many sizes ranging from 3 to 15 mm in coil diameter and 0.025 to 0.038 inch in wire caliber (Fig. 11.2). Giant coils with larger diameters are available. The catheter is positioned selectively in the vessel to be occluded. The tube containing the coil of the desired diameter is placed in the hub of the catheter. The coil is advanced through the catheter with a straight

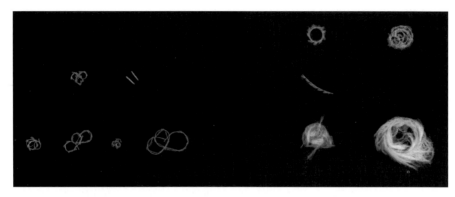

Figure 11.2 *On the left are examples of 0.018 inch platinum microcoils (Target Therapeutics, Fremont, CA). Note the attached Dacron fabric. The coils come in a wide variety of shapes ranging from straight to complex cloverleaf shapes. On the right are examples of Gianturco 0.038 inch coils and Helil 0.018 inch coils (Courtesy of Cook, Inc., Bloomington, IN).*

guidewire. The coil is carefully advanced from the distal end of the catheter under fluoroscopic control. The size of the coil is selected such that the coil can roll up within the vessel and wedge against the arterial wall, forming a solid base for thrombosis (Fig. 11.3). Coils must be placed both proximal and distal to an arterial lesion to prevent back bleeding when distal collateral flow is present. Neoplasms and AVMs are inadequately embolized by Gianturco coils because collateralization can readily occur. Gianturco coils are used to embolize arteriovenous fistulas, pulmonary AVMs, and in other situations when ligation of a large artery is desired.

Platinum microcoils were developed to embolize the lumen of aneurysms. These are 0.010 to 0.018 inch in diameter and come in a wide variety of shapes from straight to complex helical coils. Their advantage is precise delivery via microcatheters into small, peripheral aneurysms or arterial lesions. The Guglielmi detachable coil (GDC) (Target Therapeutics, Fremont, CA) is a soft platinum helical coil that is packed inside the lumen of an aneurysm and detached from the delivery wire by an electrical current. The GDC system is approved for inoperable intracranial aneurysms. Typically, five to six coils are necessary to fill the lumen of an aneurysm. Silk thread is used in a similar manner to platinum microcoils. Detachable balloons are not commercially available in the United States. Balloons have been used to treat pulmonary AVMs and occlude aneurysms. The advantage was that the embolic effect of the balloon could be tested before detachment. The disadvantage was balloon deflation with subsequent migration or recurrence.

Figure 11.3 *The diameter of the coil is chosen to correspond to the luminal size of the target vessel to embolize. On the top a 5 mm diameter coil has been placed in a 3 mm diameter vessel. This prevents the coil from assuming its configuration and leaves the coil in an unraveled state, which may protrude the end of the coil into an undesired position. In the middle, a 5 mm coil has been positioned correctly within a 5 mm diameter vessel. On the bottom, the 5 mm coil has been deployed in an 8 mm diameter vessel. The coil will embolize distally from the intended release position.*

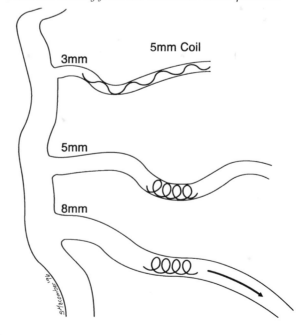

Trauma

Embolotherapy is useful in traumatic patients with pelvic hemorrhage, renal injuries, and extremity injuries. Laparotomy and evacuation of a pelvic hematoma can accelerate retroperitoneal hemorrhage and worsen shock in patients who have pelvic hematomas secondary to pelvic fractures. Surgical ligation of the internal iliac arteries is not recommended for control of pelvic hemorrhage. The proximal position of the ligature leaves all of the first order branches of this artery open to collateral flow from the large regional arteries.

Pelvic hemorrhage secondary to fractures is best treated with angiographic evaluation and embolization. The timing of pelvic fixation is best postponed to follow the embolization in unstable patients. A pelvic angiogram is used to localize the hemorrhage. Frequently the source of hemorrhage is not seen on angiography, and the side of the pelvis that has the most significant fracture is embolized. The internal iliac artery is selectively catheterized. Small Gelfoam pledgets are the preferred embolic agent. Approximately 5 to 10 of 2 to 4 mm pledgets are loaded into a 5 to 10 ml syringe filled with dilute contrast. These pledgets are injected into the proximal internal iliac artery. High flow preferentially carries the pledgets to the sources of internal hemorrhage. A single administration of pledgets is necessary in each internal iliac artery. If Gelfoam embolization does not control the hemorrhage, a Gianturco coil can be used.

Embolization for renal trauma is performed in an attempt to salvage renal function. The bleeding site is diagnosed by angiography. Superselective embolization is performed with platinum microcoils, silk thread, or Gianturco coils (Fig. 11.4). A Gelfoam pledget can be injected in an attempt to rely on the high flow rate carrying the pledget to the site of bleeding. Arterial venous fistula and pseudoaneurysms are best treated with coils.

Historically, arterial injuries were managed by ligation resulting in a high rate of limb amputation. Wartime experiences resulted in the development of techniques for arterial repair and reconstruction. Most extremity trauma is best treated by surgical repair to salvage the affected limb. The angiographic pattern is the chief determining factor for choice between surgery or embolotherapy. Embolotherapy is the treatment of choice for bleeding from small branch vessels or arteriovenous fistulas that can be catheterized. Surgical repair is warranted if the injury involves the domi-nant vessel to the extremity. Gelfoam is the preferred agent for embolization of trauma from small branch vessels. Coils are used for embolization of pseudoaneurysms or arteriovenous fistulas (Fig. 11.5).

Gastrointestinal Hemorrhage

Angiographic treatment of gastrointestinal hemorrhage has been superseded by endoscopic treatment, especially in upper gastrointestinal bleeding. Angiography still plays a limited role in diagnosis and treatment of lower gastrointestinal hemorrhage since the small bowel and blood-filled colon are difficult to examine endoscopically. The timing of the angiographic study is important because of the intermittent nature of gastrointestinal hemorrhage and the brisk rate of bleeding necessary to visualize the bleeding source. Provocative mesenteric angiography with intra-arterial vasodilatation, heparinization, or fibrinolytic administration may help localize the site of probable hemorrhage. We combine provocative mesenteric angiography with a tagged red blood cell nuclear study to optimize diagnosis of diffuse mucosal bleeding. Carbon dioxide angiography has been reported to have increased sensitivity in localizing the bleeding source.

Therapeutic options for gastrointestinal hemorrhage are vasopressin infusion and embolization. A vasopressin infusion can successfully control diffuse, mucosal bleeding such as angiodysplasia or gastritis but is labor intensive, and the bleeding can recur when the infusion is discontinued. Embolization is becoming favored, especially when a focal bleeding spot can be found and catheterized. Temporary embolization with Gelfoam can immediately control the hemorrhage and can be safely used for bleeding proximal to the ligament of Treitz. In lower gastrointestinal bleeding with a definable focus, a selective Gelfoam embolization proximal to the vasa recta can be performed. The patient is carefully monitored for ischemia.

Bronchial Artery Embolization

Bronchial artery embolization can successfully control hemoptysis. It is important to realize, however, that the treatment is palliative, and the underlying condition has not been treated. The likelihood of recurrence is

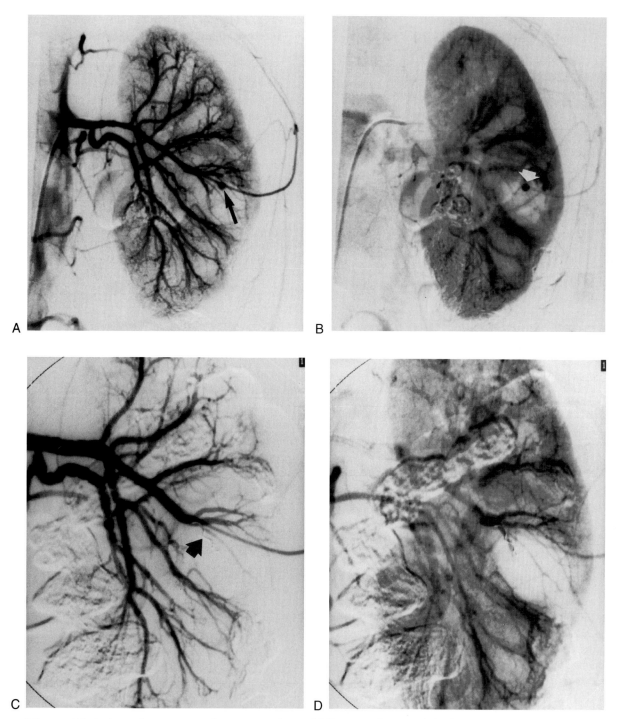

Figure 11.4 *A renal artery pseudoaneurysm formed following a biopsy. (**A**) The arteriogram demonstrated a small pseudoaneurysm in mid pole left kidney (arrow) (**B**) The pseudoaneurysm is confirmed by persistence of the contrast opacification into the venous phase (arrow). (**C**) A superselective coil embolization of the pseudoaneurysm was performed using a coaxial microcatheter system (arrow). (**D**) The capillary phase of the renal arteriogram demonstrates closure of the pseudoaneurysm and a small renal infarct. This was favored compared to the surgical option of total nephrectomy.*

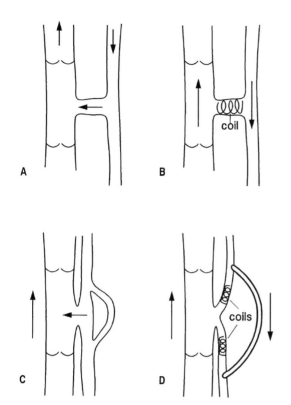

Figure 11.5 *Embolization of arteriovenous fistulas. (A) A tract exists between the feeding artery and draining vein. (B) A coil is placed within the arteriovenous fistula tract, successfully closing the fistula. The coil can be introduced from either an arterial or venous approach. A balloon occlusion catheter can temporarily block high flow through the shunt to assist in embolization. (C) Direct arterial to venous fistula with bridging collateral. (D) The fistula is bracketed by closing both the distal and proximal portions of the artery.*

high. Reported results are variable. The success rate is 80 to 90 percent in the immediate control of hemoptysis. The recurrence rate ranges from 20 to 40 percent. Bronchial artery embolization is indicated if the hemoptysis exceeds 300 ml/day or is considered life-threatening. The bleeding site is localized by bronchoscopy and confirms which vascular territory to embolize since there is a paucity of angiographic findings that definitively localize the bleeding. This is important because hemoptysis often occurs in patients with diffuse lung disease.

A good digital subtracted bronchial arteriogram is a must for diagnostic and therapeutic planning. The bronchial arteries arise from the intercostal arteries at the T3-T8 vertebral body level. Approximately 80 percent of all bronchial arteries arise at the T5-T6 level (Fig. 11.6). The intercostal and bronchial arteries are catheterized with a Cobra, Mikaelsson, or spinal catheter. Careful consideration of the arterial supply to the spinal cord must be given when the bronchial arteriogram and subsequent embolization are contemplated. The anterior spinal artery is formed from vertebral artery branches and is supplied at multiple levels by radicular branches of extraspinal arteries. A radicular branch can rarely arise from a right intercostobronchial trunk and is recognized by a characteristic hairpin loop configuration. Bronchial artery hemorrhage is rarely seen as contrast extravasation. The bronchial arteries responsible for hemorrhage are enlarged and tortuous (Fig. 11.7). There is hypervascularity and possibly systemic to pulmonary shunting present. Occasionally, small aneurysms are seen. If normal bronchial arteries are found, further angiographic search for the source of

Figure 11.6 *Bronchial artery branching variations. Most bronchial arteries arise between the T5 and T6 vertebral bodies. There may be a common bronchial trunk that gives rise to both the right and left bronchial arteries (not shown). The right intercostal bronchial trunk is more often the origin of the anterior spinal artery, which is recognized by its characteristic hairpin turn.*

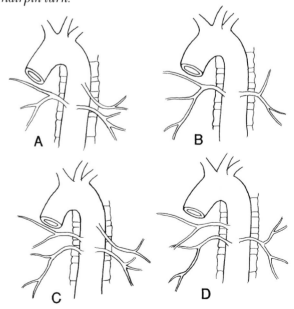

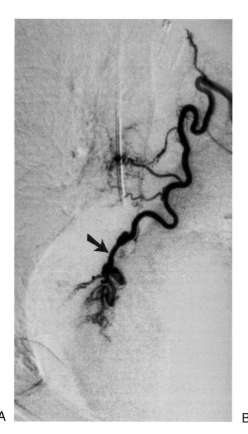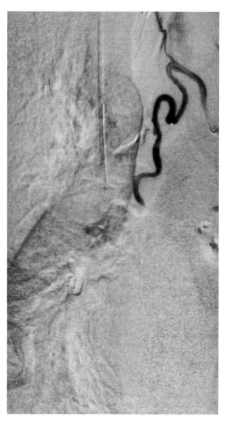

A   B

Figure 11.7 *(A) Pre-embolization right bronchial arteriogram. The vessel is tortuous and hypertrophied in size (arrow). Note the absence of contrast extravasation. (B) Postembolization arteriogram. The bronchial artery has been peripherally embolized with PVA particles. This resulted in cessation of the patient's hemoptysis. The bronchial artery trunk was preserved for potential future embolization if a recurrence occurred.*

hemoptysis is performed. Branches of the subclavian, axillary, internal mammary, and intercostal vessels occasionally supply abnormal lung parenchyma (Fig. 11.8).

It is important to embolize the distal branches of the diseased vessel and preserve the proximal trunk of the vessel. We commonly use coaxial 3 French microcatheters to achieve superselective catheter positioning for embolization. This practice preserves access to the area of bleeding if a second intervention is required and reduces the potential for spinal cord injury. The embolic agent of choice is 500 to 750 μ PVA particles or tiny pledgets of Gelfoam. PVA particles provide a permanent occlusion of the small vessels responsible for the bleeding while preserving the main vascular access into the abnormal lung.

Parathyroid Adenomas

The great majority of patients with hyperparathyroidism can have the parathyroid adenoma localized with ultrasound and removed surgically. Venous sampling and angiography are reserved for those patients who have had a previous neck exploration and have inconclusive imaging tests. The venous sampling technique is tedious and usually performed only in specialized centers. The goal of venous sampling is localization between the neck or mediastinum and the right or the left side. This helps guide angiography and transcatheter ablation. The subclavian artery is injected to identify the lesion and the arterial supply. Parathyroid

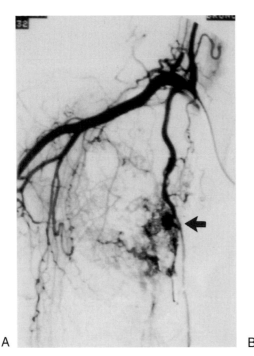 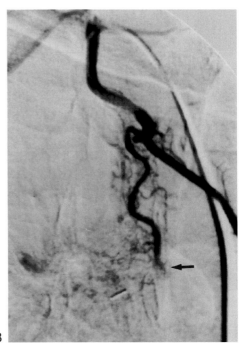

Figure 11.8 *Right internal mammary artery supplying collateral flow to the bronchial system. This resulted in hemoptysis several months following bronchial artery embolization. (A) Subclavian arteriogram showing staining and hypertrophied internal mammary arterial supply to right lung (arrow). (B) The right internal mammary collateral supply to the lung was embolized with PVA particles (arrow). This stopped the patient's hemoptysis.*

adenomas are hypervascular lesions that densely and persistently blush. Arterial supply is commonly from the inferior thyroid or internal mammary arteries. Treatment is by superselective embolization with 40 to 60 ml of contrast directly into the arterial supply to the adenoma followed by Gelfoam or coil occlusion of the main arterial supply. Alternatively, ultrasound can be used to inject alcohol directly into identifiable lesions.

Treatment of Vascular Anomalies

An understanding of the anatomy and pathophysiology of congenital vascular malformations has advanced remarkably in the last 5 years. A giant step in progress was made by Mulliken and Young who revolutionized the classification of vascular birthmarks. They advocated dividing vascular abnormalities into two distinct types: hemangiomas and malformations. Hemangiomas are benign vascular tumors. They have a predictable proliferative stage in patients between 2 weeks and 18 months of age and an equally predictable involutionary stage between 2 and 6 years. The majority of hemangiomas require no treatment because they are self-limited processes. A few hemangiomas do require treatment because of their anatomic location or their pathologic activity (platelet trapping, bleeding). The Kasabach-Merrit syndrome is bleeding induced by hemangiomas that trap platelets. This occurs during the tumor growth stage of the hemangioma and disappears when the hemangioma involutes.

An AVM has congenitally abnormal connections between arteries and veins devoid of the usual arteriolar resistance vessels or capillary beds. Vascular malformations are present at birth and grow with the patient. These often expand during adolescence, pregnancy, or after trauma. The concept of a vascular nidus is important in understanding these lesions. The nidus is the central confluence of the malformation where the shunting of arterial blood to vein occurs. The nidus can be large and spread out or may be multiple (Fig. 11.9). Obliteration of the nidus will cure the malformation. Unfortunately, this is not always possible when the nidus is large or multiple. AVMs cannot be cured by proximally blocking the arteries by embolization, surgery, or other means that supply the nidus. The stimulation to form collaterals is always available and extremely powerful. In fact, incomplete embolization or surgical ligation of the supplying arteries makes the treatment more difficult, if not impossible (Fig. 11.10).

AVM symptoms are pain, overgrowth, ischemia (steal phenomena and venous hypertension), hemorrhage, and heart failure. AVMs involving the extremities may cause leg length discrepancy, congestive heart failure, and ischemia. A multidisciplinary team of specialists is the best approach to treating these complex cases. As with any therapy, the goal is to alleviate the symptoms such as controlling the patient's pain or heart failure. Most AVMs can be managed but not always cured by embolization and sclerosis with alcohol. The treatment of AVM is staged. Large volumes of contrast are injected to completely opacify and map out the AVM. A careful search and identification of the nidus of the AVM are the goals of the diagnostic arteriogram. Magnetic resonance imaging (MRI) is a useful tool to map out vascular malformations.

The therapy is planned once the nidus or multiple nidi are identified. Therapeutic embolization options include transcatheter or percutaneous injection of alco-

Figure 11.9 *AVM of the left foot.* **(A)** *The nidus is where there is direct artery-to-venous communication (arrow). The multiplicity of lesions illustrates the difficulty in treating AVMs.* **(B)** *MRI of same patient demonstrating the hypertrophy of the left leg compared to the right. MRI demonstrates the large draining veins from the multiple AVM niduses.*

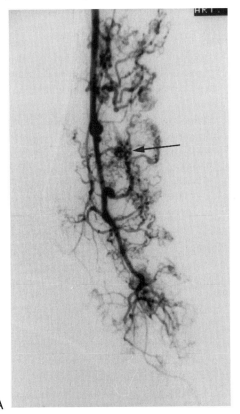

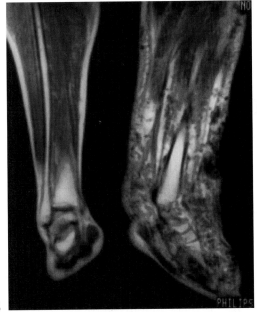

A B

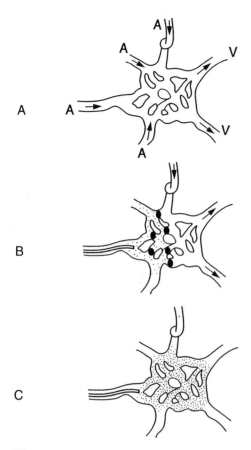

Figure 11.10 *AVM. **(A)** The direct communication between the arteries and veins is called the nidus. The nidus of ligated AVMs recruits collaterals, which are difficult to access and embolize. **(B)** Particulate embolization can deliver embolic agent into the majority of the nidus. In this situation, 90 percent of the nidus was obliterated by particles. One collateral is present, which can hypertrophy and resupply the nidus with time. **(C)** Liquid embolization is effective at treating the entire nidus. Liquid is distributed throughout the nidus resulting in total thrombosis. The drawback is the higher risk of nerve or skin damage.*

hol directly into the nidus. General anesthesia with pulmonary artery pressure measurements is recommended when using alcohol embolization. Alcohol is a potent agent and can cause skin necrosis and nerve damage. Careful injection under controlled circumstances are necessary to prevent side effects. The nidus must be directly injected and the flow pattern studied. The flow rate through the malformation with and without outflow

obstruction is estimated. Flow can be partially controlled by tourniquets or blood pressure cuffs. Stagnant flow prolongs the alcohol dwell time in the nidus. Multiple contrast injections are performed to determine the volume of alcohol necessary to just saturate the nidus.

Pulmonary AVMs occur in patients who have Rendu-Osler-Webber syndrome or hereditary hemorrhagic telangiectasia. These patients have right-to-left shunting, resulting in hypoxia and paradoxical embolization. They also have orthodeoxia, hypoxia exaggerated in the sitting or standing position, because the malformations are preferentially located in the lower lobes. This phenomenon, along with chest radiographs, is used to screen family members. There is a high incidence of cerebral vascular accidents and brain abscess, which has been underappreciated in the past. This justifies closure of the shunts with embolotherapy. Contrast enhanced spiral computed tomography (CT) is used to map the number of shunts and the angioarchitecture of the malformations. Simple malformations have an aneurysm fed by a single artery and drained by a single vein. Complex malformations have multiple feeding and draining vessels or septated aneurysms. Pulmonary AVMs are best treated by transcatheter embolization with coils or balloons in the distal feeding artery or within the aneurysm. It is recommended to treat all malformations with feeding arteries greater than 3 mm in caliber to prevent paradoxical embolization. Patients and their families are screened for recurrence or appearance of new malformations.

Venous malformations are low-flow vascular malformations. They are a collection of abnormal venous channels characterized by deficient smooth muscle. The Klippel-Trenaunay syndrome consists of port wine stains, limb hypertrophy, and venous malformations. The deep venous system is often absent. Arteriography will demonstrate normal arteries and the venous malformation will not be opacified (Fig. 11.11). The Parkes-Weber variant of Klippel-Trenaunay syndrome includes arterial malformations. The true size of a venous malformation is best demonstrated by T2-weighted MRI or by direct intralesional contrast venography. Treatment is conservative since the venous hemangioma will often regress in size with time. Embolotherapy is used when hemorrhage, severe deformity, intractable pain, heart failure, or the Kasabach-Merritt syndrome complicate the situation. Venous malformations do not respond to arterial embolization. The most effective management is direct intralesional injection of alcohol using fluoroscopic or ultrasound guidance. Tourniquets are used to slow the outflow from these lesions.

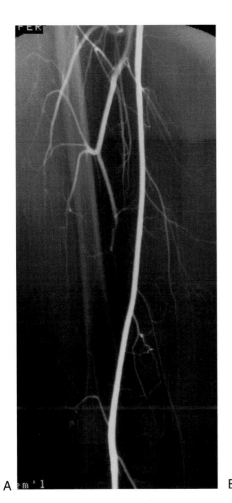

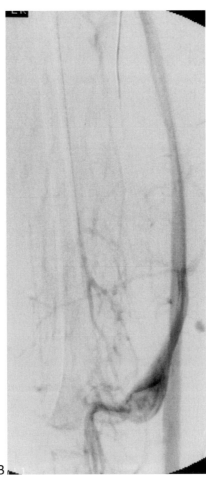

Figure 11.11 *Klippel-Trenaunay syndrome. The syndrome consists of varicose veins, hypertrophy of the limb, and port wine hemangioma.* **(A)** *Right femoral arteriogram showing normal arteries.* **(B)** *Venous phase showing aplasia of superficial femoral and popliteal veins. Venous drainage is through incompetent perforating veins feeding a hypertrophied saphenous vein. (Figure continues.)*

Varicocele Embolization

One of the primary causes of infertility in male patients is oligospermia and spermatic motility dysfunction related to the presence of a varicocele. A varicocele is pathologic dilatation of the pampiniform venous plexus caused by an incompetent valve in the internal spermatic vein. Approximately 15 percent of males develop varicoceles during puberty. It is most common on the left (about 90 percent), with only 8 percent being bilateral. About 30 to 40 percent of patients with varicoceles have reduced spermatogenesis. The surgical or embolic treatment of varicocele improves semen quality in many cases. There is a 10 percent recurrence rate in treated varicoceles due to recruitment of collateral channels. The diagnosis of a varicocele is performed using a color duplex evaluation. The examination is performed in both supine and upright positions; the patient performs a Valsalva maneuver to demonstrate the significance of the varicocele.

The technique for varicocele embolization is to catheterize the left spermatic vein with a Hopkins-type catheter from the contralateral femoral vein via a 9 French vascular sheath (Fig. 11.12). When necessary, the right spermatic vein is catheterized with a Simmons 2 catheter. Once the spermatic vein has been catheterized, a venogram is performed. Care is taken during the examination not to irradiate the testes. The venogram is used to map out the extent of collateralization and duplication of the spermatic venous system. Because of the numerous collaterals, it is advisable to place coils at several levels to completely occlude the spermatic vein (Fig. 11.13). Usually 3 to 5 mm coils are

Figure 11.11 *(Continued) (**C**) Right infrapopliteal arteriogram showing normal arteries. (**D**) Venous phase arteriogram showing hypoplasia of the deep venous system. Drainage is via the saphenous vein and superficial varicosities.*

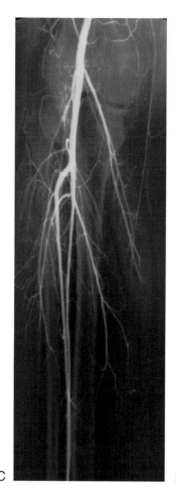

C

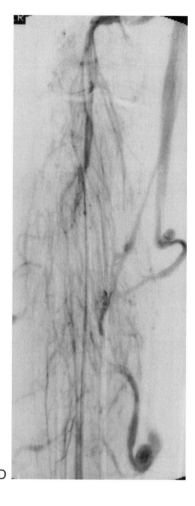

D

used. Using the 8 French Hopkins catheter as a guiding catheter, a smaller 5 French catheter or a Cragg guidewire is passed into the spermatic vein. Using this coaxial system the coils are placed first distal and then proximal within the spermatic vein. Liquid embolic agents including boiling contrast or alcohol are used when many small collaterals are present. Approximately 5 to 10 ml of boiling contrast is injected into the spermatic vein while pressure is held over the patient's groin to prevent reflux into the testicular venous plexus. A completion venogram is performed to demonstrate adequacy of the embolization.

Approximately 80 percent of patients develop an improvement in sperm count and motility. The pregnancy rate after treatment is as high as 50 percent. Side effects occur in approximately 10 percent of cases. The most common side effect is vasovagal response, pain during sclerotherapy, scrotal edema, and chemical epididymitis. Boiling contrast sclerotherapy can cause a transient paresthesia along the inner aspect of the thigh.

Pelvic Congestion Syndrome

Chronic pelvic pain is a frustrating problem that causes significant functional and psychological impairments in patients. The syndrome is defined by pelvic pain present for at least 6 months. The symptom complex has multiple etiologies, including endometriosis, infections, and ovarian vein varices. The pelvic congestion syndrome is defined by the following criteria: an ovarian vein diameter of 10 mm or greater, uterine venous engorgement,

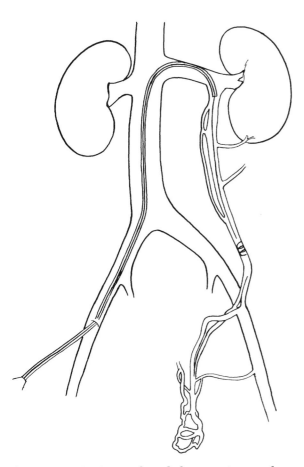

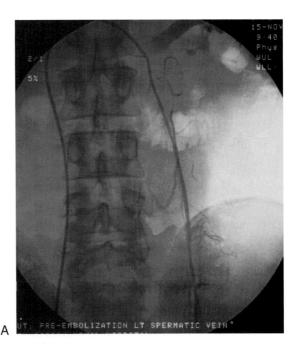

Figure 11.12 *Varicocele embolization. A curved Hopkin's catheter is used to select the origin of the left internal spermatic vein. A catheter is inserted coaxially through the Hopkin's guiding catheter into the mid to distal left spermatic vein. Coils or liquid embolic agent can be used to close the varicocele.*

congestion of the ovarian plexus, and filling of veins across the midline. Both mechanical and hormonal factors are responsible for the pain. The symptom complex can be decreased in a significant percentage of patients by interrupting the ovarian vein. The patient is initially evaluated to exclude the other causes of pelvic pain syndrome. The embolization technique is similar to male varicocele embolization. An ovarian venogram is performed to document the varices and choose the coil size. The varices are embolized using stainless steel coils. Other interventional techniques used to treat chronic pelvic pain are superior hypogastric nerve blockade and pelvic cyst drainage.

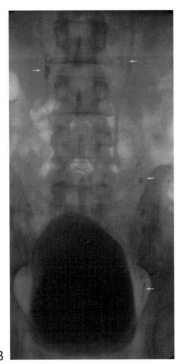

Figure 11.13 *(**A**) Left spermatic venogram through Hopkin's guiding catheter. Note the numerous collaterals and small accessory venous channels. (**B**) Bilateral coil embolization of both internal spermatic veins for treatment of symptomatic bilateral varicoceles (small white arrows).*

Obstetric Embolotherapy

Most bleeding related to normal deliveries and cesarean sections can be controlled with the usual surgical methods or the administration of oxytocin. When these methods fail, emergency embolotherapy can be life saving. Embolotherapy offers the advantage of sparing the patient's uterus for future pregnancies. Prophylactic arterial catheterization is a new approach in the management of threatened intraoperative obstetric hemorrhage. Many of these patients have abnormal placental implantations or ectopic pregnancies. This novel approach has been used successfully. The typical obstetrical embolotherapy is in a patient who has postpartum hemorrhage. This is often associated with an underlying coagulation abnormality. It is best treated by Gelfoam embolization of the uterine arteries. Several authors have reported that embolotherapy has been successful following failure to control the hemorrhage after hysterectomy. The postpartum uterine arteries are easy to catheterize selectively. Both arteries are occluded proximally with Gelfoam 2 to 4 mm size torpedoes (Fig. 11.14).

Hepatic Artery Chemoembolization

Chemoembolization combines hepatic artery embolization with simultaneous infusion of a concentrated dose of chemotherapy drugs. Malignant tumors in the liver predominantly derive their blood supply from the hepatic artery. Embolization renders the tumor cells ischemic. The blood flow arrest increases the chemotherapy drug dwell time. Tumor drug concentrations are 10 to 25 times higher than those achieved by infusion alone. Measurable levels can persist up to 1 month. Systemic drug toxicity is minimal even at high doses.

Chemoembolization is an investigational procedure requiring the approval of the institutional review board (IRB). Chemoembolization is a palliative treatment reserved for patients with liver predominant metastatic disease who are not candidates for hepatic resection. Chemoembolization is not the primary treatment for hepatic metastases, but is reserved for those patients who have had progression of tumor growth despite treatment with systemic chemotherapy. Selection criteria centers on determination of an adequate liver reserve. The bilirubin should not be elevated greater than 2 mg/dl. A recent CT scan should demonstrate that the portal vein is patent and not more than 75 percent of the liver's parenchyma is replaced by tumor.

Diagnostic arteriography always precedes chemoembolization. The initial study defines the vascular anatomy of the liver. This is done to map out any variation in the hepatic arterial supply. Portal vein patency should be reconfirmed. The chemoembolic preparation consists of cross-link collagen particles 60 to 80 μ in diameter (Regional Therapeutics, Pacific Palisades, CA). Three chemotherapeutic agents are used: doxorubicin, mitomycin, and cisplatin. Contrast medium is added to provide radio-opacity. The arterial bed is anesthetized with intra-arterial administration of 100 mg of lidocaine before injecting the chemoembolic agent. This helps lessen the embolism-provoked pain. The patient should be deeply sedated with intravenous fentanyl and midazolam (Versed). Embolization is carried out by slowly injecting the chemoembolic mixture via a Tracker catheter, which has been selectively placed within the proper hepatic artery (Fig. 11.15). The embolization is carried out until flow arrest in the target vessel occurs or the typical volume of 6 to 9 ml is administered (Fig. 11.16). Careful attention and fluoroscopic monitoring are used to ensure that inadvertent reflux of embolic material into adjacent normal vascular beds does not occur.

Treatment of the liver is generally performed in three stages at 4- to 6-week intervals. Response is monitored by liver CT scans and serum tumor markers. A CT scan is generally obtained 2 to 4 weeks after the final embolization. The hepatic metastases generally do not decrease in size but develop central low attenuation on CT scanning indicative of necrosis (Fig. 11.17).

Virtually every patient has some degree of postembolization syndrome. It usually lasts for up to 3 days and consists of right upper quadrant and shoulder pain, fever, nausea, and vomiting. Prophylactic antibiotics, narcotic analgesics, and antiemetics are given intravenously for the first 24 to 48 hours to lessen the postembolic syndrome side effects. Transient thrombocytopenia and liver dysfunction can occur as a side effect. These side effects are monitored by daily blood counts and liver function tests. Significant complications are rare and include hepatic abscess formation and fulminant hepatic failure.

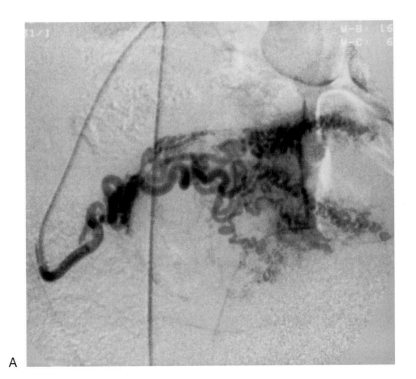

A

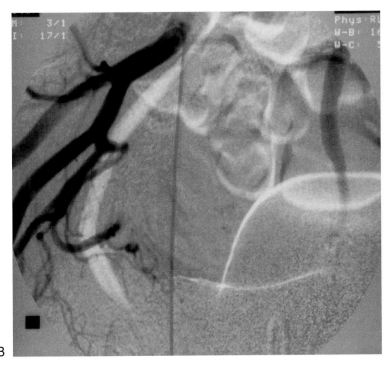

B

Figure 11.14 *Intractable post-partum hemorrhage. **(A)** Selective right uterine arteriogram. Note the enlarged hypertrophied uterine artery typical of postpartum condition. No contrast extravasation is evident. **(B)** Right internal iliac arteriogram performed following Gelfoam embolization of the right uterine artery. The left uterine artery was also embolized.*

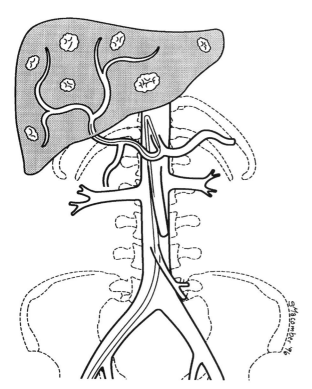

Figure 11.15 *Hepatic artery chemoembolization. Nieman visceral catheter is placed in origin of celiac access. A 3 French microcatheter is placed into the distal proper hepatic artery. The right and left hepatic arteries are infused with chemoembolic agent.*

A review of the first 75 patients treated at Northwestern showed objective response to therapy in 50 percent of patients. This was evidenced by reduction of serum tumor markers and CT evidence of tumor necrosis/shrinkage. Best responses were seen in the hypervascular neuroendocrine tumors (islet cell and carcinoid tumors). Control of symptoms is the primary objective of therapy since the life span of these patients is long regardless of treatment. The published results are disparate on the treatment of colorectal metastases and hepatomas. Lipoidal embolization has been used extensively in Japan for treatment of oriental hepatoma (Fig. 11.18). Ocular melanoma metastasis to the liver has a response rate of 46 percent, which is 10 times better than the response rate to systemic chemotherapy.

Percutaneous Tumor Injection Therapy

Percutaneous ethanol injection therapy is mainly performed in patients with hepatocellular carcinoma. It is used for small tumors ranging from 3 to 5 cm in diameter. Tumors that have satellite lesions can be injected provided there are less than three to five small satellites. Contraindications for therapy include uncontrollable ascites or marked bleeding tendency.

The tumor is evaluated by preliminary CT and ultrasonographic scans. The general guideline for total volume of injected ethanol to destroy the lesion is expressed by the equation: Volume = $4/3\ \pi(r + 0.5)^3$. The .5 cm added to the radius is a safety margin. For example, a 2 cm in diameter lesion requires 14 ml of ethanol and a 3 cm lesion requires 32 ml. In most cases, 2 to 8 ml of absolute ethanol is injected into several sites in and around the lesion in one treatment session. Multiple treatment sessions are planned to reach the intended total volume. The injections are usually performed twice per week. In large lesions, ethanol should be injected into the edges of the lesion again several months after the first treatment.

The technique involves ultrasound or CT scan guidance. We prefer the real-time imaging guidance of ultrasound but choice of imaging guidance is modified by lesion location and operator preference. The patient is given intravenous conscious sedation and local infiltrative anesthesia. A 21-gauge needle is placed into the lesion. The Bernadino needle has multiple sideholes, which evenly disperse the alcohol without having to move the needle. The absolute ethanol is injected under ultrasonographic observation and can be seen as a brightly echogenic linear focus (Fig. 11.19). The needle is left in place for several minutes to allow the tract time to close and prevent reflux of ethanol into the peritoneal cavity. In larger lesions, several needles are placed into different sites within the lesion, after which ethanol is injected.

Follow-up imaging studies are used to evaluate response to treatment. The treated tumor becomes necrotic, and the enhancement of the tumor diminishes. Serum tumor markers such as alpha-fetoprotein and carcinoembryonic antigen are used to evaluate the response to treatment. The long-term survival rates with ethanol injection compare favorably to surgery in patients with hepatocellular carcinoma. The advantage

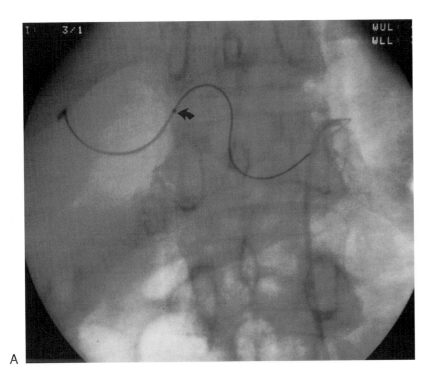

A

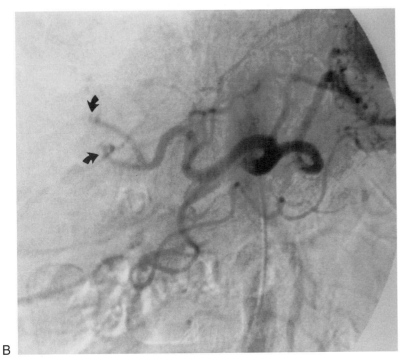

B

Figure 11.16 (A) *A 3 French microcatheter is selectively placed within the proper hepatic artery through a guiding catheter in the celiac trunk. The radio-opaque marker delineates the tip of the catheter (arrow).* (B) *Celiac arteriogram following chemoembolization. The anterior and posterior branches of the right hepatic artery are truncated in appearance from the chemoembolization (arrows).*

Figure 11.17 **(A)** *Pretreatment CT of liver showing numerous hepatic metastases from colon carcinoma.* **(B)** *Liver CT scan following three courses of chemoembolization with triple chemotherapy drugs. The hepatic metastases have changed from solid to cystic lesions.*

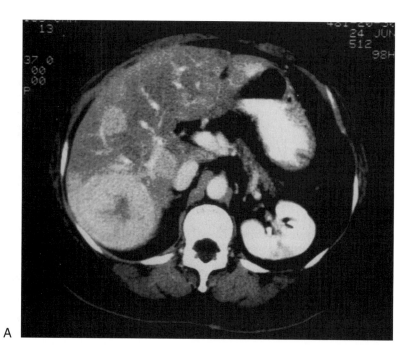

A

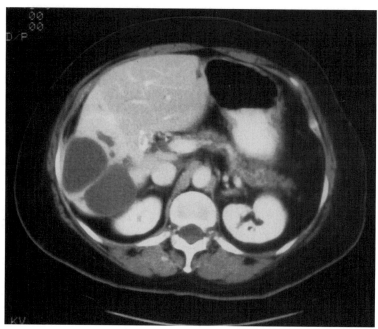

B

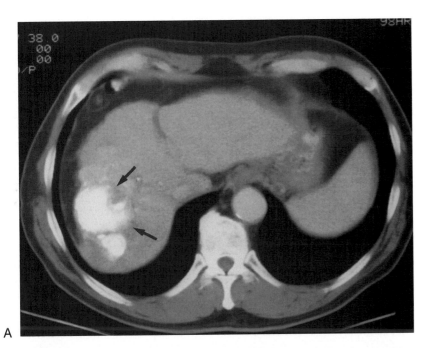

A

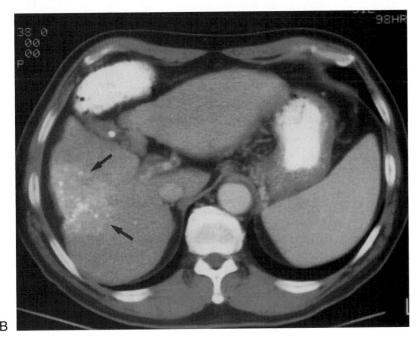

B

Figure 11.18 CT of liver following lipodiol embolization of a hepatoma. (**A**) The lipodiol densely accumulates within the hepatoma in the right lobe of the liver. The liver is cirrhotic with a nodular surface (arrows). (**B**) The lipodiol embolization agent is scattered along the margins of the hepatoma lesion (arrows).

Figure 11.19 *Ultrasound-guided alcohol hepatoma injection. Intraoperative ultrasound demonstrated nonresectability of the hepatocellular carcinoma. Ultrasound guidance was used to place multiple needles into the quadrants of the lesion and instill alcohol. (A) A 20-gauge needle has been placed into the lesion under ultrasound guidance. The white arrows outline the tumor margin. (B) Alcohol is injected as the needle is withdrawn. Injected alcohol is echogenic and readily visualized under ultrasound guidance (arrows).*

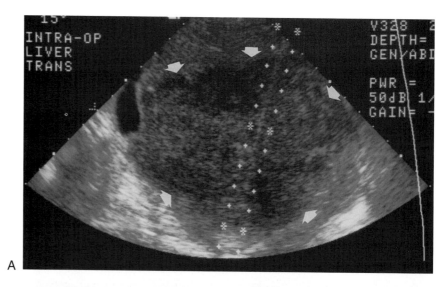

A

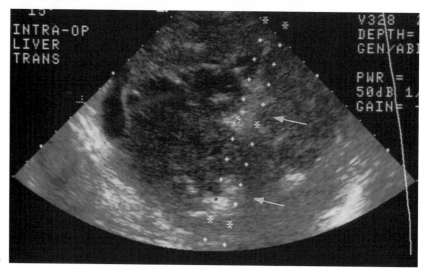

B

is that nonsurgical candidates can be offered a treatment modality paralleling the result of surgical outcomes. The 1-year survival rate is 82 percent, the 3-year survival rate is 50 percent, and the 5-year survival rate is 31 percent.

The complications are transient pain, fever, and alcohol intoxication. Most do not require special treatment. Pain can be reduced a great deal by leaving the needle in place for several minutes after injection, which prevents reflux. There can be mild changes in the liver function as seen by assay of liver function tests.

Suggested Readings

Ben-Menachem Y, Coldwell DM, Young JWR, Burges AR: Hemorrhage associated with pelvic fractures: causes, diagnosis, and emergent management. AJR 157:1005, 1991

Cauldwell EN, Siekert RG, Lininger RE et al: The bronchial arteries: an anatomic study of 150 human cadavers. Surg Gynecol Obstet 86:395, 1948

Charnsangave JC: Chemoembolization of liver tumors. Semin Invest Radiol 10:150, 1993

Coldwell DM, Stokes KR, Yakes WF: Embolotherapy: agents, clinical applications, and techniques. Radiographics 14:623, 1994

Greenwood LH, Glickman MG, Schartz PE et al: Obstetric and nonmalignant gynecologic bleeding: treatment with angiographic embolization. Radiology 164:155, 1987

Groupe D'Etude de Traitment du Carcinome Hepatocellulaire: Comparison of lipoidal chemoembolization and conservative treatment for unresectable hepatocellular carcinoma. N Engl J Med 332:1256, 1995

Guy GE, Shetty PC, Sharma RP et al: Acute lower gastrointestinal hemorrhage: treatment by superselective embolization with polyvinyl alcohol particles. AJR 159:521, 1992

Hunter DW, King NJ, Aeppli DW et al: Spermatic vein occlusion with hot contrast material: angiographic results. J Vasc Interv Radiol 2:507, 1991

Livraghi T, Bolondi L, Lazzaroni S: Percutaneous ethanol injection in the treatment of hepatocellular carcinoma in cirrhosis: a study on 207 patients. Cancer 69:925, 1992

Lukanic SP, Nemcek AA Jr, Vogelzang RL: Posttraumatic intrahepatic arterial pseudoaneurysm: treatment with direct percutaneous puncture. J Vasc Interv Radiol 2:335, 1991

Machan LS: Gynecologic interventional radiology. J Vasc Interv Radiol (suppl) 7:S273, 1996

Mitty HA, Sterling KM, Alverez M, Gendler R: Obstetric hemorrhage: prophylactic and emergency arterial catheterization and embolotherapy. Radiology 188:183, 1993

Molgaard C, Teitelbaum G, Pentecost M et al: Intraarterial administration of lidocaine for analgesia in hepatic chemoembolization. J Vasc Interv Radiol 1:81, 1990

Mulliken JB, Glowacki J: Hemangiomas and vascular malformations in infants and children: a classification based on endothelial characteristics. Plast Reconstr Surg 69:412, 1982

Mulliken JB, Young AE: Vascular Birthmarks: Hemangiomas and Malformations. WB Saunders, Philadelphia, 1988

Okazaki M, Furui S, Higashihara H et al: Emergent embolotherapy of small intestine hemorrhage. Gastrointest Radiol 17:223, 1992

Remy J, Remy-Jardin M, Wattine L, Deffontaines C: Pulmonary arteriovenous malformation: evaluation with CT of the chest before and after treatment. Radiology 182:809, 1992

Sacks BA, Pallotta J: Diagnosis and ablation of parathyroid adenomas. p. 51. In Cope C (ed): Current Techniques in Interventional Radiology. Current Medicine, Philadelphia, 1995

Shiina S, Niwa Y: Percutaneous ethanol injection therapy in the treatment of liver neoplasms. p. 3.1. In Cope C (ed): Current Techniques in Interventional Radiology. Current Medicine, Philadelphia, 1994

Sichlau MJ, Yao JST, Vogelzang RL: Transcatheter embolotherapy for the treatment of pelvic congestion syndrome. Obstet Gynecol 83:892, 1994

Soulen MC: Regional therapy of hepatic malignancies. J Vasc Interv Radiol Suppl 7:S321, 1996

Stokes KR, Stuart K, Clouse ME: Hepatic artery chemoembolization for metastatic endocrine tumors. J Vasc Interv Radiol 4:341, 1993

Uflacker R: Embolization procedures: techniques and materials. p. 17. In Uflacker R, Wholey MH: Interventional Radiology. McGraw-Hill, New York, 1991

Vogelzang RL, Nemcek AA Jr, Lyster M, Braun MA: Hepatic artery chemoembolization for treatment of hepatic malignancy: results with microfibrillar collagen and triple drug therapy. J Vasc Interv Radiol 4:61, 1993

White RI, Lynch-Nyhan A, Terry P et al: Pulmonary arteriovenous malformations: techniques and long-term outcome of embolotherapy. Radiology 169:663, 1988

Yakes WF, Haas DK, Parker SH et al: Symptomatic vascular malformations: ethanol embolotherapy. Radiology 170:1059, 1989

Yakes WF, Luethke JM, Parker SH et al: Ethanol embolization of vascular malformations. Radiographics 10:787, 1990

Young AT, Tadavarthy SM, Yedlicka JW et al: Vascular embolotherapy. p. 18. In Castaneda-Zuniga WR, Tadavarthy SM (ed): Interventional Radiology. Vol. 2. 2nd Ed. Williams & Wilkins, Baltimore, 1992

Zuckerman AM, Mitchell SE, Venbrux AC et al: Percutaneous varicocele occlusion: long-term follow up. J Vasc Interv Radiol 5:315, 1994

Interventional Venous Procedures

The scope of venous procedures has increased dramatically in the last few years. The radiologist's role has evolved from diagnostician to active participant in the therapy of venous disease. This has been made possible by creative interventionists who have applied new venous access devices, stents, and imaging guidance to solve both routine and difficult clinical problems. The most rapidly advancing areas in interventional radiology are transjugular intrahepatic portosystemic shunt, venous access, and venous thrombolysis. This section introduces these new techniques and reviews the established techniques of inferior vena cava filters, foreign body retrieval, and management of hemodialysis access.

CHAPTER 12

Venous Access MICHAEL A. BRAUN

General Principles

Venous access for delivery of fluids, blood products, and medications distinguishes modern medical care. Many medical therapies depend on reliable long-term venous access. The numbers of patients requiring venous access and the devices available for venous access continue to grow. In recent years, the role of the radiologist has evolved with regard to the care of patients requiring venous access. The initial radiologic role was treatment of the mechanical and thrombotic complications of central venous catheters. The radiologist's role in placing venous access devices has grown by using routine angiographic techniques to obtain venous access in problematic situations or by being the first to offer placement of new venous access devices. Ultrasonography and fluoroscopy provide real-time, image-guided venous access, which speeds the completion and reduces the technical complications of the procedure.

A wide variety of venous access devices are available. A provider of venous access must be familiar with the devices, applications of the devices, techniques of placement, care of devices, and management of complications. Devices are commonly requested by their proprietary names. One must be able to choose the device type, size, and lumen configuration suitable for the given clinical application.

The choice of venous access device is based on the indication, duration, and frequency of use. The indications are chemotherapy, parenteral nutrition, antibiotic therapy, transfusion, plasmapheresis, hemodialysis, patient control analgesia, hydration, and intravenous medication delivery. Continuous daily infusions of medications and fluids are best performed through an external catheter. Single lumen catheters are preferred over multiple lumen catheters whenever possible. Multiple lumen catheters require additional flushes, may have smaller lumens, and have higher infection rates compared to single lumen catheters. They are reserved for situations requiring simultaneous infusion of incompatible medications or the need for simultaneous delivery of blood products and medications. An implantable port is used when the need for access is anticipated to last longer than several months and the access is used on an intermittent basis.

Catheters may be constructed of silicon rubber or polyurethane. Silicon rubber is the most biocompatible material available. Its elasticity and flexibility make it suitable for long-term venous implantation. The same properties make these catheters difficult to push over guidewires during insertion. Polyurethane has greater tensile strength than silicon. Polyurethane catheters are stiffer than silicon and have larger internal lumens for the same outer diameter. The polyurethane material softens when intravascular and is widely used in acute care catheters. External catheters may be valved or nonvalved. The Groshong catheter has a slit valve, which acts like a vocal cord (Fig. 12.1). In the resting state, the slits are closed. Aspiration and infusion bend the cords open. Groshong valve catheters are flushed weekly with normal saline, whereas open catheters are flushed daily with heparinized saline. A Groshong valved catheter is the catheter of choice in heparin-allergic patients or patients unable to perform daily flushes. The Groshong catheter valve has a higher frequency of catheter malfunction compared to nonvalved catheters. The external tap on Groshong catheters is attached following implantation. The hub is held in place by friction and can become detached with use. Groshong catheters must be placed through peel-away sheaths and cannot be placed over a guidewire because of the valve. This is the disadvantage of Groshong catheters. Some external catheters have Dacron cuffs, which are implanted underneath the skin but outside the vein. The cuff provides an interstice for connective

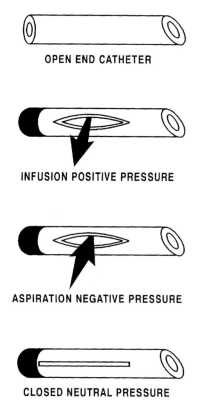

OPEN END CATHETER

INFUSION POSITIVE PRESSURE

ASPIRATION NEGATIVE PRESSURE

CLOSED NEUTRAL PRESSURE

Figure 12.1 *The Groshong valve has a three-way vocal cord type valve. The top figure is an illustration of an end hole catheter. The Groshong valve has an occluded end hole with a longitudinal slit near the distal end. The positive pressure of infusion and negative pressure of aspiration opens the valve. In the resting state, the valve is closed.*

tissue to grow into stabilizing the catheter mechanically and providing a barrier to infection. The Vita Cuff contains silver ions that slowly leach out of the cuff, providing a temporary chemical barrier to infection.

External catheters have traditionally been placed in the surgical suite using tunneled silicone rubber catheters. The tunnel is thought to provide mechanical stability and a barrier to infection. Single lumen tunneled catheters are used in patients requiring long-term total parenteral nutrition (TPN). Double lumen catheters are used for patients on short-term TPN and concomitant medications. Patients with hematopoietic malignancies or bone marrow transplants usually require multilumen devices because of the frequent necessity for simultaneous administration of multiple medications and blood products. A recent study demonstrated no difference in infection rates between tunneled and nontunneled catheters in 100 immunocompromised patients. This has lead to a decrease in the use of tunneled catheters. In patients with HIV, use of an external catheter is safer for the nursing staff than an implanted port because needles are not needed for access.

Broviac and Hickman catheters are designed for tunneled use. Broviac catheters are single lumen 2.7 to 6.6 French catheters designed for pediatric applications. Hickman catheters are available in single to triple lumen configuration in 9.6 to 14.4 French sizes. Hohn and peripherally inserted central catheters (PICC) are used for short- to intermediate-term applications. These catheters are being used increasingly in applications traditionally performed by tunneled subclavian catheters. Hohn catheters are single or double lumen 4 to 7 French silicon rubber catheters. They have both a Dacron and a Vita-cuff that is placed subcutaneously between the skin dermatotomy and vein puncture site. Hohn catheters are nontunneled. PICC catheters are single or double lumen 3 to 7 French catheters measuring from 40 to 60 cm in length. PICC lines are cost effective and vein sparing when used to replace multiple peripheral intravenous lines. They eliminate the procedural risks of central line placement (e.g., pneumothorax, arterial puncture, central venous stenosis).

Implantable ports are available in single and dual lumen configurations. Implantable ports come in various sizes for placement within the arm or chest (Fig. 12.2). The port has a plastic or titanium shell that houses a thick silicon septum. The compressed silicon septum self-seals following needle puncture and allows 2,000 punctures with noncoring Huber needles on chest wall ports and 1,000 punctures on arm ports (Fig. 12.3). Plastic reservoirs interfere less with radiologic studies than titanium reservoirs. Implantable ports require less patient care and are more cosmetic than external catheters. Implanted ports have low infection rates and require only monthly flushes. The most common use for implantable ports are in patients requiring intermittent venous access such as weekly courses of chemotherapy. Despite higher initial costs, ports become cost effective at 6 months by the elimination of dressing changes and the reduced number of heparin flushes.

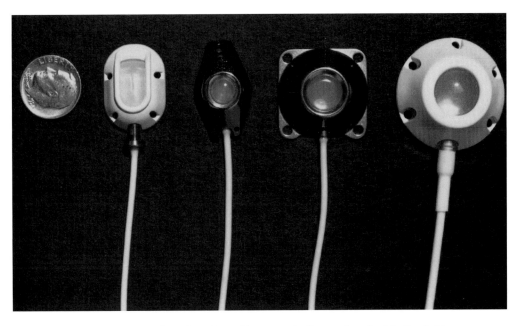

Figure 12.2 *Examples of implantable ports. Left to right: the Meditech R port, Deltec PAS port, Deltec low profile port, Cook CPC plastic Vitaport. The R port and PAS port are low profile ports for placement in the arm. The Deltec low profile port is intermediate in size for children and small adults. The CPC Vitaport is a plastic chest wall port.*

Figure 12.3 *The angle tip Huber needle does not core the silicone septum of implanted ports (right). An angled beveled needle would core the port septum resulting in leakage or blockage of the needle.*

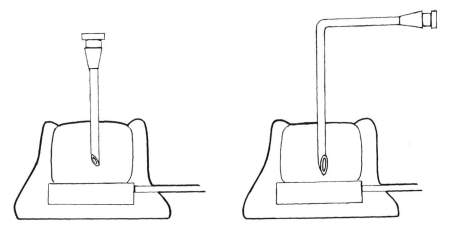

There are numerous access techniques. The standard surgical technique for placement of catheters uses anatomic landmarks. Interventional radiology techniques are sonographic or venographic guidance. Imaging guidance offers the advantage of precisely guiding a needle into the targeted vein. Imaging will determine patency and size of veins. The immediate technical complications of central line insertion are diminished considerably by imaging guidance. The veins of the upper extremity above the elbow are often spared from previous venipuncture. These veins are suitable for placement of PICC lines and peripherally implanted ports. The basilic vein is the largest vein and directly communicates with the axillary vein (Fig. 12.4). Sonographically guided puncture is advantageous in patients who have poor peripheral venous access. It eliminates the need for intravenous contrast and diminishes the risk of arterial puncture. Sonographic guidance limitations include the need for an ultrasound unit within the angiography suite and the difficulty in visualizing the needle tip.

The care of external catheters and ports is the primary determination of longevity and delayed complication rates. Strict adherence to aseptic technique when accessing catheters or ports reduces infectious complications dramatically. Prophylactic antibiotics are given before placement of tunneled or implanted ports. Meticulous surgical scrubbing of the area for implantation of the venous access device is mandatory. Duraprep solution (3M Healthcare, St. Paul, MN) is a long-lasting, broad-spectrum antimicrobial solution that forms a protective film on the skin. It is an alternative to mechanical scrubbing of the skin. This film lasts for several days and effectively kills bacteria up to 12 hours. Duraprep solution is painted onto the patient's skin in a thin, uniform manner. Once the coating is applied, the solution is allowed to dry for 2 to 3 minutes. The solution is not water soluble. All operators should scrub before placement of venous access devices. Hats and masks are mandatory for all personnel in the suite when venous access devices are implanted.

Catheter-related infections are probably the most significant and frequent complication. There are several potential sources of infection for indwelling catheters. The catheter infusate can be contaminated and seed the catheter. The skin entry site may become contaminated and allow migration of bacteria along the catheter. The catheter can be infected by an episode of bacteremia. Meticulous attention to catheter care has been shown to reduce the incidence of catheter-related infections. Wound dehiscence and nonhealing signals a potential infection. Culturing the wound or reservoir helps direct antibiotic choice. Minor erythema and induration around the port can be treated with antibiotics. Skin necrosis and exposure of the port are best treated with removal. Long-term catheters and ports are not placed in patients who are bacteremic and febrile.

Catheter-related deep venous thrombosis occurs in about 1 to 5 percent of cases. The incidence increases based on the position of the catheter tip. Precise positioning of the tip within the longitudinal lumen of the superior vena cava (SVC) near the junction of the right atrium reduces this complication significantly. A catheter positioned within the brachiocephalic vein or a catheter tip oriented toward the wall of the vessel is more likely to induce a mural thrombosis. Catheter malfunction includes luminal occlusion, catheter breakage, fibrin sheath formation, and positional catheter occlusion. Luminal occlusion and fibrin sheath formation are treated with infusion of 5,000 units of urokinase in 1 ml of saline into the catheter for 15 minutes. If the occlusion does not respond to two to three treatments, a

Figure 12.4 *Venous anatomy of upper extremity as guideline for venous access placement. The basilic vein is the largest vein. The brachial veins are paired and are immediately adjacent to the brachial artery. The cephalic vein enters into the distal subclavian vein.*

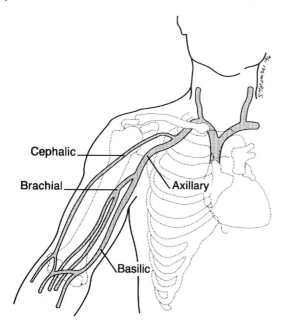

Cephalic

Brachial

Axillary

Basilic

catheter venogram is performed to define the problem. The catheter tip can be repositioned and the fibrin sheath stripped using a snare or tip-deflecting wire (Fig. 12.5). Significant catheter repositioning is best handled by catheter exchange. Tunneled catheters can be removed over a stiff Glidewire and a new catheter placed through a long peel-away sheath through the tunnel into the venous system.

Peripherally Inserted Central Catheters

PICCs were pioneered by home nurses for intermediate-term venous access. These catheters are ideal for 6-week to 3-month infusion of antibiotics, intravenous medications, pain control, and hydration but may be used longer. PICC lines can be used for chemotherapy and TPN. Whenever possible, a 5 French single lumen catheter is preferred over a double lumen catheter. The single lumen catheters require fewer flushes and have larger internal diameters, which facilitates blood draws. Double lumen catheters are reserved for cases in which incompatible medications are given simultaneously. Advantages are low initial complication rates, ease of exchange or removal, low cost, and similar performance compared to subclavian catheters. Disadvantages are the small luminal size, which makes blood products difficult to administer.

The nondominant arm is used whenever possible. If sonographic guidance is to be used, the chosen arm is scanned to assess patency, size, and location of deep venous anatomy of the proximal upper extremity. Meticulous attention to aseptic technique is used. The patient's arm is surgically scrubbed for 10 minutes; and the staff must wear masks, gowns, and surgical clothing. The use of prophylactic antibiotics is not necessary. The largest and most easily accessed vein in the patient's upper extremity is targeted. Usually this is the basilic vein, but the paired brachial veins or cephalic vein can be used. The vein is punctured midway between the elbow and axilla. This allows the external portion of the catheter to rest comfortably above the

Figure 12.5 **(A)** *Catheter venogram demonstrating occluding fibrin sheath.* **(B)** *Catheter is stripped from femoral venous insertion of goose neck snare catheter. A wire was inserted through the venous port of catheter to facilitate snaring of catheter.*

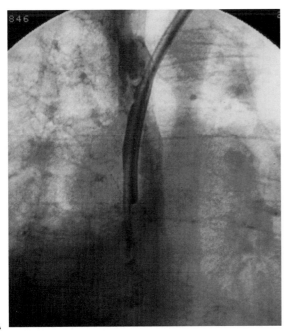

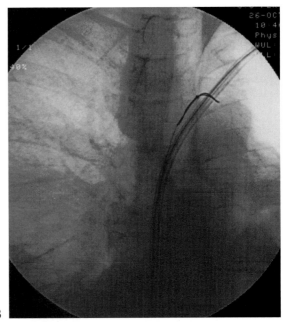

A   B

patient's elbow joint. The brachial artery is located by palpation if fluoroscopic-guided puncture is performed to avoid inadvertent arterial puncture. A tourniquet is used to maximally distend the vein.

Venipuncture can be guided with either venography or ultrasound. Venography requires a peripheral intravenous line and injection of contrast or carbon dioxide. The opacified veins are punctured under fluoroscopic guidance (Fig. 12.6). Ultrasound guidance uses a 7.5 MHz linear transducer. A vein of at least 3 mm in diameter is chosen above the elbow. The transducer is held perpendicular to the course of the vein, and a 21-gauge needle is advanced slowly toward the vein (Fig. 12.7). It can be difficult to see the needle tip. The needle tip position can be inferred by the deflection of tissue, which forms a V-shaped wave.

Venipuncture is best performed using micropuncture technique. A 21-gauge needle more readily allows single-wall puncture, which greatly facilitates subsequent guidewire passage. A 60 cm long 0.018 inch mandrel wire is advanced through the 21-gauge needle into the central venous system (Fig. 12.8). The tract is predilated with the 5 French dilator. The combined peel-away sheath and dilator are advanced over the wire into the vein. The mandrel wire is used to measure the distance from the right atrium to the venipuncture site.

The wire is marked by a clamp and is used to as a template to cut the PICC line to the appropriate length. The PICC line tip is cut with a 45° angled bevel. The bevel cut increases the surface area of the open end of the catheter and ensures that the entire length of the catheter has been removed when the catheter is pulled. The PICC line is advanced through the peel-away sheath and the tip is positioned within the SVC. The strain relief collar of the catheter is advanced underneath the skin to prevent kinking of the catheter. The catheter is secured to the patient with sutures.

The insertion site is cleansed and a transparent occlusive dressing applied over the PICC catheter. Dressings are changed daily using sterile techniques. Antibiotic ointments are avoided because their use increases *Candida* infection rates. Catheters are flushed once a day with a heparinized solution of saline both before and after each use. The catheter can be removed by simply withdrawing it from the patient and holding pressure over the entry site for 3 minutes.

Subclavian Central Venous Catheters

Hickman and Broviac catheters are large diameter, tunneled catheters traditionally used to provide long-term central venous access. The Dacron cuff buried in the subcutaneous tunnel securely anchors the catheter and is thought to provide a barrier to infection. The advantages of a tunnel have been challenged recently in several articles demonstrating equivalent infection rates between tunneled and nontunneled catheters. The Hohn (Bard Vascular Access, Salt Lake City, UT) is a 4 to 5 French single lumen and 7 French double lumen silicon rubber catheter designed for nontunneled subclavian placement. Cook TPN silicon rubber catheters are available in a wide variety of diameters and lumen configurations suitable for nontunneled subclavian placement. External catheters are preferred for administration of TPN, frequent blood sampling, frequent administration of blood products, and continuous infusions. Indications for external catheters include hemopoietic malignancies, bone marrow transplantation, and long-term TPN.

The left subclavian approach is preferred. There is less kinking of the peel-away sheath when it is placed into the more obtusely angled left brachiocephalic vein

Figure 12.6 *The basilic vein halfway between the axilla and elbow has been opacified with contrast. A 21-gauge needle has punctured the vein and a 0.018 mandrel wire is advanced into the vein.*

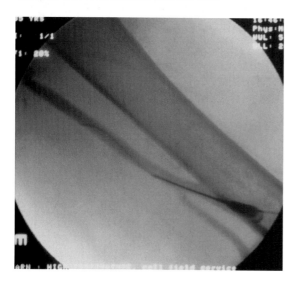

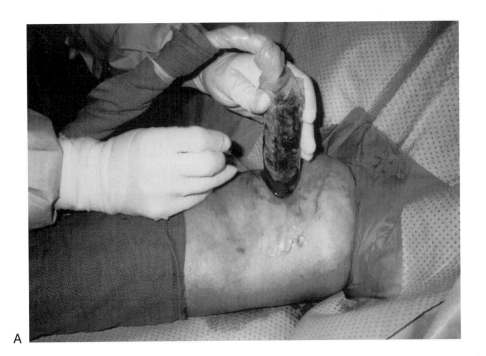

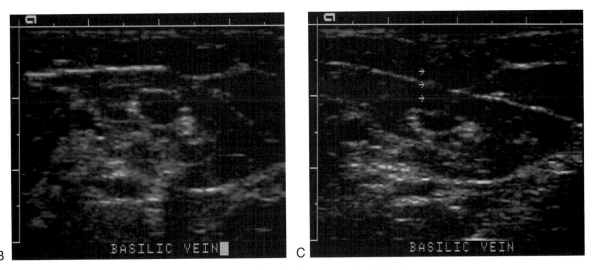

Figure 12.7 *Example of transverse ultrasound guided puncture. (**A**) A high resolution linear ultrasound transducer is held perpendicular to the coarse of the vein.
(**B**) The basilic vein is imaged in the transverse plane. The vessel is confirmed as a
vein by compressibility with the ultrasound probe. (**C**) The needle is introduced at a
steep angle to keep the needle tip in the plane of the ultrasound beam. The needle tip
can be visualized by jiggling the needle or visualizing the deflection wave caused by
needle passage (small arrows).*

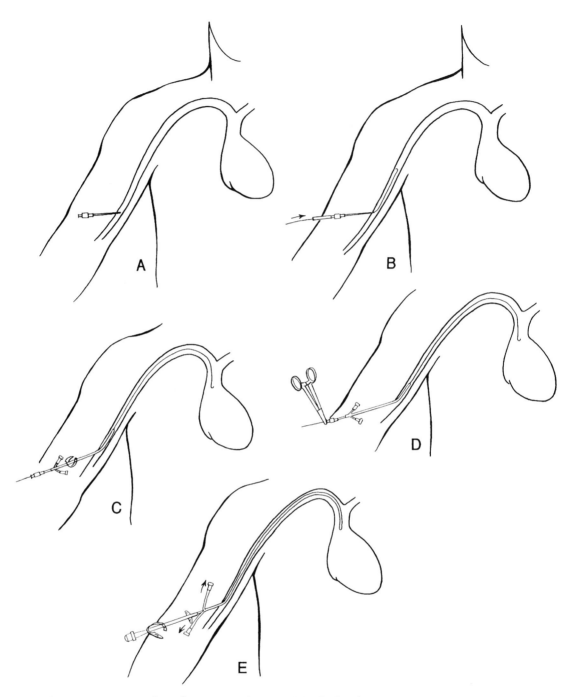

Figure 12.8 *PICC line placement technique. (A) The basilic vein is punctured with ultrasound or venographic guidance with a 21-gauge needle. (B) A 0.018 inch mandrel guidewire is introduced into the vein and central venous system. (C) The sheath-dilator is advanced over the wire with a twisting motion into the basilic vein. (D) The guidewire is used to measure the distance from the cavoatrial junction to the venipuncture site. This is marked on the wire using a hemostat and used as a template to cut the PICC line to the appropriate length. (E) The PICC line with stiffening stylet is introduced into the central venous system through the peel-away sheath. The tip is positioned at the cavoatrial junction. The peel-away sheath is removed by pulling the sheath apart.*

compared to the acute angle formed by the junction of the right subclavian vein with the right brachiocephalic vein. A left-sided catheter is easier for a right-handed individual to care for. The catheter is placed preferably in a vein that has not already had a catheter in place. If there is prior history of multiple central venous lines, a venogram or ultrasound is performed before the procedure to document patency of the vessels.

The deltopectoral groove is chosen for the entry puncture site into the subclavian vein and is marked with the marking pen. The exit site of the catheter is then chosen. In a woman, it should be at the tan line or just above the bra line to prevent irritation of the catheter by a bra strap. The exit site of the catheter is more medial compared to the puncture entry site into the subclavian vein. The exit site is chosen approximately 15 cm away from the puncture entry site to provide a tunnel of adequate length.

The patient has electrocardiogram (ECG) leads, pulse oximetry, and intravenous access established for delivery of intravenous sedation. The skin is prepared with the Duraprep surgical solution. This solution creates a film on the skin that kills bacteria for up to 12 hours. A standard femoral angiography drape is placed over the patient, and the fenestration is modified by cutting a slot in approximately the 4 o'clock position to allow access to the tunnel site. Local analgesia is infiltrated into the puncture site using a 22-gauge spinal needle.

Micropuncture technique is used because it potentially decreases puncture site complications. The 21-gauge needle provided in the Cook micropuncture set is used to puncture the left subclavian vein. A lateral puncture in the subclavian vein avoids the subclavius muscle and tendon, reducing the chance of a pinch-off syndrome. The subclavian vein is punctured distal to its entry site into the thorax between the clavicle and first rib. Venous access can be guided by anatomic landmarks, venogram, or ultrasound. Once the subclavian vein is successfully punctured, the 0.018 wire is advanced through the needle and into the SVC. A 3 cm skin incision is made to include the venipuncture site. The needle is removed and the introducer sheath is placed into the subclavian vein. The dilator and wire are removed from the introducer sheath. A 0.038 wire is placed into the SVC and threaded through the heart into the inferior vena cava (IVC) under fluoroscopic guidance. An 8 French dilator is placed into the subclavian vein. The wire is withdrawn and used as a template to measure

the distance from the distal SVC to the skin exit site. A hemostat is used to mark this position on the wire. The 8 French vessel dilator is left in place and is capped with a heplock device.

The subcutaneous tunnel is created next. The 22-gauge 3½ inch needle is used to infiltrate the tunnel tract. A small stab dermatotomy is made at the exit site of the catheter. The tunneling device is advanced from the catheter exit site to the venous entry site and is rotated to help steer and bluntly dissect through the subcutaneous tissue. The appropriate size catheter is attached to the end of the tunneling device, and the assembly is pulled through the tunnel. The catheter is positioned with its Vita Cuff and Dacron cuff placed just underneath the skin. This allows for later easy removal of the catheter. With the use of the wire template, the catheter is cut to the appropriate length once it has been positioned within the subcutaneous tunnel.

The wire is placed through the 8 French vessel dilator and advanced into the inferior vena cava. The vessel dilator is removed, and the tract is dilated with the peel-away sheath dilator. The peel-away sheath dilator is placed over the wire into the subclavian vein. The vessel dilator and guidewire are removed from the peel-away sheath, and the Hickman catheter is immediately placed into the peel-away sheath to prevent blood loss and air embolism.

The catheter is examined fluoroscopically to ascertain proper positioning. The catheter is inspected to make sure there are no kinks. At the venous entry site, the catheter often makes an abrupt turn, which kinks the catheter. Blunt dissection of the deep subcutaneous tissues will prevent this occurrence. The catheter is flushed and heparinized with the usual heparin solution of 100 U/ml of saline. The venous entry site is closed with either an interrupted suture or subcutaneous stitches.

The catheter can be removed with steady, firm traction leaving the Dacron cuff behind in the subcutaneous tunnel. Alternatively, the Dacron cuff can be removed utilizing local anesthesia and blunt dissection. Pressure is held firmly over the entry site for 5 minutes and the patient is observed for 1 hour prior to release from the hospital.

Hohn subclavian vein catheter placement technique is similar to PICC line placement. Strict sterile procedure, imaging guidance, and micropuncture technique are followed. The vein is cannulated with an 0.018 inch guidewire. The tract is dilated to the appropriate size. The distance to the cavoatrial junction is measured with the wire and the catheter cut to the measured length. A 5 mm skin incision is made and the subcutaneous tissues spread to accommodate the catheter cuffs, which are placed just under the skin. The catheter is advanced over the 0.018 inch guidewire into the central venous system. The tip is positioned in the distal cava and the cuffs buried just under the skin. The catheter suture wings are secured to the skin with 3-0 nylon suture.

Immediate procedural-related complications include pneumothorax, hemothorax, or hydrothorax. There is the potential for perforation or laceration of the vein or inadvertent arterial puncture. Other less frequent complications include induced cardiac arrhythmias, local hematomas, and brachial plexus injury. Delayed complications include catheter malposition, occlusion, fibrin sheath formation, dislodgement, or rupture. Sepsis and/or infection is a common complication, occurring in 5 to 20 percent of cases.

Chest Implanted Port Technique

Implantable ports are used for long-term, intermittent access. An implanted port consists of a reservoir connected to an infusion catheter. The port reservoir has a compressed silicon septum designed for 1,000 to 2,000 punctures with a noncoring Huber needle. Ports may be placed via central or peripheral venous access. Standard size ports are used for chest wall placement in average and large sized adults. Low profile devices are available for use within small adults and children. The P.A.S. Port (Sims-Deltec, St. Paul, MN) and the R Port (Meditech, Watertown, MA) are examples of small ports designed for extremity placement.

A single dose of an intravenous antibiotic is given immediately before the procedure. Strict adherence to aseptic technique is crucial to reduce the immediate infectious complications. The operator must wear complete surgical garb and surgically scrub for 10 minutes. The implantation site is scrubbed for 10 minutes or Duraprep is used. The venipuncture technique for port placement is similar to that used for PICC lines or subclavian lines. The catheter is placed and positioned within the central venous system.

Implantation of a port requires creation of a subcutaneous pocket. The port is positioned in a site that offers a secure base and cosmetic location. If necessary,

the port can be implanted a distance from the venipuncture access site. If this is the case, a tunnel is created between the venous access site and the port implantation site. In obese individuals or large breasted women, the port can shift inferiorly between the supine and upright positions. This must be factored into the choice of catheter length and port site location during implantation in the supine position.

The chosen pocket location is anesthetized by local infiltration of the subcutaneous tissue with lidocaine. A 4 to 5 cm skin incision is made. Blunt dissection with a hemostat is used to create the pocket. The pocket is created to have the reservoir approximately 1 cm deep to the skin and offset relative to the incision. The pocket is fashioned to snugly fit the implanted port. If the pocket is too large, the port can migrate or twirl during attempted puncture (Fig. 12.9). The catheter is cut to the appropriate length and attached to the port reservoir. The catheter attachment to the port varies among manufacturers. A secure connection is imperative. The port is fixed to the deep fascia with two sutures before the incision is closed. It is accessed and flushed before closure to determine whether the catheter attachment is secure. The pocket is closed by covering the reservoir with a layer of subcutaneous tis-

Figure 12.9 *Occluded chest wall port due to twirling or rotation of device from a loose port pocket.*

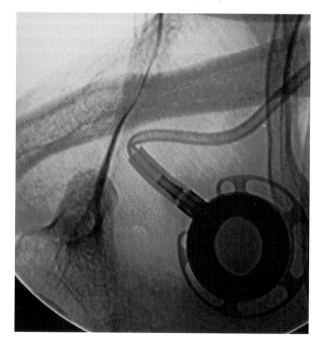

sue approximated with an absorbable suture. The catheter-to-reservoir connection is buried in the deep subcutaneous tissues so that it does not buckle under the incision. The skin incision is closed with either a subcuticular or interrupted suture technique.

Ports are removed by generously anesthetizing the reservoir region. The scar from the previous incision is incised. The catheter is removed first. Blunt and sometimes sharp dissection is necessary to free the reservoir from the surrounding fibrous capsule. The pocket is cleansed and closed in layers after port removal. Unique complications to ports are pocket infections, reservoir erosion through the skin, skin necrosis from multiple punctures, twirling of the port making access difficult, and subcutaneous extravasation of an infusion.

Upper Extremity Implanted Port Technique

Several downsized versions of chest wall ports have been produced specifically to be placed in the upper extremity. The majority of these devices have been placed in the interventional radiology suite because of the need for image guidance for venous access. Examples are the P.A.S. Port and the R Port. Pediatric-sized and low profile chest wall ports can be used and are preferable in patients with large arms. The Cath Link (Bard Access, Salt Lake, UT) is a new device that can be accessed with standard intravenous needles rather than the noncoring Huber needle. Arm ports can be used for blood sampling, chemotherapy, and antibiotic therapy. The longer length of catheter and smaller access needle size hamper rapid delivery of blood product infusions. Many patients, especially female patients, find the cosmetic results preferable compared to chest wall ports. Another advantage is the elimination of the technical risks of blind subclavian vein puncture. Disadvantages are the smaller size of the septum and the unfamiliarity of physicians and nurses with these new devices. The smaller septum size limits the septum life to 500 to 1,000 punctures compared to the 2,000 puncture life of chest wall ports. The punctures are concentrated into a smaller area of skin and smaller caliber needles are recommended (20- to 22-gauge).

Use of the patient's nondominant arm is preferred. The patency of the deep venous system in the arm is assessed using ultrasound or venography between the elbow and the axilla. The patient's upper extremity is surgically scrubbed for 10 minutes using a Betadine soap solution. The operators of the procedure must surgically scrub for 10 minutes before donning surgical garb. All personnel in the room should wear masks and hats. Before starting the procedure, 1 g cephalozin is given intravenously as prophylaxis.

The largest vein in the mid humeral region is chosen. Usually this is the basilic vein, but the paired brachial or cephalic veins can be used. Ultrasound or venographic guidance can be used to puncture the vein. The vein is cannulated using micropuncture techniques similar to placing a PICC catheter. A 0.035 Glidewire is used to place a 6 French vascular sheath within the cannulated arm vein. The catheter is passed over the Glidewire and the tip positioned at the cavo-atrial junction. The shoulder is abducted and the catheter tip observed fluoroscopically for motion before trimming the catheter. One should avoid placing the catheter tip deeply within the right atrium or proximally within the brachiocephalic veins.

The inner arm area offers the most cosmetic location for reservoir placement. One percent lidocaine is infiltrated in a fanlike manner adjacent to the venipuncture site. A 3 to 4 cm inch long transverse skin incision is made using a #15 scalpel. The stab wound of the venipuncture site is included in this incision. A subcutaneous pocket is formed by bluntly spreading the subcutaneous fatty tissue with a hemostat (Fig. 12.10). The port should be 0.5 to 1.0 cm below the surface of the skin to allow easy palpation for access. The port reservoir should fit snugly into the subcutaneous pocket (Fig. 12.11). A secure catheter to portal assembly is important. The catheter is pushed onto the portal outlet connector. The end of the catheter is advanced as close to the portal housing as possible. The catheter should be visible through the holes in the connector. The P.A.S. Port's catheter is gently pulled to seal the connector and secure the assembly. The R Port connection is secured by pulling the reservoir cannula over the catheter and twisting the cannula until a click is felt or heard. Two anchoring sutures are passed through the reservoir suture holes. The catheter and reservoir are flushed with heparinized saline. The assembly is fitted into the subcutaneous pocket. The anchoring sutures are used to secure the port to the underlying muscle fascia (Fig. 12.12). Blunt dissection is used to bury the catheter in the deep subcutaneous layer. The edges of the incision are undermined to assist in burying the catheter, but not the reservoir, in the deep sub-

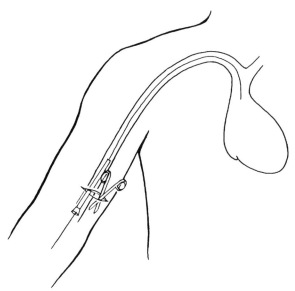

Figure 12.10 *The arm port pocket is created by using a hemostat to spread the subcutaneous tissues of the distal edge of the port implantation incision. A pocket is made to snugly fit the port. The loose subcutaneous tissues are easily dissected to create a port pocket.*

cuticular suture. An access needle is left in place if the device is planned for immediate use.

The arm port can be removed as a simple outpatient procedure. The area over the reservoir is generously infiltrated with local anesthetic. A 3 to 4 cm skin incision is made at the previous implantation incision line. The catheter is identified and removed from the patient. A combination of blunt and sharp dissection is required to free the port from the fibrous capsule. The wound is closed in layers to eliminate any dead space, and the incision is closed using interrupted sutures.

The most common complications are infections and thrombosis, which occurs in 5 to 10 percent of patients. Prophylactic antibiotic administration and careful adherence to strict aseptic practice can help lessen the immediate procedure-related infections. Minor localized infections can be treated with intravenous cephalozin or vancomycin. More serious infections require removal of the port. Low dose coumadin therapy is administered in patients with risk factors for thrombosis.

cutaneous tissues. The wound is closed in layers to protect the skin incision. The subcutaneous tissues are loosely approximated over the catheter and connector with absorbable 4-0 Vicryl suture. The skin incision is closed with interrupted 4-0 nylon skin sutures or a sub-

Hemodialysis Catheters

Vascular access for hemodialysis is a significant problem confronting nephrologists treating end-stage renal disease. Long-term vascular access is ideally provided

Figure 12.11 *Example of arm implanted port pocket. The port's catheter has been introduced through a vascular sheath. The pocket is created midway between the axilla and elbow. The port is implanted underneath the distal edge of the incision approximately 1 cm deep to the skin surface. An army-navy retractor is exposing the pocket site.*

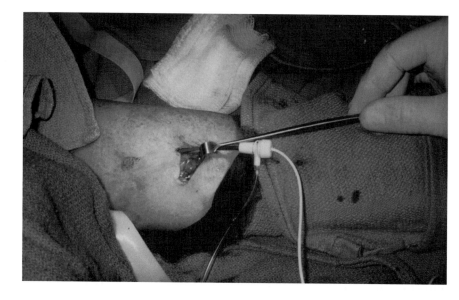

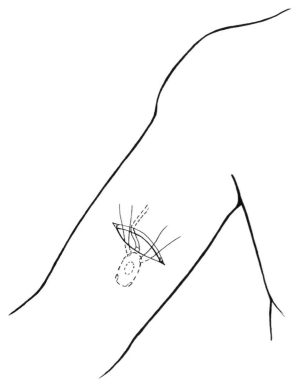

Figure 12.12 *Depiction of proper placement of a port within the upper arm. The catheter has been cut and attached to the port reservoir. Two sutures are used to secure the port to the deep subcutaneous fascia.*

by the use of native arteriovenous (AV) fistulas or synthetic AV grafts in the patient's nondominant arm. Hemodialysis catheters are predominantly used to provide temporary vascular access. They are used in

reversible acute renal failure, while AV fistulas mature, or following failure of AV fistula. Long-term hemodialysis with catheters is reserved for failures of fistulas or peritoneal dialysis. The number of catheter-dependent dialysis patients is increasing as the dialysis population ages and increases in number. Catheter-induced sepsis and thrombosis limit the life span of these devices.

Hemodialysis catheters require high flow rates. Flow rates should be greater than 200 ml/min and preferably 250 to 350 ml/min to allow an adequate dialysis. The high flow rates required of these catheters require large catheter luminal size and short catheter length. Blood is withdrawn in one lumen and returned via the other (Fig. 12.13). The proximal lumen is termed the arterial lumen in which blood is aspirated into the dialysis machine. The dialyzed blood is returned via the distal venous lumen. The catheter tips are staggered by approximately 2.5 cm. This reduces the percentage of recirculation to preferably less than 10 percent.

There are two types of hemodialysis catheters. Temporary catheters are designed for easy, bedside placement. These catheters are semistiff coaxial dual-lumen designs with tapered tips. They are not tunneled. The Vas Cath Flexicon II, Quinton Mahurkar, and Shiley catheters are examples. Long-term catheters are made of soft, biocompatible materials such as silicon rubber and polyurethane. These catheters feature side-by-side lumens with a staggered tip configuration. Permanent catheters are tunneled and have Dacron cuffs buried under the skin to anchor the device. Examples are the Vas Cath Soft Cell, Cook Uldall, Bard Hickman, and Quinton PermCath (Fig. 12.14). The catheter length ranges from 15 to 50 cm and the diam-

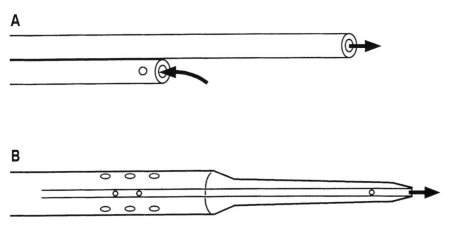

Figure 12.13 *Hemodialysis catheters. (A) Side-by-side dual lumen dialysis catheter. The distal lumen is a venous outflow and the proximal lumen is the arterial inflow. This tip configuration requires placement through peel-away sheath. (B) Coaxial dual lumen catheter can be placed over a wire. The distal tapered tip is the venous outflow and the proximal side holes are the arterial withdrawal.*

Figure 12.14 *Hemodialysis catheters. Top: Uhdall hemodialysis catheter. Second from top: Quinton Permcath. Middle: Bard Hickman hemodialysis catheter. Second from the bottom: pre-curved Vas Cath Soft Cell hemodialysis catheter. Bottom: coaxial Vas Cath Flexicon II catheter.*

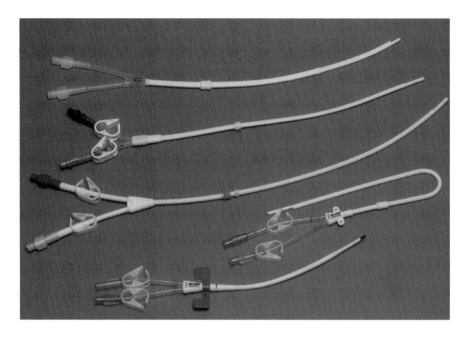

eter from 11 to 16 French. The Uldall and PermCath are 16 French oval catheters with dual round internal lumens. The Bard Hickman is a 13.5 French round catheter with dual D-shaped lumens. The Vas Cath is a 11.5 French round polyurethane catheter with dual D-shaped lumens. The Vas Cath is pre-curved to allow a 90° kink-resistant bend, which orients the staggered tips appropriately and allows the catheter exit site to be inferior to the clavicle.

The choice of temporary or long-term catheter is arbitrary. Previous recommendations are to use non-tunneled catheters for up to 4 weeks. This practice is satisfactory for patients with acute and reversible renal failure. We are preferentially placing tunneled jugular catheters in patients with chronic renal failure for periods as short as 1 to 2 weeks. The tunneled catheters are more cosmetic and have less mechanical complications than the stiff coaxial catheters. The jugular vein is preferred for hemodialysis catheter placement. The internal jugular vein allows a straighter course for placement of the dialysis catheter, with less tendency to malfunction from kinking and bony compression. The subclavian vein is a suboptimal vein for long-term hemodialysis access. The high thrombosis and stenosis rates associated with subclavian vein puncture eliminate the involved upper extremity for use as a site for an AV fistula. In patients who have had numerous prior catheters, it is often necessary to perform bilateral

upper extremity venography to document patency of the central venous system. If the SVC or brachiocephalic veins are occluded, hemodialysis catheters can be placed into the IVC via the translumbar or transfemoral routes.

Single dose antibiotic prophylaxis and meticulous sterile technique are observed. Ultrasound is used to puncture the internal jugular vein just above the clavicle. A wire is used to measure the distance from the right atrium to the venipuncture site. The appropriate length hemodialysis catheter kit is opened. Hemodialysis catheters are available in a wide range of lengths. A right jugular approach usually takes a 19 cm long catheter and the left a 23 cm long catheter. These are lengths from the cuff to the catheter tip or from the bend of the catheter to the tip of the catheter in pre-curved designs. The pre-curved Vas Cath catheters are tunneled to accommodate the distance between the cuff of the catheter and the bend in the catheter. The 180° bend of the Vas Cath allows the catheter to exit below the clavicle when placed via an internal jugular route. This is more cosmetically appealing to patients. It also helps eliminate kinking at the apex of the curve.

The technique for measuring catheter and tunnel length differs from placement of tunneled subclavian lines. Hemodialysis catheters have staggered tips that cannot be cut to adjust length. The length is chosen based on the measured length from venipuncture site to right atrium. The catheter is laid on the patient to aid in planning the length of the tunnel (Fig. 12.15). The length of the tunnel is varied to precisely position the catheter tip. Straight catheters are tunneled with a gentle bend to prevent kinking. The catheter is pulled through the tunnel and then advanced through a peel-away sheath into the central venous system. It is important to position the tip of dialysis catheters within the right atrium. This provides optimal flow. During implantation, the longer lumen is positioned adjacent to the wall of the vessel. This orientation will position the arterial lumen away from the vessel wall in the center of the vessel, which allows free aspiration of blood at the high flow rates necessary for hemodialysis. The flow rate is tested before completing the procedure. The arterial lumen must aspirate 20 ml of blood within 4 to 5 seconds. This indicates that the catheter has a flow rate of at least 240 ml/min. Hemodialysis catheters are flushed with concentrated heparin solution of 5,000 U/ml. Each lumen is flushed with its labeled priming volume. The flush is done using positive pressure technique. The clamp is closed while flushing the last bit of heparin to fully charge the lumen of the catheter with heparinized saline. This prevents reflux of blood into the catheter.

The large size and high flow rates demanded of hemodialysis catheters lead to inevitable episodes of malfunction. The catheter's performance can be affected by malposition, thrombus, or stenosis. A common malfunction is diminished blood flow. This is initially treated with infusion of urokinase 5,000 U/ml. If the urokinase does not work, a catheter venogram should be performed. The catheter venogram includes assessment of catheter tip position, luminal patency, fibrin sheath formation, venous stenosis, and positional kinking or pinching of the catheter. If an occluding fibrin sheath is discovered, stripping with a loop snare is the most successful method for removal of the fibrin "sock." Catheter lumen thrombosis is best treated by urokinase infusions, guidewire "stripping," or catheter exchange. Catheter position may prevent adequate blood flow by the catheter tip abutting the wall of the vein. A "positional" catheter requires fluoroscopic observation of the catheter during the position that causes the malfunction. Mural thrombosis can occur at the insertion site or at the catheter tip, especially if it is oriented toward the wall of a vessel. Insertion site stenosis occurs in subclavian venipuncture when the vein is punctured in the region of the thoracic outlet and pinched by the musculotendinous tissues below the clavicle. Septic complications of dialysis catheters are common. The risk of infection increases with time. The reported incidence of dialysis catheter-related sepsis ranges from 2 to 25 percent. Treatment is removal for tunnel or insertion site infections signaled by erythema or drainage. Systemic infections or fevers of unknown origin can sometimes be treated successfully with antibiotics without catheter removal in patients with limited venous access.

Translumbar Inferior Vena Cava Catheter

Patients requiring long-term central venous catheters or multiple catheters are subject to subclavian stenosis and occlusion. These stenoses are often asymptomatic and become apparent only with placement of a catheter. Aggressive treatment with angioplasty is recommended to prolong the access routes in these patients. Hemodialysis and lifelong TPN patients are likely to exhaust traditional central venous access routes, requiring alternative access routes. Novel routes of venous access are necessary in these patients with occlusions of the superior vena cava that require large diameter catheters. Translumbar IVC and transhepatic IVC routes have been developed to provide venous access in these patients (Fig. 12.16). In patients requiring medications or antibiotics, venography can sometimes identify an hypertrophied collateral vein suitable for catheterization with a PICC or Hohn catheter. Percutaneous translumbar placement of a catheter in the IVC is indicated in patients who have the need for a large intravenous access device (14 French), infected subclavian or jugular central venous catheters, or thrombosis of the subclavian veins. The transhepatic route into the IVC is a secondary choice preferable in patients with IVC filters, which would potentially interfere with a translumbar approach. Ultrasound guidance is used to cannulate the left hepatic vein from a subcostal approach.

The technique for translumbar IVC access is similar to that used for diagnostic translumbar aortography. The patient is placed supine on the angiographic table during which time the ECG monitoring device, pulse oximeter, and blood pressure cuff are applied to the patient. A peripheral intravenous line is started, and the patient is given sedation with midazolam (Versed) and fentanyl. The patient is rolled into a left-

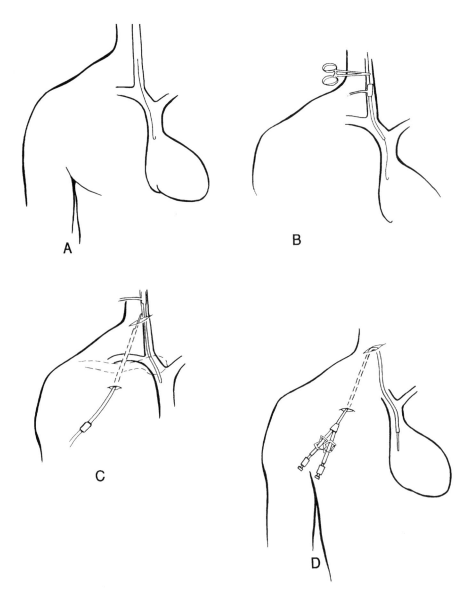

Figure 12.15 *Internal jugular tunneled hemodialysis catheter placement.*
(A) The internal jugular vein is punctured with ultrasound guidance one-third the distance between the clavicle and angle of the mandible. A wire is positioned into the distal SVC. (B) A vascular sheath is placed over the wire to preserve venous access. A guidewire is used to measure the distance from the cavoatrial junction to the venipuncture site. This calculated length plus an additional 10 to 15 cm is the minimum necessary for placing a tunneled hemodialysis catheter. A hemodialysis catheter that matches this length is chosen. (C) The catheter is laid on the patient to estimate the length and shape of the tunnel. The catheter cuff is usually placed 1 to 5 cm within the subcutaneous tunnel. The catheter is tunneled from the skin exit site to the venipuncture site using a tunneling device. The tunneling device is attached to the tip of the hemodialysis catheter, which is pulled through the tunnel. (D) The hemodialysis catheter has been pulled through the subcutaneous tunnel and placed into the central venous system through a peel-away sheath. The tip of the catheter is located at the cavoatrial junction or within the right atrium. The proximal arterial lumen should be positioned in the middle of the vein.

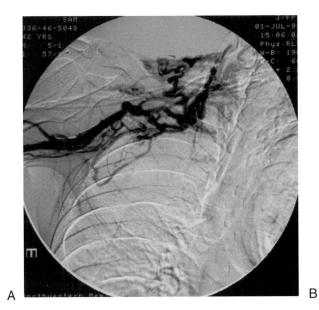

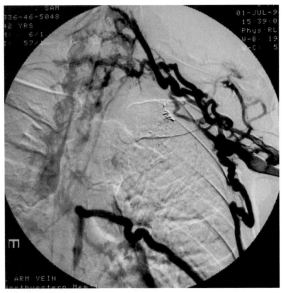

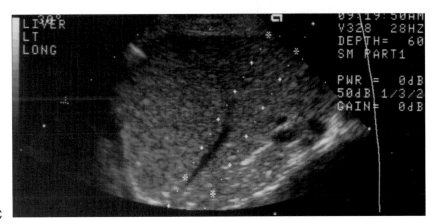

Figure 12.16 *Transhepatic venous catheter. (**A**) and (**B**) Bilateral upper extremity venograms demonstrated complete central venous occlusion. (**C**) A subcostal approach under ultrasound guidance was used to puncture the left hepatic vein. (Figure continues.)*

side-down decubitus position. With the use of a permanent marking pen, the spinous processes of the second through fourth lumbar vertebral bodies are marked (Fig. 12.17). The iliac crest is marked. A large metal instrument, such as a long scissors or sponge clamp, is used to mark the inferior end plate of the L3 vertebral body. This mark is made on the patient's right flank. The entry site is marked on the patient's side approximately one hand breadth (8 to 10 cm) to the right of the midline as marked by the spinous

processes. The entry site is slightly above the level of the iliac crest and inferior to the L3 end plate. This allows for a slight cephalad angulation of the needle, which aids in subsequent dilatation of the tract and passage of the catheter through the peel-away sheath.

The skin is prepped with Duraprep surgical solution, which is wiped on the patient's skin using a circular application process. A standard paper angiography drape is attached to the patient's side. No cloth towels are applied to the patient before attaching the surgical

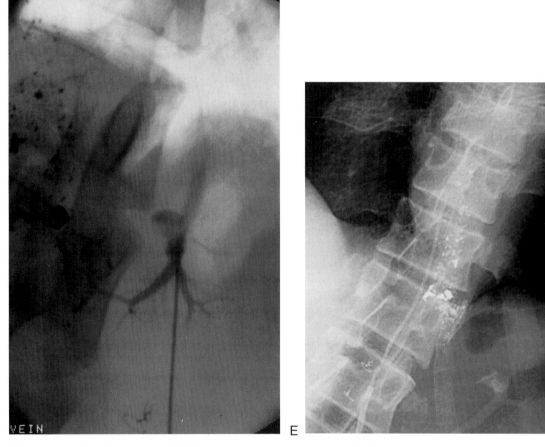

Figure 12.16 *(Continued)* **(D)** *Left hepatic venogram.* **(E)** *A Hohn catheter was placed with the tip just within right atrium.*

drape, which allows the surgical drape to adhere to the tacky Duraprep solution. The femoral angiography fenestration is modified by cutting a slot approximately 2 × 5 inches at the 2 o'clock position relative to the head of the drape. This allows for exposure of the subcutaneous tunnel, which extends superiorly to the right flank.

Fluoroscopy is used to reconfirm landmarks before making incisions. Generous local anesthesia is performed by injecting 1 percent lidocaine. An approximate 3 cm long dermatotomy is made over the skin entry site one hand breadth to the right of the midline of the lumbar spine. This incision is spread with a hemostat. Following creation of the dermatotomy, a 22-gauge spinal needle is used to anesthetize the tract toward the L3 inferior end plate. At least 20 ml of 1 percent lidocaine are used to infiltrate the entry site and tract to the IVC.

The puncture is performed under fluoroscopic control in a lateral decubitus position. The IVC is punctured using bony landmarks and translumbar aortography technique. The IVC can be targeted by a guidewire or contrast opacification to assist in fluoroscopic guidance. Alternative guidance methods are ultrasound or computed tomography (CT) scan. A 15 cm long 18-gauge Turner needle is used to puncture the IVC. In larger patients, a 20 cm long needle is required. The needle is aimed toward the inferior end plate of the L3 vertebral body. The mid portion of the L3 vertebral body is avoided to prevent an inadvertent puncture of the lumbar artery. The L3-4 disk is avoided to prevent puncturing the annulus fibrosis. The needle is advanced with a slightly cephalad angulation and is placed immediately alongside the vertebral body. The needle tract should go immediately adjacent to the vertebral body but

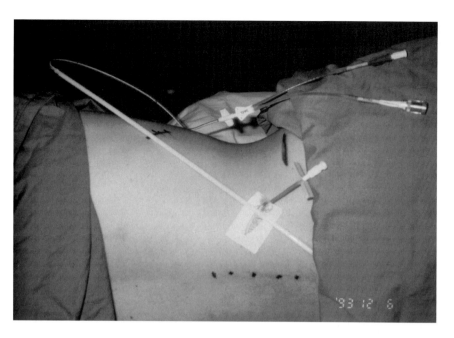

Figure 12.17 *Demonstration of the length and site of the tunnel for a translumbar IVC catheter. The patient is in the left decubitus position. The venipuncture is one hand's breadth above the spinous processes, which are marked with a dotted line. A plastic tunneling device is used to subcutaneously tunnel the catheter from the right subcostal region to the right paraspinal venipuncture site.*

should avoid the periosteum. The needle is advanced until it is approximately 3 to 4 cm anterior to the anterior margin of the L3 vertebral body. The stylet from the needle is removed and a 10 ml syringe used to provide negative suction on the needle as it is withdrawn from the tract. Free aspiration of blood indicates that the needle is positioned within the IVC. The 0.038 inch standard angiographic wire is advanced into the IVC and positioned within the SVC or subclavian veins. The tract is serially dilated with 5 and 8 French dilators. The 8 French dilator is left within the tract and confirmed to be positioned within the IVC before the wire is withdrawn from it. A cap or stopcock is placed on the 8 French dilator. The distance from the right atrium to the skin exit site is measured by placing a wire through the dilator until it is positioned within the right atrium. A hemostat is used to clamp the position on the wire corresponding to the skin entry site. This wire is set aside on the angiographic table and is used for cutting the Hickman catheter to the appropriate length.

The subcutaneous tunnel is created next (Fig. 12.18). The tract should extend superiorly along the patient's right flank for 15 to 25 cm. The exit site is in a right subcostal position in approximately the mid to distal clavicular line. Local anesthetic is infiltrated along the length of tract using the 3½ inch long 22-gauge spinal needle. A small dermatotomy is made at

the exit site of the catheter in the right flank. The tunneling device is used to create the tunnel starting from the exit site of the catheter toward the venous entry site. The catheter is connected to the end of the tunneling device and pulled through the tunnel. The Vita-Cuff is positioned just beneath the dermatotomy entry point. This facilitates future removal of the Dacron cuff and Vita-Cuff. At this point, the catheter has been pulled through the tunnel and positioned within the tunnel. The end of the catheter is coiled on the patient's back, and the 8 French dilator is present within the entry tract into the IVC. The catheter is cut to the appropriate length using the marked guidewire as a template. The guidewire is placed through the 8 French dilator and positioned within the subclavian vein or SVC. The tract is dilated to the appropriate size using the dilator within the peel-away sheath. The peel-away sheath is advanced through the tract into the IVC. The catheter is immediately advanced into the sheath as soon as the peel-away sheath dilator is removed to minimize blood loss and the potential for an air embolus. The catheter is fed through the sheath into the IVC, where the tip is positioned within the IVC at its junction with the right atrium.

The peel-away sheath has the tendency to kink at the bend between the tract and the IVC entry point. This can impede passage of the catheter through the sheath and into the IVC. It is important to preserve

Figure 12.18 IVC
catheter. (A) In left decubi-
tus position, the IVC is
punctured with an 18-gauge
needle one hand breadth
above the spine. Note the
superior angulation of the
needle. (B) A peel-away
sheath is positioned within
the IVC. The subcutaneous
tract is created with the
tunneling device. The
catheter exit site is in the
subcostal area of the right
upper quadrant anterior
abdominal wall. (C) The
catheter is pulled through
the subcutaneous tract. The
length from the venipunc-
ture site to cava is measured
and the appropriate length
of catheter inserted through
the peel-away sheath.
(D) Final position of the
IVC catheter.

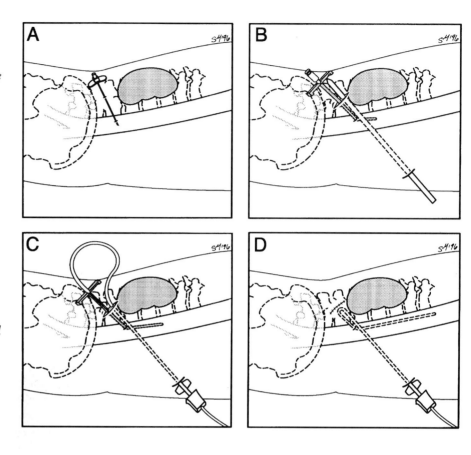

access into the IVC at this point by advancing a
Glidewire through the catheter and well into the IVC.
With the Glidewire in place the peel-away sheath can
be slowly removed. By gently withdrawing the peel-
away sheath, the kink will unfold, allowing unimpeded
passage of the catheter into the IVC.

The peel-away sheath is removed when the
catheter is positioned in the IVC within the desired
location. The catheter is flushed with saline. The
catheter is visualized fluoroscopically to ensure there
are no kinks within it. The skin incisions are closed and
the catheter flushed with heparinized saline. Care of
the IVC catheter is similar to care of a Hickman catheter. Aseptic technique is performed when handling
the catheter.

Removal of the catheter is accomplished by dis-
secting free the Dacron cuff immediately underneath
the skin at the exit site of the catheter. This requires
local infiltration with lidocaine and blunt dissection
with a hemostat. The catheter is pulled out after the

cuff is freed and pressure is applied to the subcutaneous tunnel for a few minutes. The patient is placed in
a supine position for 1 hour of strict bed rest followed
by an observation period of 1 to 2 hours before discharge from the hospital.

Complications are similar to those seen in patients
who have routine subclavian Hickman catheters. No
significant retroperitoneal hematomas or hemorrhages
have been found. Patients do report some lower back
pain and discomfort approximately 3 to 7 days after
catheter placement, which resolves with time and oral
analgesics. Mechanical complications include kinking
of the catheter, catheter tip migration into veins other
than the IVC, and dislodgement of the catheter outside the IVC. Dislodgement of the catheter tip can be
prevented by leaving a long segment of catheter inside
the IVC. Thrombotic complications of long-term IVC
catheter placement should be expected. In the University of Nebraska experience, 2 of 40 patients developed an IVC thrombosis. Both patients responded to

lysing with low dose local urokinase infusions. Fibrin sheaths forming around the catheter is a frequent occurrence, and the first 8 of 11 catheters removed had a pericatheter fibrin sheath. Infectious complications are similar to those seen with standard long-term indwelling SVC catheters. Septic complications usually occur 3 weeks after placement. Infectious complications occur in approximately 6 percent of IVC catheter placements, which compares favorably with standard subclavian Hickman catheters. One potential complication not yet observed is damage to the right ureter. The tract is intentionally created close to the vertebral bodies to avoid this complication.

Suggested Readings

Alexander HR: Vascular Access in the Cancer Patient: Devices, Insertion Techniques, Maintenance, and Prevention and Management of Complications. JB Lippincott, Philadelphia, 1994

Braun MA: Image-guided peripheral venous access catheters and implantable ports. Semin Intervent Radiol 11:358, 1994

Cardella JF, Fox PS, Lawler JB: Interventional radiologic placement of peripherally inserted central catheters. J Vasc Interv Radiol 4:653, 1993

Denny DF: Placement and management of long-term central venous access catheters and ports. AJR 161:385, 1993

Deustch LS, White GH: Central venous cannulation for hemodialysis access. p. 114. In Wilson SE (ed): Vascular Access Principles and Practice. 3rd Ed. Mosby, St Louis, 1996

Kahn ML, Barboza RB, Kling GA, Heisel JE: Initial experience with percutaneous placement of the PAS Port implantable venous access device. J Vasc Interv Radiol 3:459, 1992

Lund GB, Lieberman RP, Haire WD et al: Translumbar inferior vena cava catheters for long-term venous access. Radiology 174:31, 1990

Lund GB, Trerotola SO, Scheel PF et al: Outcome of tunneled hemodialysis catheters placed by radiologists. Radiology 198:467, 1996

Mauro MA, Jaques PF: Radiologic placement of long-term central venous catheters: a review. J Vasc Interv Radiol 4:127, 1993

Openshaw KL, Picus D, Hicks ME et al: Interventional radiologic placement of Hohn central venous catheters: results and complications in 100 consecutive patients. J Vasc Interv Radiol 5:111, 1994

Trerotola SO: Interventional radiologic placement and management of infusion catheters. p. 229. In Savader SJ, Trerotola SO (eds): Venous Interventional Radiology with Clinical Perspectives. Thieme, New York, 1996

Trerotola SO, Savader SJ, Durham JD: Venous Interventions. Society of Cardiovascular and Interventional Radiology, Fairfax, VA, 1995

CHAPTER 13

Foreign Body Retrieval   MICHAEL A. BRAUN

The prolonged use of central venous catheters can rarely result in the complication of breakage and subsequent embolization of the catheter fragment. The catheter fragment usually lodges in the central veins, the right heart, or the pulmonary arteries. Intravascular foreign bodies can cause arrhythmias, perforation, sepsis, and thrombosis. The foreign body should be removed before these complications occur. The estimated mortality is high, ranging from 25 to 60 percent. Percutaneous retrieval should be attempted whenever feasible. Foreign body retrieval techniques are used to remove lost guidewires, broken intravascular devices, missile fragments, and misplaced embolization coils. Loop snares are used to reposition catheters, strip fibrin sheaths, and snare guidewires to gain both proximal and distal control of the wire.

It is important to study the location and position of the foreign body. Choice of vascular approach to the foreign body is determined by the position of the free end of the foreign body. A vascular sheath is always used and a large 7 to 10 French size is often necessary to accommodate the snared and usually folded foreign body. Numerous retrieval devices are available. Examples are Dormia stone retrieval baskets, Curry loop snares, grasping forceps, Nitinol goose neck snares, and deflecting guidewires. Pre-shaped catheters, balloon catheters, retrieval forceps, and deflecting guidewires can be used to reposition the free end of the foreign body more favorably for snaring. The Curry snare and the Nitinol goose neck snare are the most effective means of securely grabbing the free end of a catheter fragment. Stone retrieval baskets are best used for missile fragments and embolization coils.

Most foreign bodies can readily be removed using the Nitinol goose neck snare. The diameter of the loop comes in various sizes, ranging from 5 to 35 mm. The loop makes a 90° bend relative to the shaft of the wire. This facilitates passing the loop over the free end of the catheter fragment within the tubular-shaped vascular tree. Choice of loop size depends on the caliber of the vessel or chamber in which the foreign body is located. An introducing catheter is used to guide the loop to the foreign body. Fluoroscopic triangulation is important to determine the position of the loop relative to the long axis of the free end of the foreign body. The loop snare is passed over the free end of the foreign body, and the snare is tightened to lasso the object. A hemostat is placed on the snare's wire shaft at the end of the guiding catheter. This securely holds the loop closed around the snared object. The captured foreign body and snare are removed through the vascular sheath (Fig. 13.1). Large catheter fragments or doubled up fragments are pulled into the vascular sheath, and the entire assembly is removed as a unit.

Alternative techniques can be used if the proximal free end of the foreign body cannot be snared. A frequently successful alternative is to snare the distal end of the catheter fragment. If no free ends are available for snaring, the foreign body can be repositioned into a more favorable position. Curved-tip catheters (Rösch inferior mesenteric [RIM] or pigtail) or deflecting guidewires are ideal for this purpose. Lodged foreign bodies pose a more difficult problem. A combination of a hooked catheter and a snare can be used to free wedged objects or foreign bodies without a free end. The hooked catheter tip is placed around the foreign body and the tip snared. This maneuver can be used to move the lodged foreign body into a free position. Care must be exercised to avoid a vascular tear or perforation from excess traction. The most frequent complication of foreign body removal is induced cardiac arrhythmias. Foreign bodies must be carefully removed from the heart to avoid the potential for cardiac valve or papillary muscle damage.

Figure 13.1 (**A**) *A pigtail catheter is used to favorably reposition the venous access catheter fragment in the left pulmonary artery.* (**B**) *A goose neck snare has lassoed the free end of the foreign body.* (**C**) *The securely held foreign body has been carefully removed through the heart and into the inferior vena cava.* (**D**) *The catheter fragment is pulled into a large sheath within the right femoral puncture access.*

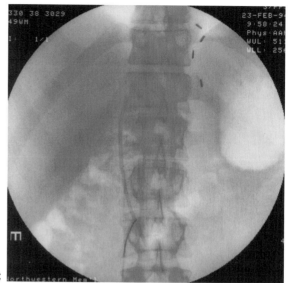

C

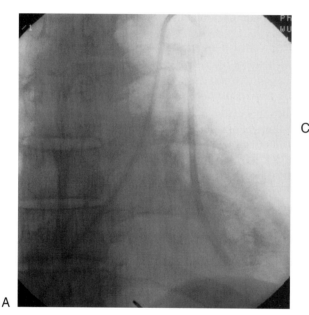

A

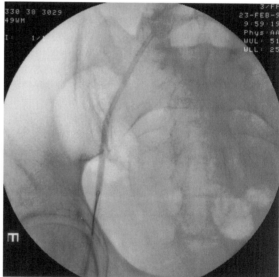

D

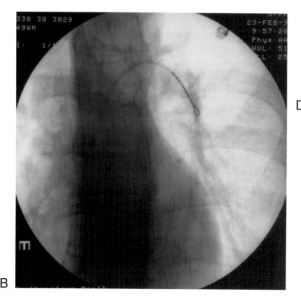

B

Suggested Reading

Yedlicka JW, Carlson JE, Hunter DW et al: Intravascular foreign body removal. p. 705. In Castenade-Zuniga (ed): Interventional Radiology. 2nd Ed. Vol. 2. Williams & Wilkins, Baltimore, 1992

CHAPTER 14

Venous Thrombolysis MICHAEL A. BRAUN

Deep venous thrombosis (DVT) is a common clinical problem whose treatment has changed relatively little in the last 35 years. Treatment for acute and chronic DVT typically consists of anticoagulation with intravenous heparin followed by oral coumadin. This standard therapy is directed at preventing propagation of the thrombosis and does not promote natural lysis of the thrombosis. Many patients tolerate acute DVT well, with the emphasis on anticoagulation therapy to prevent pulmonary embolism. The postphlebitic syndrome is the long-term sequela of DVT. The postphlebitic syndrome manifestations of venous claudication, extremity swelling, venous hypertension, and venous stasis ulcers are a source of significant debilitation, which develops only after a long latent period. These long-term symptoms are not addressed by the currently accepted therapy of anticoagulation to treat acute DVT. The ideal therapy would restore patency of the vein, spare valvular function, and prevent the complications of pulmonary embolism and postphlebitic syndrome.

The pathophysiology of venous thrombosis is still best described by Virchow's triad of endothelial injury, stasis of blood flow, and hypercoagulability of the blood. Almost all DVTs arise in the small veins of the calf, and 20 percent of affected patients continue to promulgate thrombus into the proximal deep veins. Only 5 percent of patients with calf vein DVT have symptoms. Approximately 40 to 50 percent of patients with larger, more extensive, above-the-knee DVT have signs and symptoms. DVT is characterized by three main complications: pulmonary emboli, chronic valvular insufficiency, and extremity pain and edema associated with venous hypertension. Postphlebitic syndrome is underappreciated in clinical practice because it takes many years to develop.

Most physicians lump all cases of deep venous thrombosis into a single entity based on the limited treatment options. Short segment, nonocclusive femoral thrombus is treated the same as extensive, occlusive iliofemoral thrombus. The acute and long-term consequences of these distinct conditions are different. It is useful to classify DVT into peripheral and central thromboses based on location. Central DVT includes iliofemoral, caval, and axillosubclavian venous segments. Central DVT has increased morbidity and mortality compared to peripheral. Thrombolytic therapy is best reserved for symptomatic central thromboses. Detractors of lytic therapy point to the poor reported success rates, the cost, and the increased risks involved based on studies that used peripheral or systemic infusions of streptokinase. Proponents argue that improved techniques, better patient selection, and elimination of postphlebitic syndrome give thrombolytic therapy a role in treatment of central DVT. Evidence is accumulating that catheter-directed thrombolysis techniques can successfully restore patency and preserve valve function with an acceptable risk profile. The combination of direct catheter infusion of urokinase into a central thrombosis combined with angioplasty and stenting of the inciting anatomic lesion offers a new and successful treatment option. A venous registry has been established in 40 centers across the United States. The registry's intent is to enroll prospectively successfully treated patients with urokinase fibrinolysis of iliofemoral thromboses to determine the long-term benefits of this treatment regimen. Long-term follow up is necessary to determine the reduction in the incidence of the postphlebitic syndrome.

The incidence of axillosubclavian vein thrombosis has been increasing mainly from secondary causes of thrombosis. Long-term central venous catheterizations and hemodialysis catheters are the primary etiologies. An example is oncology patients with long-term implantable ports who are at increased risk of thrombosis from the device and from the underlying hypercoagulability of their disease states. Primary thrombosis of the axillosubclavian veins occurs in young individuals who develop a DVT from a compressive anomaly in the thoracic outlet. This is termed the *Paget-Schroetter syndrome* or *effort-related thrombosis*.

Thrombolysis of axillosubclavian thrombosis is used in patients who have symptomatic conditions. Typical symptoms are arm swelling, facial edema, pain, and venous congestion. A venogram of the involved extremity is performed to document the extent of the thrombosis. The venographic access can be converted into the access site for thrombolysis. The access site vein must be large enough to accept a 5 to 6 French vascular sheath. The preferred access site is the basilic vein above the elbow. This may require ultrasound or venographic guidance to puncture. The venipuncture technique is similar to placing a peripheral inserted central catheter line. A Weinberg or angled-tip Glide catheter and a Glidewire are used to traverse the clot. Successful crossing of the thrombus is predictive of a successful outcome. A Mewissen catheter or other infusion catheter is placed into the thrombus. Urokinase is infused through the Touhy-Bourst catheter adapter. The dose is similar for peripheral arterial thrombolysis. The urokinase mixture is 1 million units in 250 ml of normal saline. The dose is 4,000 U/min for the first 4 hours followed by an infusion rate of 2,000 U/min. The progress of the thrombolysis is monitored by the patient's clinical status and venographic examina-

tions. Complete lysis generally takes 16 to 24 hours. A large thrombus burden usually requires a longer infusion period. Concomitant heparinization is performed to prevent re-thrombosis. The heparin dose is adjusted to elevate the partial thromboplastin time (PTT) to 1.5 times normal. The subsequent management following lysis is the key to the determination of a long-term success. If the venographic appearance of the vein is normal, only a short-term period of anticoagulation is necessary. Frequently, the underlying vein is abnormal, with irregularities and residual stenoses. This is best treated with angioplasty or stenting to prevent re-thrombosis (Fig. 14.1). For catheter-induced thrombosis it is usually necessary to remove the central catheter.

Patients with iliofemoral DVT are at significant risk for developing postphlebitic syndrome and frequently do not symptomatically respond to anticoagulation alone. Patient selection for catheter-directed therapy includes patients who have documented lower extremity venous thrombosis from the popliteal vein to the inferior vena cava. Preferably the thrombosis is limited to the iliofemoral venous segment. The thrombosis must be symptomatic. Contraindications include active bleeding, intracranial disease, recent eye operation

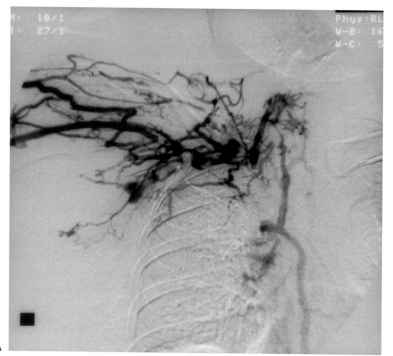

Figure 14.1 *Superior vena cava (SVC) syndrome.* **(A)** *Right upper extremity venogram demonstrating total venous occlusion of right brachiocephalic and SVC. (Figure continues.)*

A

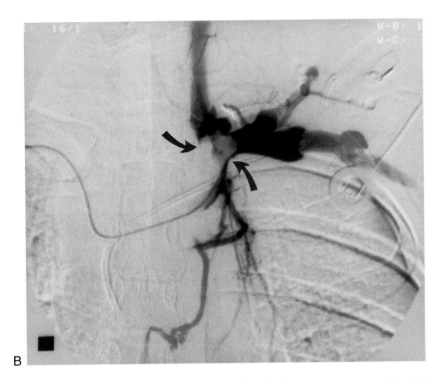

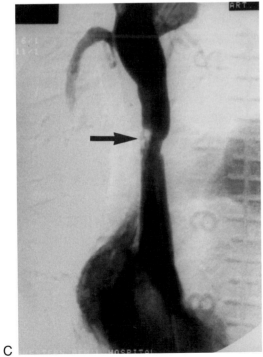

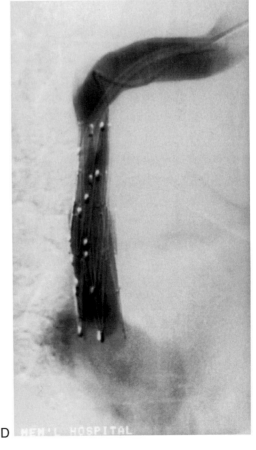

Figure 14.1 *(Continued)*
*(B) Left upper extremity veno-
gram demonstrating acute
thrombosis of left brachiocephalic vein. Arrows denote distal extent of thrombus. (C) An
overnight infusion of catheter-
directed thrombolysis dissolved
the caval occlusion and uncovered a high grade stenosis of the
mid SVC (arrow). (D) The stenosis did not respond to angioplasty alone, and a Gianturco Z-
stent was used to buttress open
the caval stenosis. This relieved
the patient's SVC syndrome
symptoms.*

B

C

D

(3 months), recent operation (less than 10 days), pregnancy, and recent delivery. Phlegmasia cerulea dolens (painful blue inflammation) is a rare and severe complication of iliofemoral DVT. There is a high association with a malignancy-induced hypercoagulable state. Extensive venous thrombosis causes arterial insufficiency from venous hypertension and increased pressures in the microcirculation. There is massive edema, a bluish discoloration of the extremity, and arterial ischemia. Prompt treatment is necessary before venous gangrene occurs, which is usually irreversible.

The symptomatic iliofemoral occlusive thrombosis is best approached from the popliteal or lessor saphenous vein. This allows the shortest route with the best mechanical advantage to push the guidewire through the iliofemoral thrombus working with the flow of the valves. Other approaches are the contralateral femoral or jugular vein (Fig. 14.2). Direct puncture into the

Figure 14.2 (A) An infusion catheter was placed within the left proximal femoral vein thrombosis from the jugular approach (arrow). (B) The popliteal vein was punctured, and an infusion catheter was placed in the distal superficial femoral vein (arrow). This maximizes the length of the thrombus infused. The infusion is through a 5 French multisidehole catheter at 2,000 U/hr divided between the two catheters. Most lyses can be achieved with administration of 5,000,000 units of urokinase. (Courtesy of Robert Beres, St. Luke's Medical Center, Milwaukee, WI.)

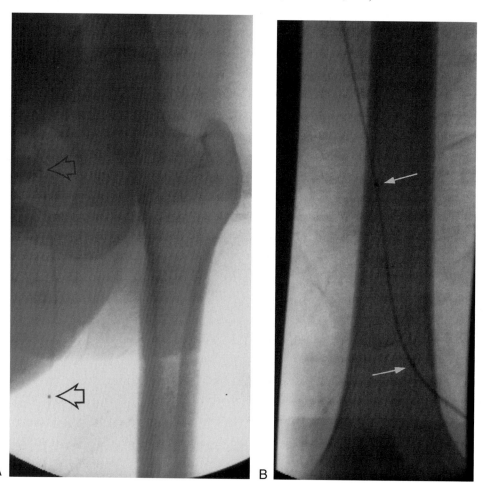

A   B

thrombus is avoided. Steerable catheters and Glide-wires are used to traverse the thrombus. If the thrombus cannot be crossed initially, an overnight infusion of urokinase may soften the clot and permit guidewire and catheter traversal. Urokinase is delivered with infusional techniques directly into the thrombus using a single infusion catheter or a coaxial infusion catheter and infusion guidewire system. It is recommended to mechanically disrupt the clot with angioplasty to expedite the thrombolytic therapy. Concomitant heparin is administered to maintain the PTT at 1.5 times normal. The fibrinogen level is maintained above 100 mg/dl. Follow-up venography is performed daily to assess the amount of thrombolysis and reposition the infusion catheter as necessary. Three days of thrombolytic therapy is considered maximal. In general, if the vein is completely free of thrombus, no furthers interventions are necessary, except for careful anticoagulation (Fig. 14.3). For the first 6 weeks following successful thrombolysis, it is crucial to keep the anticoagulation at 1.5 times normal to prevent rethrombosis. In patients who have had symptoms for 4 weeks or longer, there is an organization of the underlying thrombus and damage to the vein. Following a successful thrombolysis, the vein remains markedly narrowed and irregular. These damaged veins will not remain open if left

Figure 14.3 *Left iliofemoral venous thrombolysis. **(A)** Left leg venogram demonstrating extensive thrombosis of left iliofemoral vein. Note tram track sign (arrows). **(B)** There is complete occlusion of the superficial femoral artery and significant thrombus within the profunda femoris (arrow). (Figure continues.)*

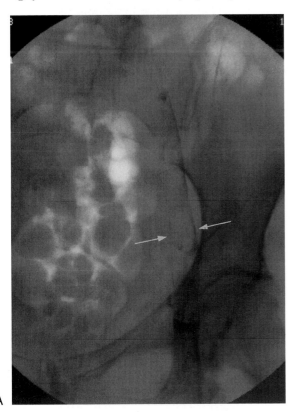

A

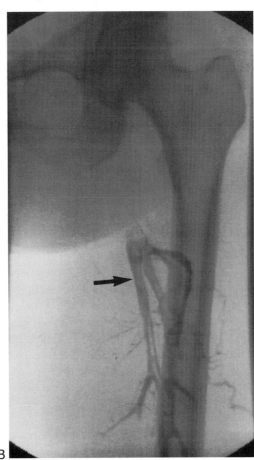

B

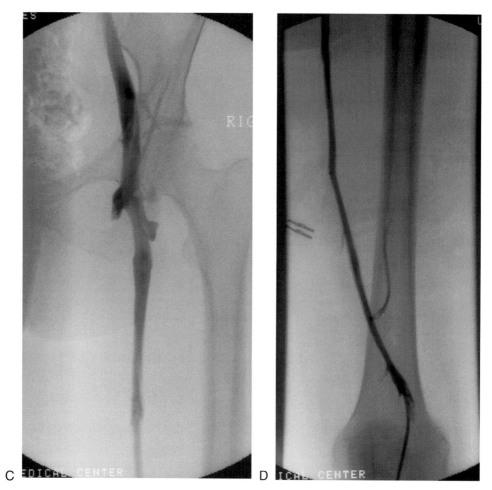

Figure 14.3 *(Continued)* **(C)** *A total of 4,000,000 units of urokinase were used to dissolve the iliofemoral thrombosis from a popliteal venous approach. The left femoral and iliac vein are patent.* **(D)** *The distal superficial femoral vein is patent following infusion. (Courtesy of Robert Beres, St. Luke's Medical Center, Milwaukee, WI.)*

untreated. Further intervention consists of placement of endoluminal stents. The current recommendation is to pre-dilate venous stenoses before placing stents. Stents are used above the inguinal ligament. Wallstents are used for long segment stenoses and in locations that utilize its flexibility. Palmaz stents are used for short segment stenoses.

A successfully treated patient requires long-term follow-up to assess the results and monitor for rethrombosis. This includes duplex ultrasound examinations at 6 weeks, 6 months, and 1 year. The duplex examination should measure the rate of flow through the segments of stented veins. A flow greater than 30 cm/second is considered adequate to prevent rethrombosis. If the flow is less than 30 cm/second, the stented and thrombolyzed venous segment is considered at high risk for re-thrombosis. These patients should be considered for creating of a distal arterial venous fistula. Anticoagulation is recommended for at least 4 to 6 months after successful lysis. A caval filter is not necessary during the treatment unless the patient has had recurrent pulmonary embolism.

Suggested Readings

Comerota AJ: Thrombolytic therapy for acute deep vein thrombosis. p.175. In Comerota AJ: Thrombolytic Therapy for Peripheral Vascular Disease. JB Lippincott, Philadelphia, 1995

Druy EM: Thrombolytic therapy for secondary axillosubclavian vein thrombosis. p. 209. In Comerota AJ (ed): Thrombolytic Therapy for Peripheral Vascular Disease. JB Lippincott, Philadelphia, 1995

Kumpe DA, Durham JD, Mann DJ: Thrombolysis and percutaneous transluminal angioplasty. p. 239. In Wilson SE (ed): Vascular Access Principles and Practice. 3rd Ed. Mosby, St Louis, 1996

Machledar HI: Thrombolytic therapy for acute primary axillosubclavian vein thrombosis. p. 197. In Comerota AJ (ed): Thrombolytic Therapy for Peripheral Vascular Disease. JB Lippincott, Philadelphia, 1995

Semba CP: Venous thrombolysis. J Vasc Interv Radiol Suppl 7:337, 1996

Semba CP, Dake MD: Iliofemoral deep venous thrombosis: aggressive therapy using catheter-directed thrombolysis. Radiology 191:487, 1994

CHAPTER 15

Management of Hemodialysis Access   MICHAEL A. BRAUN

More than 100,000 patients in the United States undergo long-term hemodialysis. Maintaining hemodialysis access requires the cooperative efforts of nephrologists, interventional radiologists, and surgeons. Successful management of chronic renal failure means that patients will require several arteriovenous (AV) fistulas in their lifetime, potentially exhausting the routine sites available. Interventional radiology techniques are important in the surveillance, maintenance, and salvage of hemodialysis access. Successful interventional strategies maximize access longevity and preserve veins for use as future access sites.

There are three types of vascular hemodialysis access: dual lumen catheters, native arteriovenous fistulas, and prosthetic bridge grafts. Hemodialysis catheters are the treatment of choice for acute renal failure and temporary hemodialysis access. Catheters can immediately be used for hemodialysis. The long-term use of external catheters is limited by the complications of infection, thrombosis, and stenosis. Native AV fistulas are considered the optimal vascular access. The Brescia-Cimino fistula is an end-to-side or side-to-side connection between the cephalic vein and the radial artery at the wrist (Fig. 15.1). The fistula requires a maturation period when the venous outflow dilates and develops thick walls capable of withstanding multiple venipunctures and resisting thrombosis. Once functioning, the native fistulas have the lowest complication rate and highest patency among vascular access alternatives. The 3-year patency rate is 60 to 70 percent, with some grafts surviving for 10 years. The major disadvantage is that not all patients have sufficient arteries or veins suitable for creation of an AV fistula. Prosthetic bridge grafts use a 6 to 8 mm diameter conduit of polytetrafluoroethylene (PTFE) to connect an artery to a vein. The graft may make a loop between adjacent artery and vein anastomoses or may make a straight bridge between distant anastomoses. Prosthetic bridge grafts are the majority of new vascular accesses created (80 percent). The 1-year patency rate of a PTFE graft is approximately 70 percent; the 2-year rate is 50 percent. The most common reason for a PTFE graft failure is thrombosis from progressive luminal narrowing at the venous anastomosis from intimal hyperplasia.

Preoperative venography is important in the evaluation of an upper extremity that has had a prior central venous line. The incidence of subclavian stenosis is clinically underestimated due to the lack of symptoms following placement of a subclavian central line. A prospective study by Surratt et al. demonstrated a 40 percent incidence of a subclavian stenosis in patients with prior temporary subclavian hemodialysis catheters. These clinically silent subclavian stenoses may cause venous hypertension and arm swelling after a fistula is created.

Hemodialysis access surveillance is a strategy to prolong graft patency by identifying stenoses before thrombosis occurs. Clinical screening methods are the physical examination, dialysis pressures, dialysis flow rates, and recirculation percentages. Loss of the palpable graft thrill, reduced dialysis flow rates (< 400 ml/min), and increased recirculation (> 15 percent) are clinical signs of a stenosis that warrant venographic investigation. Sullivan et al. advocate using a ratio of the pressure in the graft compared to the systemic pressure as a method of detecting a graft stenosis. A ratio of less than 0.4 has a 91 percent sensitivity in predicting a graft stenosis. Duplex sonography and contrast venography are used based on clinical suspicion of impending graft failure. Ultrasound is useful for confirming thrombosis,

Figure 15.1 *Examples of surgically created AV access. (A) Cimino-Brescia AV fistula. The radial artery is connected to the cephalic vein at the level of the wrist. (B) Loop forearm prosthetic bridge graft. The arterial anastomosis is on the medial aspect of the elbow into the brachial artery. The venous anastomosis is into the antecubital, basilic, or cephalic vein on the lateral aspect of the elbow. (C) Straight forearm graft. A straight prosthetic bridge graft extends from the distal radial artery to the basilic vein at the elbow. (D) Straight bridge graft between the brachial artery at the elbow and the axillary vein.*

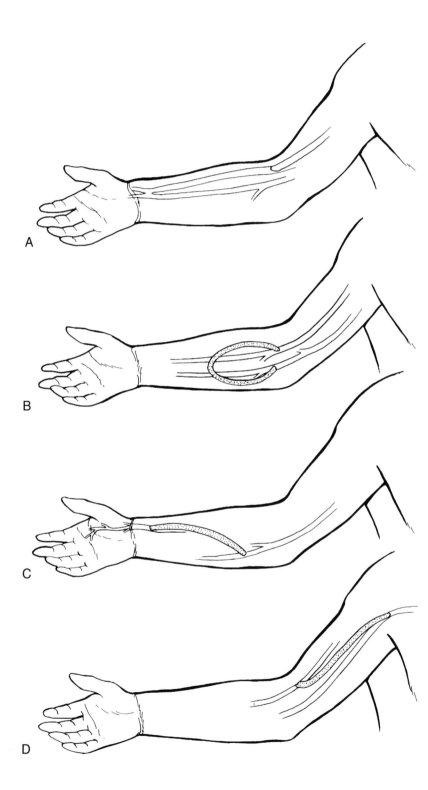

kinks, stenoses, and pseudoaneurysms but is limited in visualizing central stenoses and is time consuming to perform. AV fistulograms can be performed through dialysis graft access needles and provide a comprehensive assessment of the situation. The venous outflow is first examined by injections of 5 to 20 ml of contrast. The central veins including the superior vena cava must be evaluated. Complex angled views of the anastomoses may be necessary to unfold overlapping vessels. A tourniquet or blood pressure cuff is used to temporarily occlude venous outflow, allowing contrast to reflux past the arterial anastomosis. This is important in cases of steal phenomenon and poor arterial inflow. Only rarely is upper extremity arteriography required.

Angioplasty of graft stenosis is the treatment of choice and can add up to 1 year of access life span. Comparison of balloon angioplasty to surgical revision for treatment of graft stenosis documented equally effective results in terms of secondary graft patency. Angioplasty was less costly and preserved the venous outflow. The 1-year patency for intragraft stenosis is 18 percent, venous anastomotic stenosis is 40 to 50 percent, and central vein stenosis is 20 to 35 percent. Comparison of stented stenosis and angioplastied stenosis showed no significant difference in patency rates. Stents are best used for angioplasty failures from elastic recoil. In cases of intimal hyperplasia, stents may have worse results than angioplasty.

Graft thrombosis is usually caused by a venous anastomosis stenosis in the majority of the cases but can be caused by hypotension, dehydration, and compression. Early graft failures within 3 weeks of creation are technical failures best treated by surgical revision. Pharmacomechanical thrombolysis is highly effective in the primary management of thrombosed dialysis grafts. This method relies on a combination of pulse sprayed urokinase thrombolysis with mechanical disruption of any residual clot with an angioplasty balloon. The patient is premedicated with diphenhydramine hydrochloride, 50 mg, and acetaminophen, 2,000 mg, orally. The type of graft is determined by records and configuration of scars and needle puncture marks. The graft is punctured by palpation or ultrasound guidance. Micropuncture technique is preferred. The venous and arterial limbs are punctured in a retrograde fashion. The puncture sites are spaced to allow overlap of the infusion catheters. Two multisidehole infusion catheters are placed in a criss-crossing configuration within the graft (Fig. 15.2).

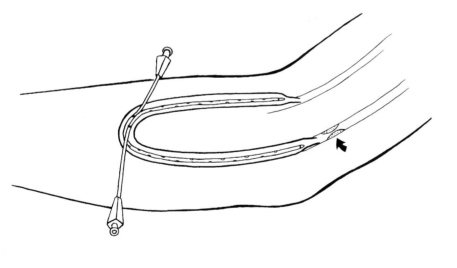

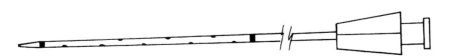

Figure 15.2 *Criss-crossing infusion catheters have been placed in the apex of a forearm loop graft to cover the entire length of the graft. Note that the arterial anastomosis is usually narrower than the wider venous anastomosis. A stenosis is present at the venous anastomosis causing the graft to fail (arrow). The bottom depicts a multisidehole infusion catheter. These catheters are placed over a wire with the wire occluding the distal end hole. Infusion is via a Y connector.*

One catheter is directed toward the arterial limb, and the other is placed in the venous limb. Appropriate length catheters are positioned to infuse the entire length of the graft. A 20 ml mixture of 250,000 units of urokinase, 5,000 units of heparin, and saline is prepared. This mixture is pulse sprayed in volumes of 0.5 to 1.0 ml directly into the thrombus via both catheters over 10 to 20 minutes. The catheter directed toward the venous anastomosis is removed over a guidewire and a short 7 French sheath placed into the graft. The venous anastomosis stenosis is dilated with a 6 to 8 mm balloon catheter to establish outflow (Fig. 15.3). Residual clot within the graft is macerated with the balloon catheter. This usually results in re-establishment of flow through the graft. Sometimes a small plug of thrombus remains at the arterial anastomosis. This must be gently angioplastied and any thrombus fragments coaxed into the graft to avoid arterial emboliza-

tion. A completion fistulogram is performed and the central venous outflow carefully examined for a distant stenosis. The vascular catheters or sheaths can be replaced with similar sized hemodialysis catheters for immediate hemodialysis.

The advantage of thrombolysis over surgery for treatment of graft thrombosis is that the thrombolysis technique allows immediate postprocedure hemodialysis, maximizes graft life spans, eliminates the need for a temporary hemodialysis catheter, and preserves veins as sites for future fistulas. The most common complication of transcatheter therapy, perigraft hemorrhage, is managed with manual compression with a Gelfoam pledget and a surgical sponge pad. Arterial embolization can result from clot fragmentation at the arterial anastomosis by catheter or guidewire manipulations. Care must be taken when approaching this anastomosis.

Figure 15.3 *(A) Criss-crossing thrombolysis infusion catheters have been placed into a loop forearm graft. The thrombus was dissolved with pulse spraying 250,000 units urokinase and 5,000 units heparin into the thrombus over 10 minutes. (B) Post-thrombolysis fistulogram demonstrating long segment stricture of the venous anastomosis (arrows). (Figure continues.)*

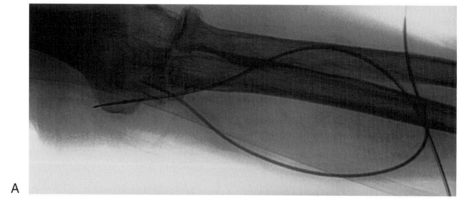
A

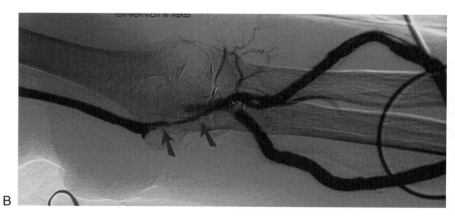
B

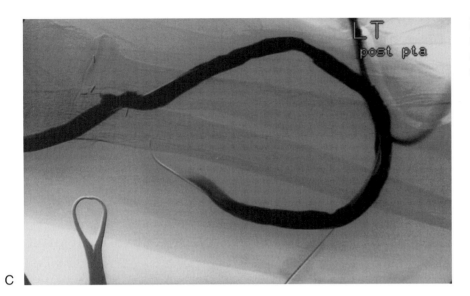

C

Figure 15.3 (*Continued*) (*C*) *An 8 mm angioplasty eliminated the venous anastomotic stricture.*

Suggested Readings

Cohen MA, Kumpe DA, Durham JD: Thrombolytic therapy and angioplasty for treatment of clotted and failing hemodialysis access. p. 329. In Comerota AJ (ed): Thrombolytic Therapy for Peripheral Vascular Disease. JB Lippincott, Philadelphia, 1995

Gray RJ, Horton KM, Dolmatch BL et al: Use of Wall-stents for hemodialysis access related venous stenoses and occlusions untreatable with balloon angioplasty. Radiology 195:479, 1995

Kanterman RY, Vesely TM, Pilgrim TK et al: Dialysis access grafts: anatomic location of venous stenosis and results of angioplasty. Radiology 195:135, 1995

Schwartz CL, McBrayer CV, Sloan JH et al: Thrombosed dialysis grafts: comparison of treatment with transluminal angioplasty and surgical revision. Radiology 194:337, 1995

Sullivan KL, Besarab A, Bonn J et al: Hemodynamics of failing dialysis grafts. Radiology 186:867, 1993

Surratt RS, Picus D, Hicks ME et al: The importance of the preoperative evaluation of the subclavian vein in dialysis access planning. AJR 156:623, 1991

Vorwerk D, Guenther RW, Mann H et al: Venous stenosis and occlusion in hemodialysis shunts: follow-up results of stent placement in 65 patients. Radiology 195:140, 1995

CHAPTER 16

Transjugular Intrahepatic Portosystemic Shunt MICHAEL A. BRAUN

Portal hypertension decompression through a percutaneously established communication between the hepatic and portal veins was first conceived of by Rösch in 1969. The technique was first applied to humans in 1982 by Colapinto. The communication was made durable by the advent of expandable metallic vascular stents to maintain the patency of the tract between the portal and hepatic veins. This concept of creating a fistulous tract between the branches of the hepatic and portal veins has been termed transjugular intrahepatic portosystemic shunt (TIPS).

Portal hypertension is the result of obstruction of the portal venous outflow. This can occur at many different sites either within or outside of the liver. Normal portal pressure is between 5 and 10 mmHg and is usually 3 to 6 mmHg greater than right atrial pressure. Mild portal hypertension is 10 to 15 mmHg, moderate is 15 to 20 mmHg, and severe is greater than 20 mmHg. Varices do not develop until the gradient is 12 mmHg. Portal hypertension is associated with splenomegaly, ascites, hepatic encephalopathy, and coagulopathies.

The treatment of life-threatening variceal hemorrhage in patients with portal hypertension secondary to cirrhosis is difficult. The only definitive therapy is liver transplantation, but the shortage of donor organs makes this therapy prohibitive for most patients. Operative portosystemic shunting has the lowest rate of re-bleeding. Reported mortality rates exceed 50 percent in most series describing the results of emergency portosystemic shunts. This high mortality rate has made nonoperative management the recommended initial therapy. Endoscopic treatments of sclerotherapy or variceal banding are successful in controlling acutely bleeding esophageal varices in 90 percent of patients. More than 50 percent of patients re-bleed because sclerotherapy does not address the underlying problem of portal hypertension. Sclerotherapy cannot treat bleeding gastric or gastrointestinal varices. Mechanical tamponade of esophageal varices with a Sengstaken-Blakemore tube and pharmacologic vasoconstriction with vasopressin or somatostatin are temporizing methods of conservative treatment.

The TIPS procedure is an attractive alternative to surgically created portosystemic shunts because of the lower morbidity and mortality. TIPS effectively decompresses the portal hypertension, and the shunt diameter can be tailored in size to reduce the portosystemic gradient to a safe level. TIPS shunts are created to prevent variceal re-bleeding and treat cases refractory to endoscopic therapy. Indications for TIPS include medically intractable ascites, bridge to transplantation, and significant variceal hemorrhage that does not respond to medical management and endoscopic sclerotherapy. The relative indications for TIPS are treatment of hepatorenal syndrome, Budd-Chiari syndrome, and portal vein occlusion. The long-term efficacy and role of TIPS have yet to fully evolve. The initial enthusiasm given to TIPS shunts has been tempered by the high incidence of stenoses complicating TIPS shunts and the potential worsening of hepatic encephalopathy.

The Child-Pugh classification system was created in the 1950s to assess the patient's prognostic risk for undergoing a portosystemic shunt (Table 16.1). The classification system is valuable for stratifying patients according to risk to determine the prognosis and select patients for treatment. The risk factors are the clinical findings of ascites, encephalopathy, nutritional status, and the laboratory data of bilirubin, albumin, and prothrombin time (PT). A good risk patient (Child's class A) has essentially normal clinical and laboratory data.

Table 16.1 *Child's classification of cirrhosis*

Criteria	A	B	C
Serum bilirubin (mg/100 ml)	< 2.0	2.0–3.0	> 3.0
Serum albumin (g/100 ml)	> 3.5	3.0–3.5	< 3.0
Ascites	None	Easily controlled	Not easily controlled
Encephalopathy	None	Minimal	Advanced
Nutrition	Excellent	Good	Poor

Child's class B patients have mild derangements of their laboratory values and no evidence of hepatic encephalopathy. Child's class C patients have hepatic encephalopathy, ascites, and marked elevations in the laboratory values. A Child's class C patient has bilirubinemia of greater than 3, hypoalbuminemia, and mildly elevated PT. Child's class C patients who have variceal hemorrhages have a very high surgical mortality rate following portosystemic shunt creation of up to 80 to 90 percent.

Two complete TIPS sets are available. The Ring set (Cook, Inc., Bloomington, IN) is a modified Colapinto transjugular needle biopsy kit. The kit includes an angled-tip vascular access sheath, Colapinto needle, Colapinto needle protective 9 French catheter, selective catheters, and guidewires. The Colapinto needle is used to create the tract between the hepatic and portal vein. The 16-gauge Colapinto needle has an angled tip with reverse bevel to facilitate passage through the 9 French catheter. The arrow on the needle hub indicates the direction of the needle curve. The Rösch set (Cook, Inc., Bloomington, IN) replaces the Colapinto needle with a Rösch-Uchida transjugular needle. This flexible needle trocar catheter system is designed to pass easily through the fibrotic liver.

The most difficult step in performing a TIPS is creating the tract between the right hepatic vein and the right portal vein. The portal vein should be imaged before the procedure to confirm patency. Several techniques have been used to aid and direct portal vein puncture. Most authors have used blind puncture, directing the Colapinto needle anteriorly and inferiorly. Several unique techniques have been advanced to aid in portal vein catheterization. Examples are wedged portography with contrast and carbon dioxide, percutaneous portal vein catheterization, hepatic artery catheterization with portography, nasobiliary stent, and ultrasound guidance. The technique developed at Northwestern was percutaneous portal vein catheterization via a patent paraumbilical vein. A search is made for a recanalized paraumbilical vein with ultrasound just above the umbilicus. The paraumbilical vein is catheterized using ultrasound-guided micropuncture technique. A 5 French pigtail catheter is placed within the portal vein to aid in targeting the portal vein during creation of the TIPS tract (Fig. 16.1).

The initial step is to puncture the right internal jugular vein. The angled-tip 10 French sheath combined with the 9 French sheath are guided into the right or middle hepatic vein over a guidewire. The right hepatic vein is preferred. The Colapinto needle is advanced through the sheath over a guidewire. It helps to puncture the right hepatic vein centrally near the junction of the 11th rib and vertebral body. The Colapinto needle is rotated to aim inferior and anterior toward the anticipated location of the portal vein (Fig. 16.2). The needle is jabbed into the liver parenchyma approximately 3 to 4 cm. There is significant resistance to passage of the needle through cirrhotic liver due to the periportal fibrosis induced by cirrhosis. A 10 ml syringe partially filled with contrast is attached to the needle. The needle is slowly withdrawn while suction is applied. When blood is aspirated, a small amount of contrast is injected to ascertain position of the needle within the portal venous system. A guidewire is passed into the portal vein. If the guidewire is directed into the distal portal venous tree, the floppy tip Bentson guidewire is buckled to reverse its direction into the central portal vein. The needle and sheath are advanced over the guidewire dilating the parenchymal tract and seating the sheath into the parenchymal tract. A 5 French pigtail catheter is placed into the portal vein. Pressures are measured in the portal vein and right atrium. This establishes the portal gradient. A transjugular portogram is performed using an injection rate of 10 ml/sec for 30 ml of total contrast (Fig. 16.3).

The parenchymal tract is dilated to 8 mm in diameter with an angioplasty balloon. The length of the tract is estimated, and an appropriate length 10 to 12 mm diameter Wallstent is placed across the tract and deployed to bridge the fistula created between the portal and hepatic veins. It is necessary to dilate the stent once it is employed within the parenchymal tract. Portal pressures and portography are performed to assess the position and hemodynamic result of the stent. One

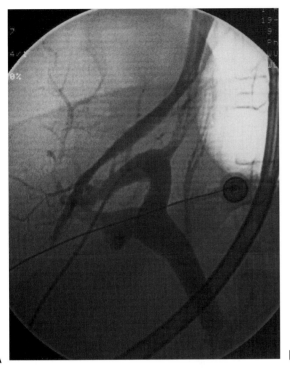
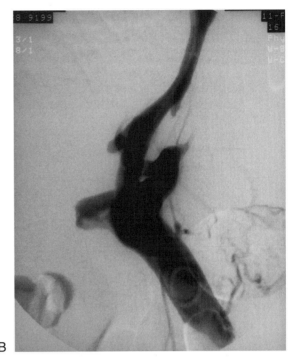

A   B

Figure 16.1 *(**A**) Simultaneous right hepatic venogram and paraumbilical por-*
togram. This lateral view demonstrates the relative positions of the right hepatic
vein and portal vein. In this case, the needle was directed inferior and slightly
*anterior to create a TIPS shunt. (**B**) Same patient showing successful creation of a*
TIPS shunt. Note the diversion of flow through the shunt and the reduction in
flow in the distal branches of the portal vein.

advantage of TIPS is the ability to optimize the size of the shunt. The goal is to reduce the gradient sufficiently to eliminate variceal hemorrhage without diverting flow entirely from the liver (Fig. 16.4). If the portosystemic gradient is > 15 mmHg and varices are visualized on the portogram, the stent can be dilated to 10 or 12 mm in diameter. If the gradient remains borderline elevated (12 to 20 mmHg), the residual varices can be selectively catheterized and embolized with Gianturco coils or Gelfoam. If a gradient greater than 20 mmHg remains, a second TIPS shunt can be created to further lower the portal hypertension.

The morbidity and mortality compares favorably with operative portosystemic shunts. The direct procedural mortality is estimated to range between 2 and 5 percent. The 30 day mortality ranges from 40 to 45 percent depending on the patient's underlying risk factors. Following a successful TIPS procedure, the patient is

carefully monitored for the hemodynamic changes following decompression of portal hypertension. The TIPS shunt elevates the right atrial filling pressures, and pulmonary edema is a potential complication. Post-TIPS fevers occur in up to 10 percent of patients. TIPS shunts are preferably placed in patients who have no signs of infection.

Hepatic encephalopathy and shunt stenosis are the long-term complications that can occur as a consequence of TIPS. Hepatic encephalopathy is reported to occur in 15 to 25 percent of patients. It usually can be controlled medically with lactulose or oral antibiotics. The long-term durability of shunts is limited by the high incidence of stenosis. The stenosis usually occurs in the hepatic venous side of the stent. Approximately 50 to 75 percent of shunts undergo stenosis or occlusion. Stenoses are surveyed for by frequent re-evaluation of the TIPS shunt with ultrasound and venography.

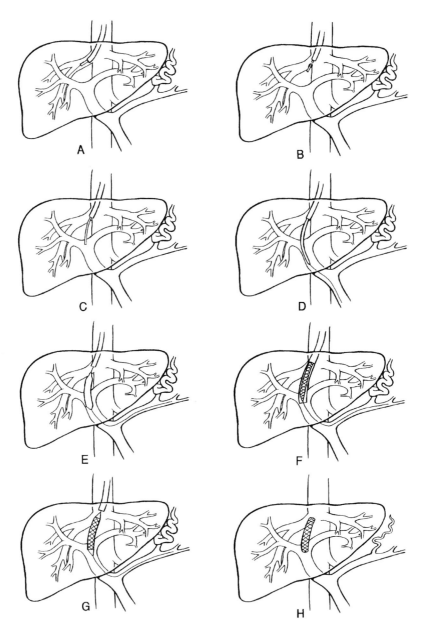

Figure 16.2 *TIPS procedural steps. (A) The 10 French angled tip sheath is inserted over the catheter and guidewire into the right hepatic vein. (B) The Colapinto needle is inserted over the wire into the right hepatic vein through the protective sheath. The needle is aimed anteriorly and inferiorly. (C) The needle is inserted 3 to 5 cm into the liver parenchyma. The syringe is attached to the needle, and the aspiration of blood confirms the position within the portal vein. (D) A guidewire is inserted into the portal vein. The sheath is inserted into the parenchymal tract. A 5 French pigtail catheter is placed into the portal vein. Contrast portography and pressure measurements are made. (E) The parenchymal tract is dilated to 8 mm in diameter. (F) The appropriate length Wallstent is positioned across the parenchymal tract. (G) The Wallstent is dilated to 8 mm in diameter. Repeat pressure measurements and portography are performed. (H) Successful decompression of portal hypertension with elimination of coronary vein varices. (Modified from Zemel G, Katzen BT, Becker GJ et al: Percutaneous transjugular portogyatemic shunt. JAMA 266: 390, 1991, with permission.)*

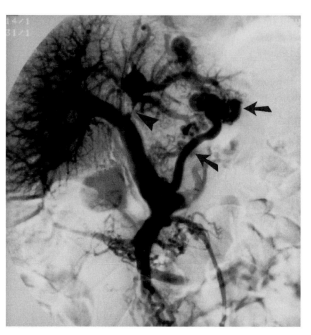

Figure 16.3 *Transhepatic portogram demonstrating large coronary vein feeding gastric and esophageal varices (arrows). Note tight stenosis in left portal vein (arrowhead).*

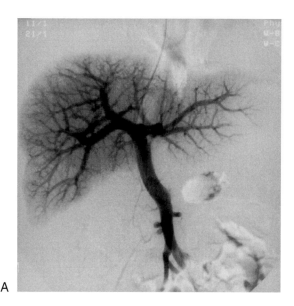

A

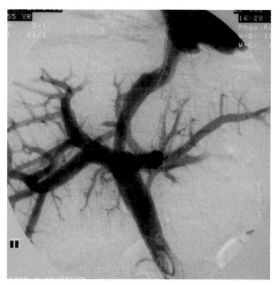

B

Figure 16.4 *(A) Transhepatic portogram in patient with intractable ascites. Note absence of variceal filling and relative normal appearance of portal vein branches. (B) An 8 mm TIPS shunt was created between portal vein and right hepatic vein. The flow through the shunt has diminished the capillary staining of the portogram compared to the pre-shunt study.*

The strictures are treated by balloon angioplasty and placement of additional stents. The strictures are usually due to neointimal hyperplasia. This problem is the greatest challenge to the long-term durability of TIPS. Other complications include separation, dislodgement, or migration of the stents.

After placement of the TIPS, a baseline duplex and color ultrasound of the shunt are performed. The duplex ultrasound is repeated at 3-month intervals. The maximum velocity through the shunt should be carefully analyzed by duplex ultrasound. The flow should be 100 to 300 cm/sec. A stenosis is suspected if the maximum velocity decreases by 25 percent compared to the baseline study or the maximum velocity is less than 60 cm/second. Secondary ultrasound findings of a TIPS stenosis is reaccumulation of ascites and re-formation of portosystemic collaterals. At 6-month intervals, transjugular portography is performed with hemodynamic pressure measurements to further assess patency and function of the TIPS shunt.

It is well documented that liver function deteriorates from flow diversion through the shunt. This is seen following both TIPS and surgical portosystemic shunts. It is thought to be secondary to the diversion of flow through the shunts with deprivation of flow into the liver. In most patients, with time the hepatic artery compensates loss of flow to the liver from the shunt. A small percentage of patients may undergo further hepatic decompensation. In these cases the shunt is closed by embolization or thrombosis.

The placement of TIPS shunts in patients who have undergone liver transplantation can optimize care of patients who have liver failure. Liver transplantation candidates require precise positioning of the TIPS shunt. TIPS shunts that extend into the main portal vein or the inferior vena cava may interfere with the surgical anastomoses required during liver transplantation. It is critical to place a totally intrahepatic TIPS shunt in candidates for liver transplantation.

Suggested Readings

Colapinto RF, Stronell RD, Birch SJ et al: Creation of an intrahepatic portosystemic shunt with a Grüntzig balloon catheter. Can Med Assoc J 126:267, 1982

Coldwell DM, Ring EJ, Rees CR et al: Multicenter investigation of the role of transjugular intrahepatic portosystemic shunt in management of portal hypertension. Radiology 196:335, 1995

Foshager MC, Ferral H, Nazarian GK et al: Duplex sonography after transjugular intrahepatic portosystemic shunt (TIPS): normal hemodynamic findings and efficacy in predicting shunt patency and stenosis. AJR 165:1, 1995

Kerlan RK, LaBerge JM, Gordon RL, Ring EJ: Transjugular intrahepatic portosystemic shunts: current status. AJR 164:1059, 1995

LaBerge JM, Durham JD: Portal Hypertension: Options for Diagnosis and Treatment. Society of Cardiovascular and Interventional Radiology, Fairfax, VA, 1995

LaBerge JM, Ring EJ, Gordon RL et al: Creation of transjugular intrahepatic portosystemic shunts with the Wallstent endoprosthesis: results in 100 patients. Radiology 187:413, 1993

Rees CR, Niblett RL, Lee SP, et al: Use of carbon dioxide as a contrast medium for transjugular intrahepatic portosystemic shunt procedures. J Vasc Interv Radiol 5:383, 1994

Radosevich PM, Ring EJ, LaBerge JM et al: Transjugular intrahepatic portosystemic shunts in patients with portal vein occlusion. Radiology 186:523, 1993

Richter GM, Noeldge G, Roeren TK, Kauffmann GW: Five-year results of TIPS: technical standard and long-term clinical efficacy. J Vasc Interv Radiol 5:20, 1994

Ring EJ, Lake JR, Roberts JP et al: Percutaneous intrahepatic portosystemic shunts to control variceal bleeding prior to liver transplantation. Ann Intern Med 166:304, 1992

Rösch J, Hanafee WN, Snow H: Transjugular portal venography and radiologic portocaval shunt: an experimental study. Radiology 92:1112, 1969

Savader SJ, Trerotola SO: Venous Interventional Radiology with Clinical Perspectives. Thieme, New York, 1996

Zemel G, Becker GJ, Bancroft JW et al: Technical advances in transjugular intrahepatic portosystemic shunts. Radiographics 12:615, 1992

Zemel G, Katzen BT, Becker GJ et al: Percutaneous transjugular portosystemic shunt. JAMA 266:390, 1991

CHAPTER 17

Inferior Vena Cava Filters

MICHAEL A. BRAUN

The indications for an inferior vena cava (IVC) filter are pulmonary embolism or deep venous thrombosis in a patient with a contraindication to anticoagulation and recurrent pulmonary embolism despite adequate anti-coagulation. Relative indications include prophylactic placement before major surgery and placement in trauma patients or other patients who are considered at high risk for pulmonary embolism. A free-floating thrombus within the iliac or femoral vein is considered high risk for embolization and a relative indication.

Five filter devices are currently available for use: (1) the stainless steel Greenfield filter, (2) the titanium Greenfield filter, (3) the Vena Tech filter, (4) the Bird's Nest filter, and (5) the Simon Nitinol filter. The choice of which filter to insert depends on the size of the cava, route of insertion, physician familiarity, and availability of the device. All the currently available filters can be inserted percutaneously. The ease and safety of percutaneous filter insertion have resulted in a more liberal and frequent reliance on these devices. Filters should be inserted only with appropriate forethought and evaluation of the patient's clinical situation. An inferior cavogram is performed before every filter insertion to ensure patency of the IVC and determine position of the renal veins. A ruler is placed along the left side of the lumbar vertebral bodies to assist in fluoroscopic deployment of the filter.

The Greenfield filter is an inverted cone-shaped device (Fig. 17.1). The apex of the filter cone is placed within the laminar flow region of the IVC. The filter is designed to trap emboli greater than 3 mm in diameter. It is secured to the IVC in a planar fashion. The Greenfield filter has the longest follow-up of all the filters, and its performance is considered the yardstick by which all other filters are judged. It has the highest patency rate. Filter tilting of greater than 15° may cause inadequate filtration or indicate perforation of the caval wall.

There are three models of Greenfield filters. The stainless steel Greenfield requires a 24 French sheath

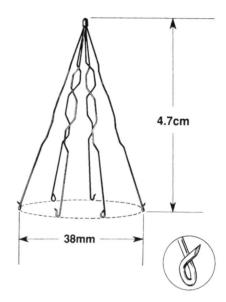

Figure 17.1 *The titanium Greenfield filter is a cone-shaped filter with six legs. The pre-curved hook fixes the legs to the caval wall and provides a wide base to minimize perforation. (Courtesy of Meditech, Watertown, MA.)*

insertion, which has traditionally been done via a surgical cutdown. The stainless steel Greenfield has the longest follow-up and performance results accumulated thus far. A 12 French over-the-wire stainless steel and 12 French titanium Greenfield systems are available for percutaneous insertion. The Greenfield filter is introduced through either a jugular or femoral approach. A 12 French combined sheath dilator is inserted and positioned relative to the renal veins. From the femoral approach, the sheath is placed just above the renal veins. The dilator is removed and the sheath flushed and locked to its hub. The carrier catheter with the pre-loaded titanium Greenfield filter is inserted into the sheath. The tip of the carrier capsule is positioned at the intended implantation site, which is just below the level of the lowest renal vein. The sheath is retracted by gently pulling it back until the hub of the sheath meets the luerlock connector at the distal end of the handle. When the sheath is retracted and locked to the handle, the carrier capsule will be fully extended beyond the distal end of the sheath. A fluoroscopic confirmation of the position of the device relative to the renal veins is made. Any final adjustments of the position of the filter's location are made. The filter is deployed by unlocking the tab on the handle and slowly sliding the tab down the release track. This automated device retracts the capsule containing the Greenfield filter and releases it into the intended position (Fig. 17.2). The position is confirmed by a follow-up cavogram and the sheath is subsequently removed.

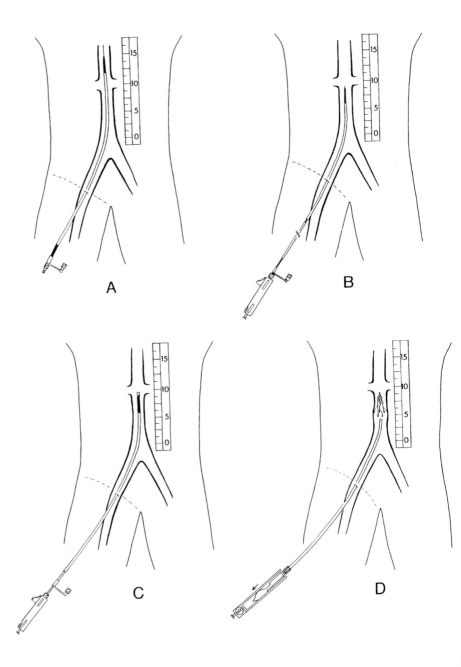

Figure 17.2 *Greenfield filter technique.* **(A)** *The cavogram and ruler are used to mark the position of the renal veins. The introducer sheath and dilator are advanced over the wire beyond the implantation site.* **(B)** *The carrier capsule containing the pre-loaded titanium Greenfield filter is introduced through the sheath to the implantation site.* **(C)** *The sheath is connected to the handle of the carrier capsule. The luerlock connection is secured. The filter in the carrier capsule now extends above the sheath tip. Final positioning is confirmed by fluoroscopy.* **(D)** *The filter is released by sliding the tab on the carrier capsule handle.*

The Vena Tech filter is an inverted cone design that has side struts attached to the cone legs (Fig. 17.3). The Vena Tech filter engages the wall of the IVC in a cylindrical fashion. The side struts are designed to align the cone within the center of the vena cava. The struts reduce the incidence of caval penetration. The Vena Tech filter can be introduced from a femoral or jugular approach. It can be deployed in vena cavas measuring up to 28 mm in diameter. It is introduced through a 12 French sheath. The radio-opaque marker of the sheath is placed in the anticipated position of the filter's apex. It is usually positioned 5 mm below the lowest renal vein. The external marker collar on the sheath is advanced to visually mark the sheath's position relative to the groin puncture site. The inner dilator of the sheath is removed. The pre-flushed syringe containing the filter is attached to the sheath and the filter injected. The filter is advanced through the sheath with the blunt end of the pushing catheter. The pushing catheter contains a pre-marked line to indicate that the filter is in the immediate predeployment position. The position of the filter is confirmed fluoroscopically before release. The Vena Tech is released by a pin-and-pull technique. The pushing catheter is held firmly in position while the outer sheath is smoothly withdrawn (Fig. 17.4). Following filter deployment, a cavogram is performed to document the filter's position.

The Bird's Nest filter is a random mesh of filtration wire that is placed into the lumen of the cava (Fig. 17.5). The mesh does not require the precise coaxial placement that cone-shaped filters require. The Bird's Nest filter can be placed in cava up to 40 mm in diameter, which is the device's major advan-

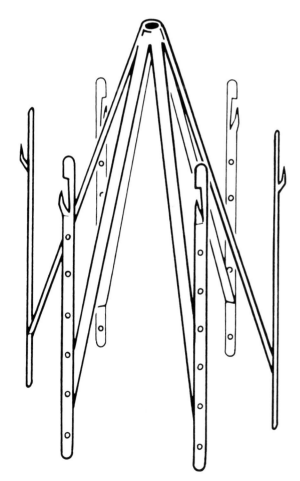

Figure 17.3 *The Vena Tech filter. The filter has a cone shape with attached side legs to center the device and prevent caval perforation. (Courtesy of B. Braun, Evanston, IL.)*

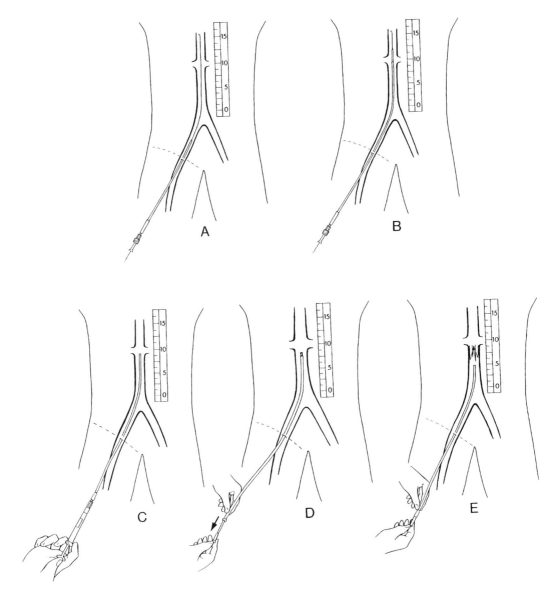

Figure 17.4 *Vena Tech deployment. (**A**) The delivery sheath and dilator are introduced over a guidewire. (**B**) The tip of the sheath is positioned 5 mm below the renal veins. (**C**) The dilator and wire are removed. The filter is loaded into the sheath by injecting via the loading syringe. The filter must be loaded in the proper orientation for femoral or jugular deployment. (**D**) The blunt end pushing device advances the filter through the sheath to the implantation site. The position is confirmed before release. Release is by pin-and-pull technique. The pushing catheter is held stationary while the outer sheath is withdrawn. (**E**) The pin-and-pull technique releases the filter at the implantation site. A contrast injection confirms position.*

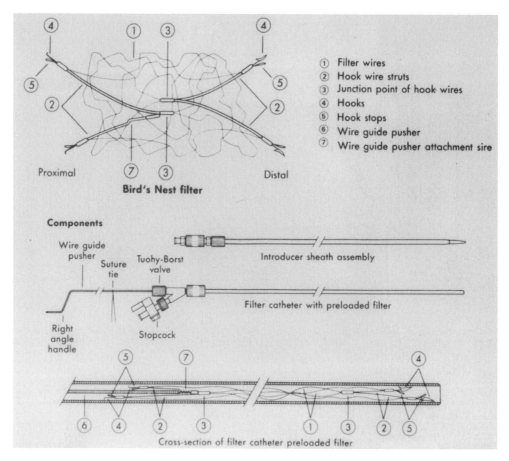

① Filter wires
② Hook wire struts
③ Junction point of hook wires
④ Hooks
⑤ Hook stops
⑥ Wire guide pusher
⑦ Wire guide pusher attachment sire

Proximal   Distal

Bird's Nest filter

Components

Wire guide pusher

Suture tie

Tuohy-Borst valve

Introducer sheath assembly

Right angle handle

Stopcock

Filter catheter with preloaded filter

Cross-section of filter catheter preloaded filter

Figure 17.5 *Bird's Nest filter. Filtration is by a free formed wire mesh in the vessel lumen anchored by proximal and distal hook wire struts. (Courtesy of Cook, Inc., Bloomington, IN.)*

tage. The other choice for megacavas is bilateral common iliac cone-shaped filters. The disadvantage of the Bird's Nest is the complex maneuvers required to deploy the device. A 12 French sheath dilator system is placed into the cava, preferably from the right common femoral vein. The sheath dilator system is advanced to the level of the renal veins. The dilator is removed and replaced by an 11 French pre-loaded introducer catheter, which contains the Bird's Nest apparatus. The 11 French introducer catheter is advanced fully into the 12 French sheath and locked in place. The proximal renal struts are exposed and positioned below the renal vein orifices. With the pusher wire fixed in its stationary position, the sheath assembly is withdrawn to the dark mark on the pusher wire. This motion releases

the proximal struts to engage into the wall of the infrarenal IVC. These proximal struts are set into the wall of the cava with a 1 to 3 mm forward-and-backward motion. The introducer and sheath assembly is slowly withdrawn 1 to 5 cm. This exposes the filtration wires, which are compacted into the cava by slowly advancing the catheter assembly. This forward-and-backward motion is repeated until the entire filtration wire is deployed within the cava. The distal struts of the Bird's Nest filter are then released. The juncture points of the distal struts are positioned so that they overlap with the proximal struts slightly. With the guidewire pusher fixed, the catheter assembly is withdrawn until the distal struts are released and become anchored into the cava wall. The guide-

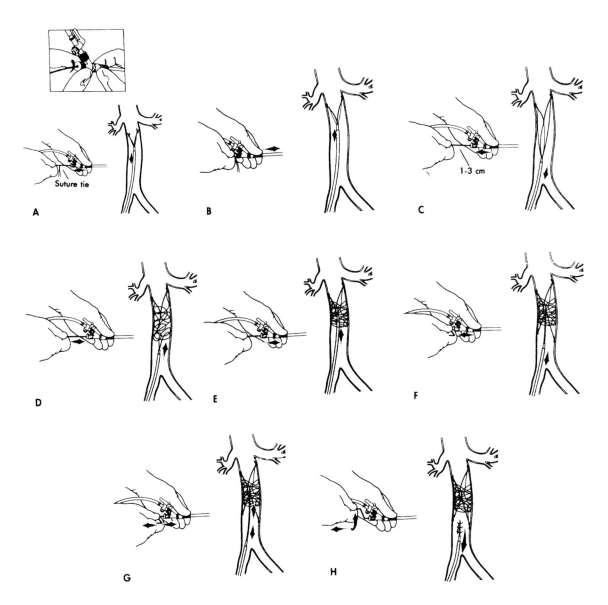

Figure 17.6 *Gianturco Bird's Nest filter.* **(A)** *The 12 French sheath/dilator is positioned below renal veins. The dilator and guidewire are removed. The 11 French introducer catheter is advanced into the sheath and locked into position. The proximal struts are released by loosening the hemostasis valve and withdrawing the sheath catheter assembly to the mark.* **(B)** *The proximal struts are anchored into the wall with a tiny forward backward motion.* **(C)** *The catheter sheath assembly is withdrawn over the pusher wire 1 to 5 cm.* **(D)** *The filter wires are discharged by advancing the guidewire pusher into the catheter sheath assembly. The guidewire pusher is advanced until the proximal junction point of the distal struts is visualized in the distal end of the catheter sheath.* **(E)** *The entire wire guide and catheter/sheath assembly is advanced until the proximal side struts are slightly overlapped.* **(F)** *The distal struts are released by withdrawing the catheter sheath over the stationary wire guide pusher.* **(G)** *The distal struts are anchored into the wall by the tiny forward backward motion.* **(H)** *The wire guide pusher is released from distal struts by rotating the pusher 10 to 15 turns in a counterclockwise direction. (Courtesy of Cook, Inc., Bloomington, IN.)*

wire pusher is released from the Bird's Nest filter apparatus by counterclockwise rotation of the guide-wire pusher handle. Disengagement between the guidewire pusher and the Bird's Nest filter is signaled by slight release or jumping of the assembly. The guidewire pusher is withdrawn into the catheter assembly and removed from the patient (Fig. 17.6). A completion venogram is performed.

The Simon Nitinol filter represents an attempt to further downsize the size of the deployment sheath. It is introduced through a 9 French catheter. The filter uses nitinol wire, which has thermally activated shape memory. Nitinol is malleable when it is perfused with cold saline and stiffens into a pre-formed shape when exposed to body temperature. The filter consists of a proximal 28 mm pedal-shaped dome formed by multiple overlapping wire loops. The dome is fixed to the caval wall by six diverging legs fitted with terminal hooks (Fig. 17.7). This represents two filtration mechanisms formed by the dome of the filter and the diverging legs. Tilting of the filter does not adversely affect the filtration efficacy. The filter is best deployed in an infrarenal position within the IVC. It can be deployed from a femoral, jugular, or antecubital approach. The 9 French introducer catheter is positioned within the cava below the level of the lowest renal vein. Cold saline was initially recommended to be infused into the side port of the introducer system to soften the nitinol wire but is no longer considered necessary. Two filter device delivery systems are available. The original system housed the pusher wire in a hoop, and a ratcheting maneuver

was used to advance the filter through the delivery sheath to the deployment location. The dome of the filter can be formed in the cava before releasing the filter's legs. This allows for exact fluoroscopic position of the device within the infrarenal IVC. The filter is released by a backward motion of the catheter storage assembly while the pusher is held stationary (Fig. 17.8). The newer delivery system uses a nitinol wire to push the filter through the delivery sheath. The wire advances the filter to the end of the 9 French catheter, which is marked with radio-opaque markers. The filter is released by pinning the wire handle and pulling the delivery sheath (Fig. 17.9). The 9 French catheter is withdrawn and a postdeployment cavogram performed.

No perfect filter exists. Complications have been documented for all filters. Each design has advantages and disadvantages. Ideally, a physician should be familiar with the deployment of several or all of the different devices. The choice of the device can be dictated by each clinical situation. The majority of filters are placed into an infrarenal IVC. Occasionally, thrombus lines the IVC. In this case, a suprarenal IVC filter is recommended (Fig. 17.10). Some investigators recommend suprarenal placement for pregnant women or young females to avoid compression by a gravid uterus. Temporary filter designs are being investigated. The major complications of IVC filters include insertion site thrombosis, caval thrombosis, recurrent pulmonary embolism, and filter migration. Patients who receive a filter for recurrent pulmonary embolism should be maintained on an anticoagulation regimen.

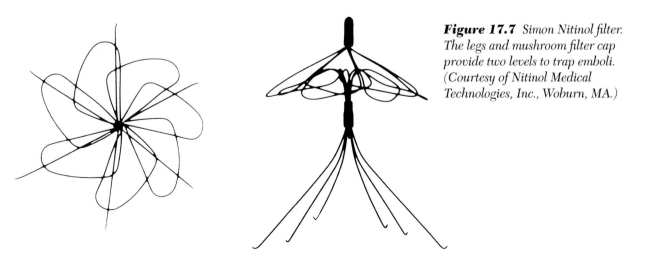

Figure 17.7 *Simon Nitinol filter. The legs and mushroom filter cap provide two levels to trap emboli. (Courtesy of Nitinol Medical Technologies, Inc., Woburn, MA.)*

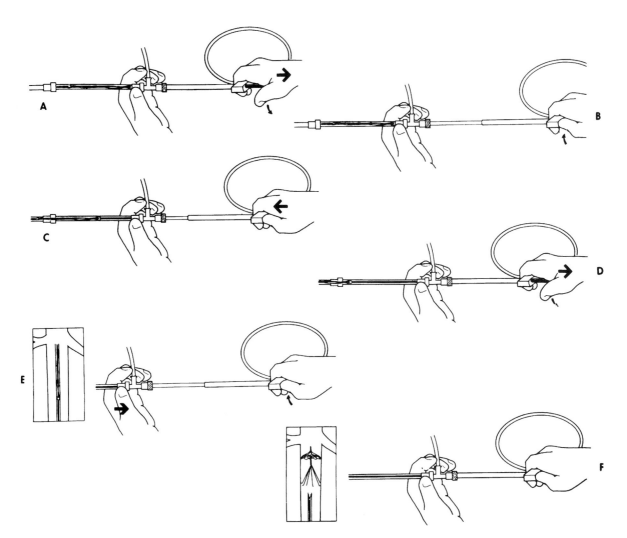

Figure 17.8 Simon Nitinol filter with ratcheting device. (**A**) The 9 French introducing catheter is held stable with the left hand. The right hand is used to retract the hoop ratcheting device. (**B**) The right thumb fixes the wire pusher in place. (**C**) The ratchet loop is pushed forward toward the introducing catheter, which is held stable with the other hand. This advances the filter through the introducing sheath. (**D**) The pusher wire is released, and the loop handle is extended. This process is repeated until the filter is positioned at the implantation site in the cava. (**E**) The final filter position is confirmed by fluoroscopic landmarks. The filter is released by pinning the pusher wire and loop storage assembly while withdrawing the sheath. The mushroom portion of the filter cap can be initially released and repositioned as necessary. (**F**) The filter is completely released when the side legs are exposed to engage the caval wall. (Courtesy of Nitinol Medical Technologies, Inc., Woburn, MA.)

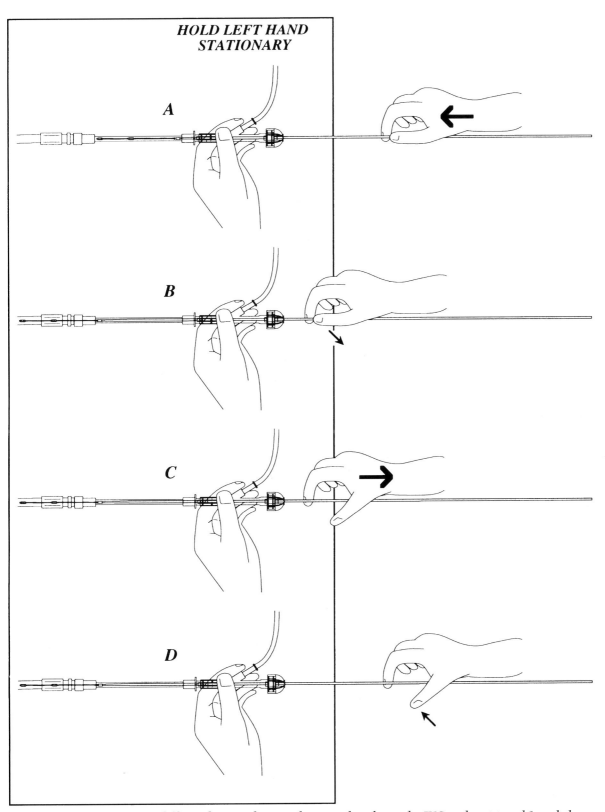

Figure 17.9 *Simon Nitinol filter. The introducer catheter is placed into the IVC and positioned 1 cm below the level of the lowest renal vein. The filter storage tube is attached to the introducer catheter, which is already in the vein. (A) The filter is advanced into the introducer catheter by moving the Nitinol pusher wire forward. (B-D) The wire is released and the hand repositioned on the wire to readvance the wire. (Figure continues.)*

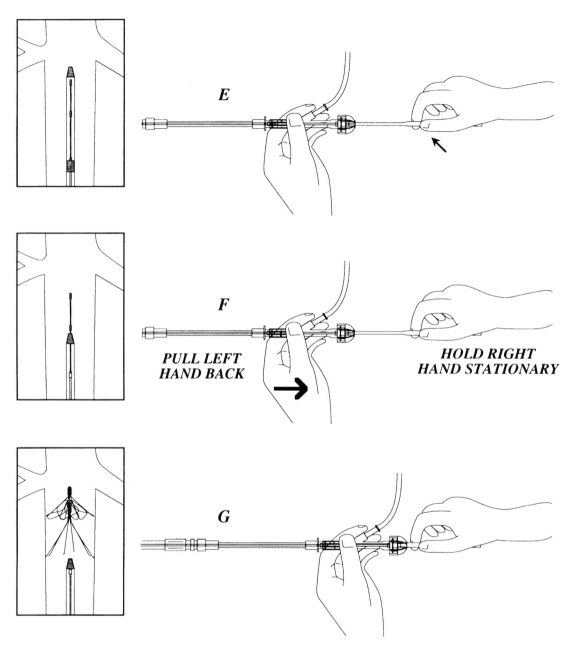

Figure 17.9 *(Continued)* *(E)* *The filter is positioned between the radio-opaque markers on the introducer catheter. (F) The filter is released by pinning the pusher wire stable and pulling the sheath over the pushing wire. (G) The pin-and-pull maneuver has released the filter below the renal veins.*

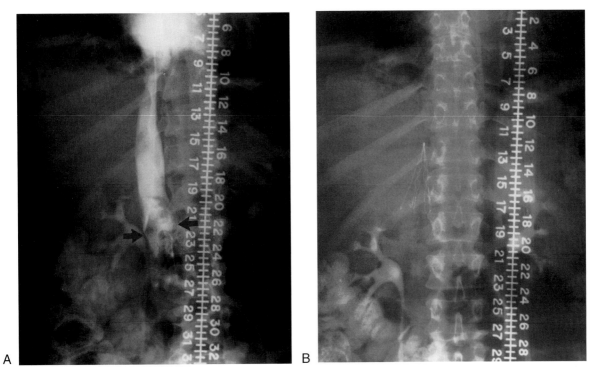

Figure 17.10 *(A) The IVC was filled with thrombus to the level of the renal veins, causing recurrent episodes of pulmonary embolism (arrows). (B) A Greenfield filter was placed in the suprarenal segment of the cava. The planar insertion of the Greenfield filter legs with the wall of the cava minimizes branch vessel overlap and provides a secure attachment.*

Suggested Readings

Dorfman GS: Percutaneous inferior vena cava filters. Radiology 174:987, 1990

Ferris EJ, McCowan TC, Carver DK, McFarland DR: Percutaneous inferior vena cava filters: follow-up of seven designs in 320 patients. Radiology 181:851, 1993

Grassi CJ: Inferior vena cava filters: analysis of five currently available devices. AJR 156:813, 1991

Greenfield LJ, Procter MC, Cho KJ et al: Extended evaluation of the titanium Greenfield vena cava filter. J Vasc Surg 20:458, 1994

Kandarpa K, Archibald GR: Percutaneous inferior vena cava filter placement. p. 579. In Kim D, Orron DE (eds): Peripheral Vascular Imaging and Intervention. Mosby, St Louis, 1992

Murphy TP Dorfman GS, Yedlicka JW et al: LGM vena cava filter: objective evaluation of early results. J Vasc Interv Radiol 2:107, 1991

Roehm JOF, Johnsrude IS, Barth KH, Gianurco C: The Bird's Nest inferior vena cava filter: progress report. Radiology 168:745, 1988

Rose BS, Simon DC, Hess ML, Van Aman ME: Percutaneous transfemoral placement of the Kimray-Greenfield vena cava filter. Radiology 165:373, 1987

Simon M, Athanasoulis CA, Kim D et al: Simon nitinol inferior vena cava filter: initial clinical experience. Radiology 172:99, 1989

Vesely TM: Technical problems and complications associated with inferior vena cava filters. Semin Interv Radiol 11:121, 1994

Nonvascular Interventional Procedures

Image-guided acquisition of tissue is a safe and accurate method of obtaining pathologic confirmation of disease processes. The fundamental techniques of image-guided biopsy form the basis of the more complex abdominal and chest interventional procedures. Percutaneous abscess drainage and gastrostomy tube placement are well established in the medical community. The application of percutaneous drainage techniques to the pleural space is a growing area of interventional radiology and requires a knowledge of pleural space physiology to manage chest drainage catheters. The last two chapters provide a basic review of biliary and genitourinary interventional procedures supplemented by a concise update of newer procedural innovations.

Image-Guided Biopsy

MICHAEL A. BRAUN
ALBERT A. NEMCEK, JR.

Image-guided biopsy and diagnostic fluid aspiration are frequently performed procedures that have high levels of accuracy (80 to 90 percent) and low complication rates (< 2 percent). Percutaneous needle biopsy can diagnose primary versus metastatic malignancy, tumor recurrence, diffuse parenchymal disease, or infection. Most biopsies are performed to establish a cellular diagnosis of malignancy before embarking on chemotherapy or radiation therapy in nonresectable patients or patients with metastatic or recurrent disease. Small collections of pleural fluid or ascites can be sampled for diagnostic aspiration using imaging guidance. The etiology of diffuse liver or renal parenchymal disease can be accomplished with ultrasound-guided core biopsies of these organs. Most biopsies are performed on an outpatient basis. The procedure is explained to the patient, and the patient is given instructions on breath holding and position. Anxiety can be relieved and cooperation improved by good physician–patient rapport and mild intravenous sedation when necessary. The major contraindication is an uncorrectable coagulopathy. This is screened for by history and coagulation studies. Since most biopsies are elective procedures, a coagulation disorder should be evaluated and corrected before performing the biopsy.

Each procedure has several steps: A lesion or organ is identified as amenable to biopsy, a needle path is plotted, a method of guidance to this target is chosen, a needle or other device is chosen to obtain the tissue or fluid, and the material is sampled and processed for pathologic review. The films should be reviewed before biopsy to plan the procedure and to rule out normal variants, pseudolesions, and benign lesions such as hepatic hemangiomas. On occasion, review of films leads to the suggestion of a noninvasive method for establishing a confident diagnosis. Selecting an optimal path to a target involves consideration of technical ease and safety. In general, the shortest path to the lesion that crosses the fewest and least critical structures is best. If more than one lesion is present, the largest and most accessible is chosen. Interposition of most solid abdominal organs along the needle path is not a contraindication to prohibit biopsy. As with biopsy of splenic lesions themselves, transsplenic biopsy is controversial but has been used. Transgression of bowel should be avoided if possible. The presence of ascites does not adversely increase the risk of biopsy.

The interventional radiologist should decide which modality to use in guiding the biopsy. The needle can be guided to the target lesion by fluoroscopy, ultrasound, or computed tomography (CT). Ultrasound and fluoroscopy have the advantage of real-time guidance of the needle towards a lesion. This is a significant advantage in sampling lesions affected by respiratory motion (e.g., lung and dome of liver). Fluoroscopy and ultrasound-guided biopsies tend to be less time consuming and a more efficient means of performing a biopsy when these means are feasible. The size, location, and depth of the lesion determine the best means for guidance. The majority of lesions can be biopsied under CT guidance, especially deep and small targets such as retroperitoneal lymph nodes and adrenal gland masses. CT guidance is the easiest method to learn and probably is the most reliable in the majority of cases. When a lesion is accessible by either CT or ultrasound, however, we prefer the real-time guidance of ultrasound over CT.

Fluoroscopic-guided biopsy is used for pulmonary nodules, ureteral strictures, and biliary stenoses. The biliary tree or ureter can be opacified with contrast and fluoroscopy used to target an obstructing lesion or stenosis. A C-arm is necessary for rapid triangulation and complex angulation to guide the needle. The C-arm is rotated to determine the shortest and easiest path to the target. The needle is passed parallel to the fluoroscopy beam toward the target. Rotating the C-arm to different obliquities will ascertain the depth of the needle relative to the target lesion. Real-time imaging can be used to make fine adjustments to account for target motion or mobility.

Ultrasound has the advantage of continuous visualization of the needle course toward the target. The speed, portability, cost effectiveness, and lack of ionizing radiation make ultrasound a preferred technique. The disadvantages are that the technique requires a longer learning curve than CT and the needle tip can be difficult to visualize. The two methods of ultrasound guidance are freehand or detachable biopsy guide. Freehand method is used for superficial biopsies of thyroid nodules or breast lesions. A high-frequency linear array transducer is used to guide a needle toward the lesion. The needle and probe are controlled by the same operator. The needle is advanced in the transverse or longitudinal plane along the beam path toward the lesion. The narrow beam width requires a steep angulation of the needle to maintain the needle tip in the visualized field. Subtle manipulations and corrections of the beam plane and needle path are necessary to direct the needle into the lesion. Deeper lesions can be approached with the freehand method, but the technique is more difficult, requiring triangulation of the needle passage with the probe beam visualization of the path and target. Ultrasound manufacturers have developed biopsy guides and electronic delineation of the needle tract, which greatly facilitates sampling of deep lesions. Most biopsy guides are sterile attachments designed for specific probes. A sterile biopsy condom is placed over the transducer. The guide is attached to the probe (Fig. 18.1). The target is lined up in the electronic path. The skin is anesthetized and nicked with a scalpel. The needle is introduced through the slot in the guide, which directs the needle along the predetermined path. Real-time imaging is used to target the lesion and place the needle directly within the lesion (Fig. 18.2). Visualization of the needle tip under ultrasound can be difficult and can be improved in several ways. The position of the needle tip can be inferred by the deflection wave caused by the displacement of tissues. Jiggling the needle or stylet can help visualize the needle tip. Dedicated ultrasound biopsy needles with echogenic needle tips or screw-tipped stylets slightly improve visualization.

CT is best suited for small and deep lesions, especially those involving the retroperitoneum and presacral space. The needle tip can be unequivocally demonstrated, and surrounding structures can be avoided. The target lesion is scanned using 10×10 mm or smaller cuts. The CT slice that is best centered on the target lesion is selected. A perpendicular path to the lesion is the easiest to perform. An angled approach is used to avoid inter-

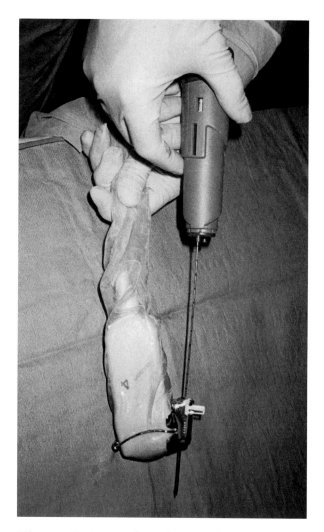

Figure 18.1 *A condom ultrasound-guided biopsy. The ultrasound probe is covered with a sterile condom and the sterile metal biopsy guide attachment is snapped on the probe. A plastic barrel-shaped needle guide is inserted into the metal biopsy guide attachment. The plastic barrel needle guide is available in 14- to 22-gauge needle sizes. The automated biopsy gun needle is inserted through the biopsy guide, which directs the needle along the electronic delineation of the path toward the target lesion.*

posed structures such as bone and vessels. The depth of the lesion and the path angle are measured. The skin entry site can be measured from the midline if the CT is equipped with external laser light beams. Alternatively, a radio-opaque grid is used to determine the skin entry

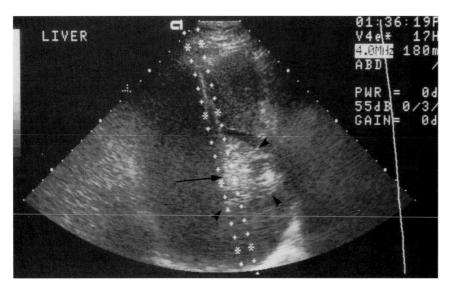

Figure 18.2 *The electronic needle pathway is aligned on the mass in the dome of the right lobe of the liver. The mass is outlined by arrowheads. The tip of the needle is present within the echogenic mass (arrow).*

site. The skin entry is prepped and draped in the usual fashion. The skin is infiltrated with lidocaine, and a small dermatotomy is made with a stab-type scalpel. The needle is properly angulated and advanced to the appropriate depth. The patient is coached to breath hold during the needle passage. The depth on the needle is marked with a piece of sterile tape or plastic depth marker. The estimation of a complex angle is improved by spotters assisting the needle operator to gauge the angulation. A lateral or anteroposterior scout film is used to image the needle. The needle tip is then imaged using a 5 to 10 mm thick CT slice. The needle tip is recognized by the characteristic streak artifact. If the initial needle pass misses the target, it is left in place to aid in correcting the angle of the second needle passage. If the needle is within the lesion, we advocate performing a tandem needle biopsy. A second needle is placed along a parallel course to the needle within the lesion. In this way multiple samples of the lesion can be rapidly obtained without having to perform interval scans (Fig. 18.3). Coaxial technique also reduces the risks and procedural time of the biopsy. A guiding needle is placed to a depth that will guide smaller coaxially placed needles into the target.

Three varieties of needles are available: aspiration needles, small-gauge biopsy needles, and large-gauge cutting needles. The Chiba needle is an example of an aspiration needle. It is also referred to as a skinny needle because of its thin walls and flexibility. The Chiba needle has a stylet and simple flat bevel tip. Small-gauge biopsy needles are modifications of aspiration needles

with serrated tips or side-cutting ports. The tip design is an important factor in tissue acquisition (Fig. 18.4). Studies have shown that the Franseen needle with a cutting tip performs better than the Chiba needle with a flat bevel. The Franseen needle has a serrated tip and either a 20- or 22-gauge needle is used in the majority of abdominal biopsies. It has been suggested that side-cutting needles, such as the Wescott, perform better in softer tissues, whereas end-cutting needles perform better in firmer tissues. Large-gauge cutting needles range in size from 14 to 20 gauge and are intended to obtain a core of tissue for histopathologic review. These are used for parenchymal biopsies or evaluation of lymphoma. The Biopty (Bard, Covington, GA) is the best known device. The spring-loaded device throws a side-notched inner trocar needle forward immediately followed by an outer cutting needle. The specimen is trapped in the side notch of the inner needle. Other automated Tru-Cut devices manually advance the inner trocar needle and use a spring to fire the outer cutting needle. The Temno (Bauer, Italy) is an example. The Temno device handle is smaller than the other automated guns.

The sample is collected by connecting a 10 to 20 ml syringe directly to the hub of the needle. Negative aspiration is applied as the needle is jiggled to and fro within the lesion. The amplitude of each stroke should be greater than 3 to 4 mm. This threshold was determined experimentally. Specimen weight increases linearly with increased suction applied to the needle, as long as there is simultaneous needle movement into

Figure 18.3 *CT biopsy retroperitoneal lymph node. (**A**) The patient is scanned in prone position and needle path chosen by scanning the area of interest with a grid. (**B**) The first needle was successfully placed into the edge of the lymph node. A tandem needle is placed alongside this needle to quickly acquire multiple specimens without interval scans. Note the presence of the two needles that follow the same path (arrow).*

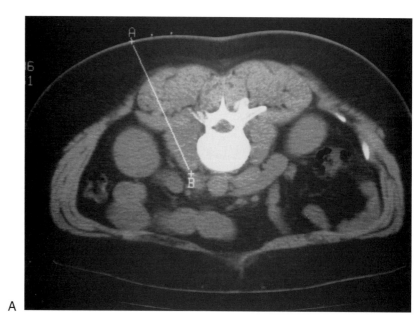

A

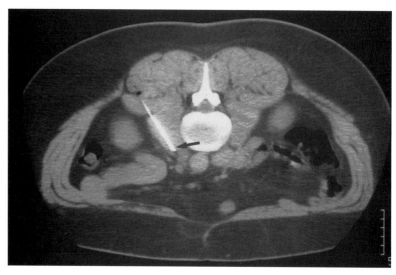

B

the tissue. Many practitioners advance the needle with a rotary or screwing motion while performing aspiration biopsy. This practice has not been experimentally proven. As soon as a flash of tissue fluid or blood is seen within the hub of the needle, the suction is released and the needle removed. The sample is immediately processed by gently depositing the specimen onto glass slides or cell block solution. If the specimen clots within the needle, the needle stylet can be used to extrude the specimen from the needle's lumen. There are some reports that nonaspiration technique for fine needle biopsy may work well in certain situations (i.e., thyroid and breast). This technique relies on capillary action in which fluid or semifluid material flows into the lumen of narrow needles. It reduces the contamination of the specimen with blood. In routine abdominal biopsy, the aspiration technique is superior to nonaspiration.

The amount of tissue and its pathologic quality figure in the evaluation of the yield of biopsy. The more tissue obtained leads to a higher diagnostic yield. The number of needle passes increases the diagnostic yield

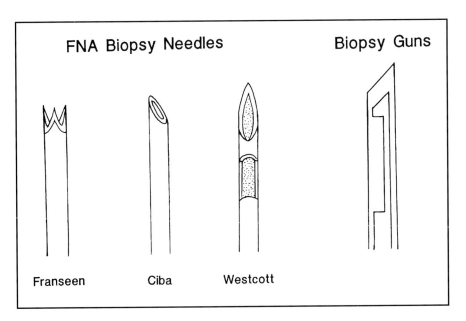

Figure 18.4 *Biopsy needle types. The Franseen biopsy needle has a serrated cannula tip. The Westcott biopsy needle has a specimen side notch, which is exposed by removing the stylet. The Chiba needle has an angled bevel tip. Core biopsies are performed using automated specimen notch-type needles. The stylet has a specimen notch and is fired first into the target lesion. The outer cannula cuts the core of tissue, which is collected within the specimen notch of the stylet needle.*

but follows the law of diminishing returns. In general, two to four 20-gauge needle passes will obtain a diagnostic specimen in 80 to 90 percent of cases.

Core specimens are important in the diagnosis of lymphoma and in diagnosing diffuse parenchymal disorders involving the liver and kidney. Twenty- or 18-gauge cores of involved lymph nodes are adequate for the subtyping of lymphoma. Three specimens usually suffice. Core-type biopsies are best performed using automated biopsy guns. Percutaneous liver biopsies are usually a 16-gauge core biopsy of the left lobe using a subcostal ultrasound-guided approach. Percutaneous renal biopsies of both native and transplanted kidneys are 14-gauge specimens under ultrasound guidance. The automated Tru-Cut needle is advanced to the periphery of the lesion to be sampled. The trocar needle is thrust forward into the lesion, followed by the outer cutting needle. The typical needle excursion is 2 to 2.5 cm long. This should be accounted for when positioning the needle tip.

Transjugular liver biopsies are performed in patients who have diffuse liver disease and concomitant coagulopathy, thrombocytopenia, portal hypertension, or ascites. Transjugular liver biopsies are performed in conjunction with wedged hepatic pressures and venograms. Percutaneous biopsy with tract embolization is an alternative when a focal lesion needs to be sampled. Several devices are available for obtaining transjugular biopsies. The traditional device is the Colapinto needle, an 18-gauge needle with a curved tip that can be passed over a 0.038 inch guidewire through a long 9 French guiding sheath. It is directed into the liver via the right or middle hepatic vein. The needle excursion into small, cirrhotic livers is limited to prevent capsular perforation. The specimens obtained from this device are usually small fragments. Multiple passes are usually required to obtain an adequate volume of specimen. Automated devices have been developed because of dissatisfaction with this device. Cook, Inc. (Bloomington, IN) makes a long automated 19-gauge biopsy gun, which obtains 19-gauge cores from a transjugular introduction through a sheath. The automated gun more reliably obtains core samples rather than fragmented tissue pieces. The specimen should be at least 1 cm long to be adequate for comprehensive diagnosis. A third transvenous biopsy method uses a grasping forceps designed for endoscopic biopsy. The flexible nature of the grasping forceps allows a femoral approach. Small 2 to 3 mm chunks are obtained using this device. If possible, the grasping forceps is used to create a tunnel into the liver to obtain both superficial and deep pieces of hepatic tissue.

The major complication of biopsy is hemorrhage. The risk of hemorrhage varies with the size of the biopsy device used and the vascularity of the organ sampled. The mechanism of injury can be laceration of an artery or vein along the target course of the needle passage, oozing from the lesion biopsied, or formation of a pseudoaneurysm in a vascular organ such as the kidney. The risk of hemorrhage increases when the patient has an underlying abnormality of coagulation. The use of screening laboratory values to determine the risk of subsequent hemorrhage is controversial. Recent studies based on economic analysis have questioned the need for screening laboratory values in patients. It is suggested that the history is often the best screening criterion. Based on the history, laboratory tests can be tailored to the underlying medical problem. There are no threshold values to determine safe performance of a biopsy. Each case must be analyzed individually and the risks weighed against the potential benefits in light of the alternative scenarios for making a confident diagnosis. Similarly, there is no standard for observing the patient postbiopsy. The minimum should be 30 minutes to 1 hour. High-risk patients should be monitored longer.

Suggested Readings

Charboneau WJ, Reading CC, Welch TJ: CT and sonographically guided needle biopsy: current techniques and new innovations. AJR 154:1, 1990

Dahnert WF, Hoagland MH, Hamper UM et al: Fine needle aspiration biopsy of abdominal lesions: diagnostic yield for different needle tip configurations. Radiology 185:263, 1992

Gamble P, Colapinto RF, Stronell RD et al: Transjugular liver biopsy: a review of 461 biopsies. Radiology 157:589, 1985

Gazelle GS, Haaga JR: Biopsy needle characteristics. Cardiovasc Interv Radiol 14:13, 1991

Hopper KD, Abendroth CS, Sturtz KW et al: Automated biopsy devices: a blinded evaluation. Radiology 187:653, 1993

Kinney TB, Lee ML, Filomena CA et al: Fine-needle biopsy: prospective comparison of aspiration versus nonaspiration techniques in the abdomen. Radiology 186:549, 1993

Mewissen MW, Lipchik EO, Schreiber ER et al: Liver biopsy through the femoral vein. Radiology 169:842, 1988

Nemcek AA, Jr: Imaging-guided sampling of abdominal and pelvic lesions: current issues. p.139. In Gore RM (ed): Syllabus for Categorical Course on Gastrointestinal Radiology. American College of Radiology, Reston, VA, 1991

Parker SH, Hopper KD, Yakes WF et al: Image-directed percutaneous biopsies with a biopsy gun. Radiology 171:663, 1989

Silver B, Matalon TAS: Techniques of percutaneous tissue acquisition. p. 1543. In Gore RM, Levine MS, Laufer I (eds): Textbook of Gastrointestinal Radiology. Vol. 2. WB Saunders, Philadelphia, 1994

Zins M, Vilgrain V, Gayno S et al: US-guided percutaneous liver biopsy with plugging of the needle track: a prospective study in 72 high-risk patients. Radiology 184:841, 1992

CHAPTER 19

Abdominal Drainage MICHAEL A. BRAUN

Paracentesis

The removal of peritoneal fluid may be performed for diagnostic or therapeutic purposes. Ultrasound guidance is used to aspirate small amounts of ascitic fluid and minimize the risk of complications. The most common causes of ascites are cirrhosis and cancer. Other causes are tuberculosis, congestive heart failure, spontaneous bacterial peritonitis, pancreatic disease, biliary leakage, and renal failure.

Ultrasound is used to scan the abdomen and choose the safest route to the largest accumulation of fluid. Large collections of ascites can be marked with ultrasound and drained separately. Smaller collections require real-time imaging guidance. The skin is cleansed with Betadine. Local anesthetic with lidocaine is performed. Diagnostic paracentesis is performed with an 18- or 20-gauge intravenous needle used to aspirate 50 to 100 ml of fluid. Therapeutic paracentesis is performed with an angiocath or a 5 French pigtail catheter. The pigtail catheter expedites removal of a large amount of fluid. The needle or catheter can be connected to a vacuum bottle to quickly evacuate the fluid. Diagnostic paracentesis specimens are sent for culture and sensitivity, Gram stain, cytology, cell count, protein, and amylase.

The complications of paracentesis are hemorrhage and perforation of bowel. Avoiding the epigastric vessels is the best way to minimize hemorrhagic complications. If a large volume paracentesis is performed, an intravenous line should be present to facilitate the correction of intravascular volume depletion. Some advocate administration of albumin to patients undergoing large volume paracentesis to prevent intravascular volume depletion. The administration of albumin is controversial and expensive.

Abdominal Abscess Drainage

Percutaneous abscess drainage was one of the initial procedures that created the field of interventional radiology. Untreated abdominal abscesses are invariably fatal, and the surgical mortality rate is approximately 20 percent for a single abdominal abscess. Image-guided percutaneous abscess drainage has negligible mortality and eliminates the morbidity of surgery. Percutaneous drainage causes less contamination of adjacent structures, has no incision to heal, and does not require a general anesthetic. Percutaneous drainage is curative in most cases. In noncurative cases, decompression of the abscess is often pivotal in reversing the systemic septic effects of the abscess, justifying its use as a temporizing measure.

An abscess is a collection of pus contained by the abscess wall and adjacent structures. The dependent location of the subphrenic space and pelvic cul de sac make these areas typical locations for abscesses. As the abscess grows, its mass effect and displacement of adjacent structures usually creates a favorable window for percutaneous drainage. Most abscesses are generally diagnosed and drained under computed tomography (CT) guidance. The CT findings of abscesses are a round fluid collection with a contrast-enhancing capsule. A fine bubbly gas distribution or air–fluid level is seen in approximately half the cases. Differentiation from fluid-filled loops of bowel may require additional enteral contrast and delayed scans. Diagnostic needle aspiration is an important tool for confirmation of an abscess and identification of the causative organisms. Most intra-abdominal abscesses are polymicrobial. The sole disadvantage of CT guidance is the absence of real-time imaging to guide subsequent catheter and guidewire manipulations. If the abscess is readily visualized by ultrasound, it is preferable to perform the

193

procedure in the angiography suite under combined fluoroscopic and ultrasonographic guidance. Ultrasound can be used for bedside drainage of an abscess in critically ill patients.

The best access route is the shortest, safest tract. Care should be taken to choose a route that avoids bowel, spleen, major vessels, and the pleural space. Physical factors and patient comfort should be kept in mind when choosing a site for percutaneous drainage. A direct posterior approach is seldom optimal because of the subsequent potential kinking of the tube, which can occur when the patient lies in the supine position. Catheters can be placed through the stomach to reach an abscess, although this is not preferable. If the stomach is transgressed, the patient should receive nothing by mouth. Major abdominal visceral organs such as the liver and kidney can be transversed to provide drainage. Pelvic abscesses can be drained using a transgluteal approach under CT guidance. In the transgluteal approach, the needle is placed through the greater sciatic notch into the abscess cavity. The tract is made close to the sacrum above the sacrospinous ligament to avoid the sacral nerve plexus and vessels (Fig. 19.1). Suspected hepatic echinococcal disease

should be approached carefully because of the danger of peritoneal spillage with subsequent shock.

The drainage catheter may be placed using Seldinger or Trocar technique. Seldinger technique is used for deep abscess locations or when needle passage is near vital structures. In Seldinger technique, the fluid collection can be punctured with a 21-gauge micropuncture kit or an 18-gauge trocar stylet needle. A small amount of fluid is aspirated to confirm needle placement within the abscess cavity. The 21-gauge micropuncture kit has a transitional dilator/sheath, which is used to upsize from a 0.018 inch to a 0.038 inch wire. The 0.018 inch mandrel wire is inserted through the 21-gauge needle. The needle is removed and the sheath–dilator system is advanced over the mandrel wire. The dilator and stiffening cannula are removed from this sheath–dilator. The 0.018 inch wire is left in place. A super-stiff 0.038 inch wire can be placed alongside the 0.018 inch mandrel wire and coiled within the abscess cavity (Fig. 19.2). The sheath and mandrel wire are removed. The tract is dilated to the appropriate size. A drainage pigtail catheter is placed into the cavity. The 18-gauge trocar stylet needle saves the intermediate step of the transitional dilator/sheath. The abscess cavity is punctured with the 18-gauge needle. A

Figure 19.1 *Transgluteal drainage of an appendiceal abscess. The needle is placed close to the coccyx to avoid the neurovascular bundle and pyriformis muscle.*

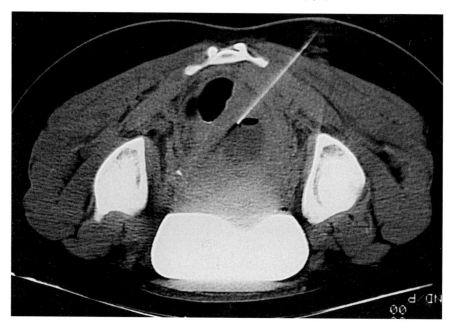

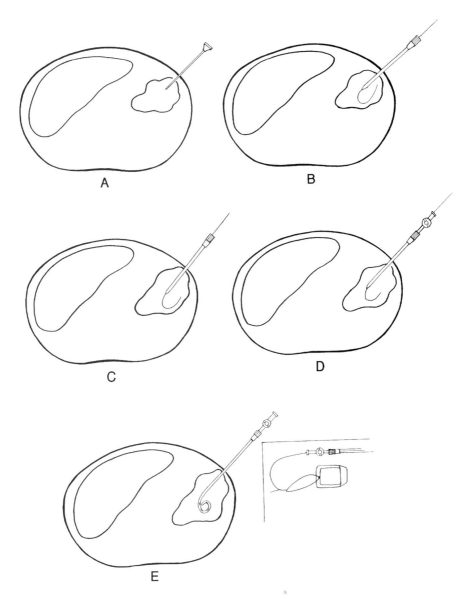

Figure 19.2 *Seldinger technique abscess drainage. (**A**) A 21-gauge needle is placed into the abscess drainage under image guidance. (**B**) A 0.018 inch guidewire is coiled in the abscess cavity. The sheath dilator is passed over the 0.018 inch guidewire. (**C**) The 0.018 inch guidewire has been removed. The stiffening metal cannula and dilator from the sheath dilator has been removed. A stiff 0.038 inch guidewire is passed through the sheath into the abscess cavity. (**D**) The drainage catheter and stiffening metal cannula are advanced over the guidewire into the cavity. (**E**) The pigtail is formed and secured by the suture locking mechanism.*

0.038 super-stiff guidewire is introduced through the 18-gauge needle, the tract is dilated, and a drainage catheter is placed. Trocar technique is suitable for large, accessible abscesses and is analogous to an intravenous needle. The catheter/trocar needle is pushed to the estimated depth, and the catheter is fed off the trocar needle and coiled in the cavity (Fig. 19.3).

Small unilocular abscess cavities are drained with 8 to 10 French locking pigtail catheters. The string inside the catheter is pulled tight, which forms and secures the pigtail loop. The locking screw on the hub of the catheter is turned 180° to secure the pigtail loop. The string is then cut flush with the catheter hub (Fig. 19.4). Larger abscesses are drained with 12 to 14 French pigtail catheters. Single lumen catheters are favored over sump catheters. Multiple, nonconnected abscesses require multiple catheters.

The abscess cavity is completely evacuated of its contents at the time of the initial drainage. A small contrast injection can be performed to document catheter

Figure 19.3 *Trocar abscess drainage.*
(A) The drain is mounted on a stiffening metal cannula with a diamond pointed stylet needle. This is inserted under imaging guidance into the abscess cavity.
(B) The catheter is disconnected from the metal stiffening cannula and stylet needle. The cannula is pinned and the catheter is fed off the cannula into the cavity.
(C) The pigtail catheter is secured with the suture locking mechanism.

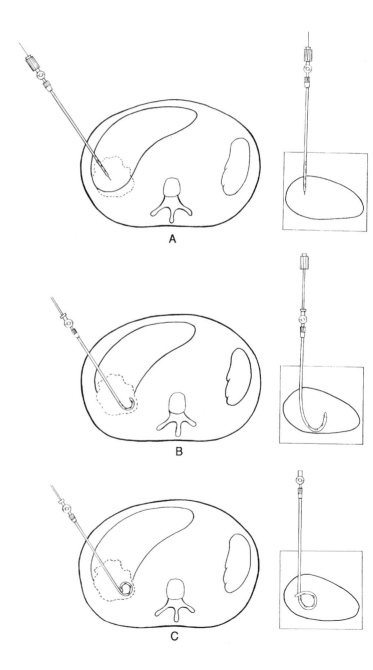

A

B

C

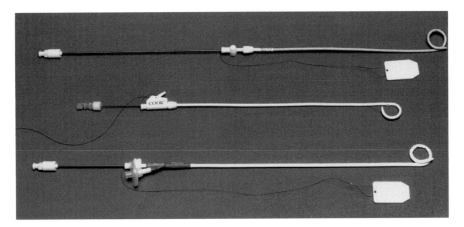

Figure 19.4 *Drainage catheters. The top catheter is a Meditech 10 French all purpose drain. The suture is connected to a tab, which is pulled to form the pigtail. The tab is used to turn the screw, which locks the suture-tethered pigtail in place. The middle catheter is a Cook 10 French drain catheter. The suture is pulled tethering the pigtail in locked configuration. The suture is fixed by depressing the lever locking suture in place. The bottom catheter is a Meditech dual lumen sump drain. The sump drain vents the cavity, preventing the walls from being collapsed into the drainage holes on the pigtail catheter. A filter on the sump drain prevents inadvertent contamination of the cavity.*

and sidehole position within the cavity. The cavity is not lavaged, and a large volume of contrast should not be injected to avoid bacteremia. Specimens should be sent for Gram stain, complete blood count, and culture and sensitivity. The patient is placed on intravenous antibiotics and the catheter connected to either bulb suction or gravity drainage. A sinogram of the cavity is scheduled after 24 to 72 hours of drainage. The initial sinogram is performed to assess abscess cavity size and confirm location of the catheter within the cavity. Additional sinograms are performed at 3- to 5-day intervals. Fistulas may not be evident until late in the course of the drainage when inflammation in the abscess wall subsides, opening the orifice of the fistula.

Patients with drains in abscesses are visited daily while in the hospital. Clinical response is monitored by following the temperature curve and white blood cell count. Patients can be managed as outpatients with drainage tubes. They are given return visit appointments to the Interventional Radiology Service before discharge. The patients are given instruction on basic tube care, dressing changes, and skin hygiene. The patient or caregiver is requested to record the tube's daily output. Patients who are scheduled for a tube

check are treated as a clinic-type visit. They are questioned about any fevers or tube-related pain. They are asked whether there is any pericatheter fluid leakage, which implies obstruction of the tube. A sinogram is performed to assess the drain's position and cavity size. Estimated daily tube drainage, drain manipulation, and drain removal are recorded on the films taken during the tube check. Most successful abscess drainages are accomplished within 1 to 2 weeks in uncomplicated cases. Abscess drainage catheters remain in place until the drainage either ceases or is less than 10 ml/day and a sinogram shows complete collapse of the cavity.

Enteric Abscesses

Enteric abscesses originate from a bowel perforation. Examples are intra-abdominal abscesses secondary to appendicitis, diverticulitis, Crohn's disease, and post-bowel surgery. The presence of these abscesses implies communication between the bowel and the cavity. These abscesses cannot be cured until the communication from the gastrointestinal tract has closed. A fistula should be suspected when there is greater than 50 ml/day of drain output following 48 hours of drainage. A sinogram (tube check) is performed by slowly injecting dilute water-soluble contrast under fluoroscopic control. The size of the cavity is estimated from the amount of contrast injected. The configuration and size of the cavity are assessed in multiple views. Occult fistulas are seen as areas of beaking of the abscess cavity. Overdistention of the cavity is avoided to prevent intraperitoneal spillage and bacteremia. The fistula is usually not seen on the initial sinogram. When the inflammation within the abscess subsides, the fistula becomes obvious on contrast injections. The fistula becomes easier to visualize as the size of the abscess cavity decreases. Factors that interfere with fistula closure include distal bowel obstruction, malignancy, radiation, poor nutrition, and epithelialization of the fistula tract.

Fistulas are divided into low and high output. Low output fistulas generally close within 2 to 6 weeks with adequate drainage. High output fistulas have greater than 200 ml/day of output and are often due to duodenal or proximal small bowel perforations. High output fistulas are challenging to manage. It is important to place the patient on bowel rest and provide nutritional support via hyperalimentation. Reduction of pancreatic and biliary secretions by placing the patient on somatostatin helps reduce the fistula output. High output fistulas are treated by placing a catheter across the fistula tract into the bowel. This promotes healing and granulation of the fistula tract.

Diverticulitis describes a broad range of disease from local inflammation to perforation with abscess formation. Diverticular abscesses have been surgically treated with three-staged operations to (1) drain the abscess and divert the colon, (2) resect the involved colon, and (3) reanastomose the colon. Initial percutaneous drainage of the abscess can effectively treat the abscess and allow an elective colon resection and anastomosis.

Pancreatic Fluid Collections

Pancreatitis can be complicated by sepsis, abscess formation, and pseudocyst formation. Pancreatic pseudocysts and abscesses are problematic to treat due to the large amount of necrosis induced by the pancreatitis and the potential communication with the pancreatic duct. The overall success rate in curing pancreatic fluid collections is less than that achieved in draining enteric abscesses. Pancreatic abscesses are probably the most difficult percutaneous drainage problem challenging radiologists. Often, a combination of surgical and percutaneous drainage is required. The palliative effects of percutaneous drainage can allow optimization of the patient's clinical status, thus allowing operative drainage and debridement. Pancreatic abscesses frequently require multiple catheters. When thick necrotic tissue is seen on sinograms, large Thal-quick catheters can be used to percutaneously debride the necrotic tissue and debris. This can be accomplished by irrigation through large chest tube-type catheters or by using an alligator-type grasping forceps introduced percutaneously (Fig. 19.5). Careful evaluation of sinograms to assess for the amount of debris within cavities and communication with the pancreatic duct is essential for success.

The drainage of pancreatic pseudocyst has an approximate 85 percent cure rate. Small pseudocysts less than 4 cm and large, asymptomatic cysts can be managed expectantly. Drainage is considered when the pseudocyst is symptomatic, infected, or enlarging. Pseudocysts associated with chronic pancreatitis are less likely to resolve spontaneously, lowering the threshold for drainage. Direct routes into the pseudocyst or, if possible, a transgastric approach is preferred. The transgastric route is the equivalent of a cystogastrostomy, and a double J stent is available for internal drainage. The percutaneous drainage catheter should remain in place until the communication with the pancreatic duct closes. This frequently requires long-term drainage for 3 to 15 weeks.

Necrotic Tumors

Necrotic tumors that become infected secondarily can be treated by percutaneous drainage. The presence of the tumor impedes the body's natural immune response to eradicate the abscess. Long-term drainage is common, since the cavity will not collapse until the tumor is successfully treated with systemic chemotherapy or irradiation. Sclerosis with alcohol can be used to collapse the cavity.

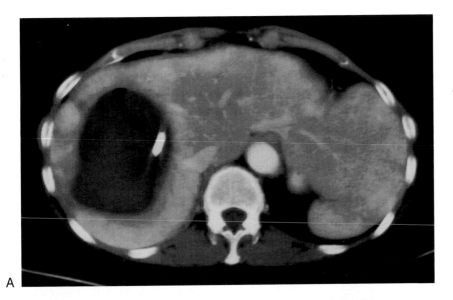

A

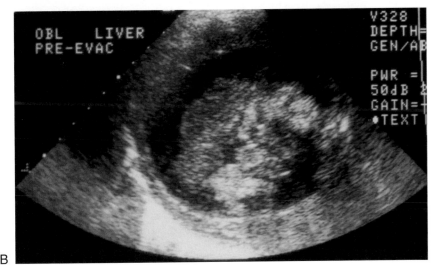

B

Figure 19.5 *Biloma.*
(A) Liver CT scan showing low-density fluid collection with pigtail drain in it. The fluid collection did not decrease in size following percutaneous drainage and percutaneous biliary diversion. (B) Ultrasound of bilioma shows echogenic debris within the bilioma surrounded by a rim of fluid. Intracavitary urokinase diminished the amount of debris by approximately 25 percent. The patient remained symptomatic. (Figure continues.)

Miscellaneous Abdominal Drainage

Hepatic and splenic abscesses arise from hematogenous spread of infection. Solitary, unilocular cavities are successfully drained with a single catheter (Fig. 19.6). Multiple cavities require multiple catheters or aspirations, depending on the cavity size. Hepatic abscess related to biliary obstruction necessitates decompression of the biliary tree. Bilomas occur after hepatic surgery or trauma. Drainage is indicated when infection is suspected. The biliary tree may need to be drained to divert bile flow. A nuclear medicine biliary scan can be used to demonstrate the bile leak. The drainage catheter is left in the bilioma until the communication from the bile duct seals. Most hepatic amebic abscesses are managed with metronidazole (Flagyl). Some amebic abscesses are refractory to medication and can be drained by percutaneous methods. The spleen is drained with an 8 French catheter to minimize bleeding complications. Splenic subcapsular collections, abscesses, and septic

Figure 19.5 *(Continued)* **(C)** *A 24 French chest tube was placed into the cavity using Seldinger technique. An alligator clamp was used to percutaneously debride the solid material within the cavity. This emptied the cavity and allowed the cavity to collapse in size.*

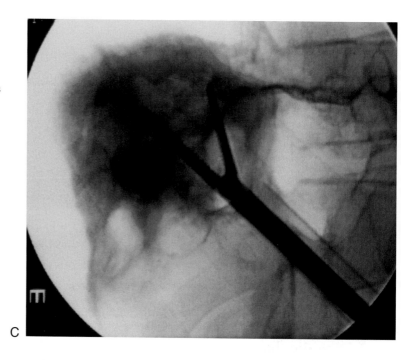

C

infarctions have been treated successfully with percutaneous drainage (Fig. 19.7).

Percutaneous drainage can be applied to a wide variety of pathologic conditions. The strategy for treatment of tubo-ovarian abscesses is medical treatment with broad-spectrum antibiotics. In patients who fail conservative treatment, percutaneous drainage is curative and spares the reproductive capability. Post-traumatic or postoperative infected hematomas can be drained percutaneously. The liquefied component of the hematoma is relatively easy to drain. The thick organized hematoma is refractory to simple drainage. Debridement with intracavitary urokinase has been successful in further debulking the clot and evacuating the hematoma. The dosage regimen is similar to empyema treatment (see Ch. 20). Urinomas occur after trauma, surgery, or renal transplantation. As with bilomas, the urinary tract is catheterized to divert flow of the urinary stream. The urinoma may close with percutaneous nephrostomy if the urine leak is small. For larger leaks, ureteral stenting is performed to expedite healing of the leak without formation of a stricture (see Fig. 22.5).

Lymphoceles occur after surgery or lymph node dissections. Percutaneous drainage is performed for symptomatic or infected lymphoceles. Lymphoceles frequently require prolonged periods of drainage ranging from 4 to 6 weeks. The lymphocele can be sclerosed with Betadine or alcohol if a course of prolonged drainage fails. A sinogram of the cavity is performed to assess the volume of the cavity and exclude any fistulous communications. A small volume of absolute alcohol is injected into the cavity for 1 hour to sclerose and collapse the walls of the cavity. The cavity is drained until the output is negligible and the cavity is collapsed around the pigtail catheter.

Percutaneous Gastrostomy

The three gastrostomy techniques are surgical, percutaneous endoscopic (PEG), and percutaneous image-guided. Surgical gastrostomy has been replaced by percutaneous methods because of surgery's higher costs and procedure-related complications. PEG placement offers additional diagnostic capabilities and was less expensive than other methods as reported by Wollman et al. Radiologic placement was slightly more successful and had fewer complications. A percutaneous gastrostomy is used when an endoscope cannot be passed into the stomach or when the abdominal wall cannot be

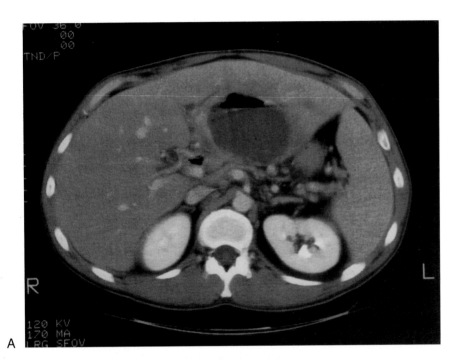

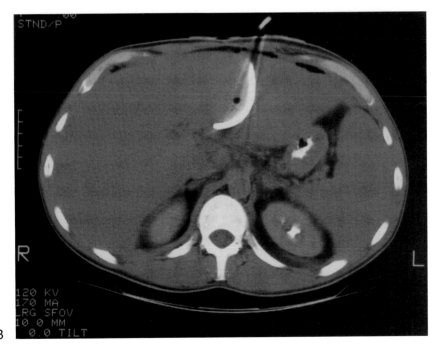

Figure 19.6 (A) Left lobe of liver abscess in patient with Crohn's disease. Note air fluid level (arrowheads). (B) A 10 French pigtail was placed subcostally into the abscess and the fluid aspirated. CT scan demonstrates complete evacuation of the abscess immediately after tube placement.

Figure 19.7 *A 25-year-old with cardiac valve complicated by splenic abscess. (****A****) Large subcapsular splenic abscess (arrowheads). (****B****) The abscess resolved and the spleen significantly decreased in size after 6 days of drainage.*

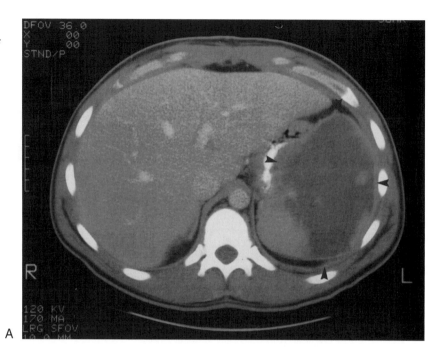

A

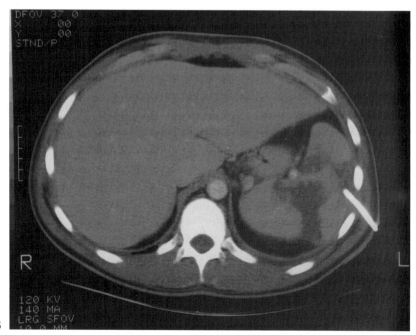

B

transilluminated. The indications are for long-term nutritional support or gastric decompression. Direct enteric nutrition avoids the vascular access problems, hepatic toxicity, and higher risk of infection associated with parenteral nutrition. Patients requiring gastrostomy are usually in poor medical health, and the 30-day reported mortality rate from all causes averages 15 percent. Gastrostomies can be placed in postpartial gastrectomy patients. The presence of moderate to marked ascites requires a gastroplexy and serial post-placement paracentesis to prevent leakage.

The patient receives nothing by mouth before gastrostomy placement. A nasogastric tube is passed into the stomach, and the stomach is distended with air. Intravenous glucagon is administered to decrease gastric peristalsis. Ultrasound is used to map out the position of the spleen and left lobe of the liver relative to the stomach. The colon can be opacified by administration of oral contrast the night before. Alternatively, the transverse colon and splenic flexure can be delineated by injecting a small amount of contrast or air per rectum.

A subcostal approach to the left of the midline is chosen. The inferior epigastric artery runs along the lateral third of the rectus abdomini muscles and is avoided. The stomach is reinflated with air to optimize the window for placement of the gastrostomy tube. A gastropexy is performed using three Brown/Mueller T-fasteners, which are placed into the stomach in a triangular configuration approximately 3 cm apart. The T-fasteners are pre-loaded within a needle that is jabbed into the stomach using a quick, sharp thrust (Fig. 19.8). Air is aspirated to confirm position within the stomach. The T-fastener is released from the needle, and the stomach wall is gently retracted up to the anterior wall of the abdomen (Fig. 19.9). The gastropexy is intended to minimize the complication of gastric leakage.

An incision is made in the middle of the T-fastener triangle. An 18-gauge arterial access needle is passed into the stomach angling toward the gastric outlet. This facilitates conversion to a gastrojejunostomy. A super-stiff wire is coiled within the stomach and the tract is dilated. The gastrostomy catheter is placed through a peel-away sheath (Fig. 19.10). The balloon on the catheter is inflated and gently retracted toward the anterior abdominal wall to prevent gastric outlet obstruction (Fig. 19.11). The catheter is secured to the skin and a molnar disk is attached to the tube to prevent internal migration. The T-fasteners are removed in 10 to 14 days.

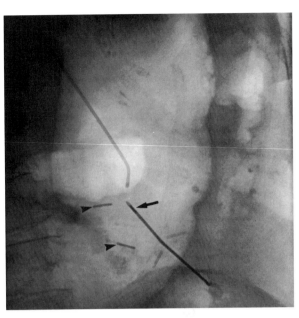

Figure 19.8 *An angle-tip guide catheter was used to negotiate a tight esophageal stricture to maximally distend the stomach with air. Two T-fasteners have been placed into the stomach (arrowheads). The third T-fastener is being inserted in a triangular configuration to perform a gastropexy. The needle is advanced through the subcutaneous tissue and jabbed through the anterior stomach wall (arrow). Air inflation confirms position within the stomach.*

We prefer larger caliber 16 to 20 French gastrostomy tubes for long-term feeding. Bard gastrostomy catheters are silicone catheters with multiple lumens intended for long-term use. Smaller caliber pigtail catheters or large lumen venous access lines are alternative devices that can be used for gastric decompression and feeding. Large caliber tubes are less likely to be occluded by crushed medications and foods. Smaller caliber tubes require more expensive liquid medications.

The feeding gastrostomy can be used on the first day after placement. A plain film of the abdomen is obtained to exclude free air before using the gastrostomy. If the patient has pain or peritoneal signs, a sinogram of the gastrostomy tube is performed in the lateral position to assess for any potential leak between the stomach and peritoneal cavity. Complications are infrequent and include peritonitis, gastrointestinal hemorrhage, leakage, superficial infection, and tube malfunction.

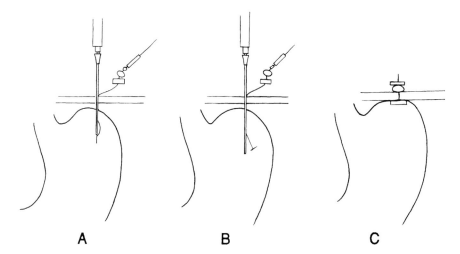

A   B   C

Figure 19.9 *T-fastener technique. (**A**) The Brown-Mueller T-fastener is pre-loaded in a slotted needle tip. The needle is inserted into the lumen of the stomach. (**B**) The syringe plunger advances the needle stylet and deploys the T-fastener. (**C**) The needle is withdrawn. The T-fastener is used to retract the stomach wall to the anterior abdominal wall and is secured by tying the suture strings on the fastening button.*

Alternative gastrostomy tubes include gastric buttons and push-type tubes. The gastric button is a silicon tube that stents open the fistulous communication between the stomach and skin. It is placed after the gastrostomy site has matured and is used predominantly in children. It eliminates the need for the catheter to be hanging out of the child's body. The gastrostomy button closure is opened and a feeding catheter placed into the stomach by the caregiver. The pull-type tubes are placed during the PEG procedure. During this procedure a wire is placed from the percutaneous transabdominal route through the stomach and esophagus exiting the patient's mouth. The tube is loaded on the oral end of the wire and is pushed into the stomach and out the percutaneous access. The flared disk of the push-type tubes eliminates the need for an intragastric balloon. There is the risk of oral flora contaminating the gastrostomy tract.

The choice of gastrostomy or gastrojejunostomy is controversial. A feeding gastrostomy allows bolus feedings, which are more physiologic than constant infusion feedings. A gastrostomy tube is easier to place and is potentially larger in diameter than a gastrojejunostomy. A gastrojejunostomy tube is indicated in patients who have poor gastric emptying or gastroesophageal reflux.

The percentage of patients with gastroesophageal reflux is disputed. Many practitioners prefer gastrojejunostomies to gastrostomies to prevent the complication of aspiration pneumonitis. Percutaneous gastrostomies are converted to a gastrojejunostomy by using a steerable guidewire and angle-tip catheter to cannulate the duodenum. Placing the patient in an left posterior oblique (LPO) position facilitates guidewire passage through the pylorus into the duodenum. A gastrojejunostomy catheter is advanced into the jejunum over the guidewire through a peel-away sheath. Several manufacturers make gastrojejunostomy tubes. We prefer triple lumen, silicon rubber tubes with proximal stomach and distal stomach ports (see Fig. 19-10F).

Percutaneous jejunostomies are placed in patients who have had previous gastrectomies and require long-term enteric nutrition. Surgical jejunostomies can be placed using laparoscopic techniques. Radiologic techniques rely on either CT or fluoroscopy to puncture the jejunum. The percutaneous puncture of the jejunum is difficult because of the mobility of the small bowel. The proximal jejunum is punctured and T-fasteners are used to perform a jejunopexy. Single lumen Hickman catheters or self-retaining pigtail catheters can be used for the jejunostomy.

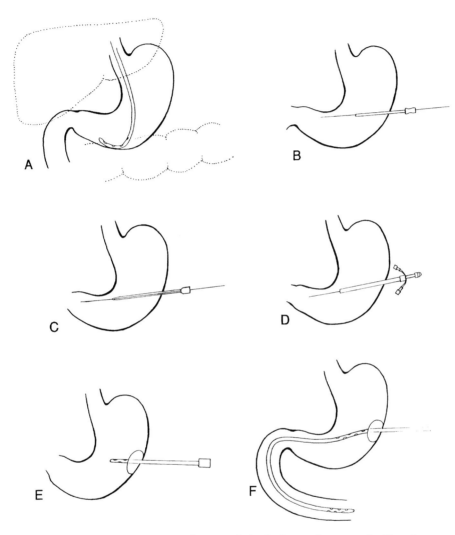

Figure 19.10 *Gastrostomy technique.* **(A)** *The liver edge is marked by ultrasound. The colon is carefully visualized by air or contrast examination. The stomach is distended with air insufflation through a nasogastric tube.* **(B)** *A needle is placed into the stomach with the tip of the needle oriented toward the pylorus. A wire is coiled within the stomach.* **(C)** *The tract is dilated.* **(D)** *A peel-away sheath is placed into the stomach over the wire.* **(E)** *The gastrostomy tube is placed into the stomach through the peel-away sheath. The balloon is inflated and used to retract the anterior gastric wall to the abdominal wall.* **(F)** *A feeding gastrojejunostomy tube is placed over a wire that has been negotiated into the duodenum. The tube has a lumen for gastric decompression and jejunal feeding. A balloon is inflated in the stomach and gently retracted toward the abdominal wall.*

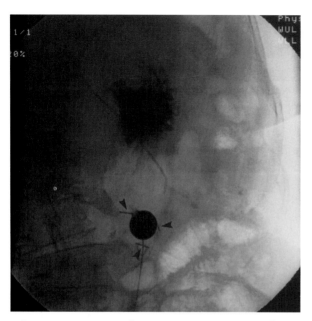

Figure 19.11 *Completion gastrostomy picture showing balloon inflated and pulled back toward the anterior abdominal wall. The three gastropexy T-fasteners are in place (arrowheads). A small contrast injection confirms position within the stomach. The contrast within the gastrostomy balloon was subsequently removed and replaced with saline.*

Suggested Readings

Bell SD, Carmody EA, Yeung EY et al: Percutaneous gastrostomy and gastrojejunostomy: additional experience in 519 procedures. Radiology 194:817, 1995

Borge MA, Vesely TM, Picus D: Gastrostomy button placement through percutaneous gastrostomy tracts created with fluoroscopic guidance: experience in 27 children. J Vasc Interv Radiol 6:179, 1995

Gray RR, Ho C-S, Yee A et al: Direct percutaneous jejunostomy. AJR 149:931, 1987

Kerlan RK, Jeffrey RB, Pogany AC, Ring EJ: Abdominal abscess with low-output fistula: successful percutaneous drainage. Radiology 155:73, 1985

Lambiase RE: Percutaneous abscess and fluid drainage: a critical review. Cardiovasc Interv Radiol 14:143, 1991

Lambiase RE, Deyoe L, Cronan JJ, Dorfman GS: Percutaneous drainage of 355 consecutive abscesses: results of primary drainage with 1-year follow-up. Radiology 184:167, 1992

Lee MJ, Rattner DW, Legemate DA et al: Acute complicated pancreatitis: redefining the role of interventional radiology. Radiology 183:171, 1992

Mueller PR, Saini S, Wittenberg J et al: Sigmoid diverticular abscesses: percutaneous drainage as an adjunct to surgical resection in 24 cases. Radiology 164:321, 1987

Olson DL, Krubsack AJ, Steward ET: Percutaneous enteral alimentation: gastrostomy versus gastrojejunostomy. Radiology 187:105, 1993

Schuster MR, Crummy AB, Wojtowcycz MM, McDermont JC: Abdominal abscesses associated with enteric fistulas: percutaneous management. J Vasc Interv Radiol 3:359, 1992

van Sonnenberg E, D'Agostino HB, Casola G et al: Percutaneous abscess drainage: current concepts. Radiology 181:617, 1991

vanSonnenberg E, Wittich GR, Casola G et al: Percutaneous drainage of infected and noninfected pancreatic pseudocysts: experience in 101 cases. Radiology 170:757, 1989

Wollman B, D'Agostino HB, Walus-Wigle JR et al: Radiologic, endoscopic, and surgical gastrostomy: an institutional evaluation and meta-analysis of the literature. Radiology 197:699, 1995

Chest Biopsy and Drainage

MICHAEL A. BRAUN

Pleural drainage and chest tube management have long been the proprietary knowledge of thoracic surgeons. Treatment of pleural diseases with interventional methods requires knowledge of pleural physiology, pleural drainage systems, and chest tube care. Familiarity with these principles will allow the interventional radiologist to become comfortable with managing routine chest drainage. Interventional techniques offer the advantage of precise imaging guidance and less chest wall trauma. The goals of pleural drainage are the removal of air, fluid, or blood from the pleural space and the re-expansion of the underlying lung. Percutaneous drainage catheters combined with enzymatic therapy can effectively treat pleural fluid collections traditionally considered drainable only by large bore chest tubes. Image-guided catheter drainage can be used to treat pneumothoraces, empyemas, hemothoraces, and malignant effusions.

Pleural Space Anatomy and Physiology

The pleura is a thin, serous membrane that consists of a single layer of mesothelial cells. The parietal pleura lines the inside surfaces of the chest wall, the mediastinum, and the diaphragm. The visceral pleura covers all the surfaces of the lungs including the interlobar fissures. The pleura has an extensive lymphatic drainage system. The parietal pleural lining the mediastinum contains numerous stomata that drain directly into the mediastinal lymphatic vessels. The stomata are important for removal of excess fluid, blood cells, and protein from the pleural space.

The pleural space is bathed by a small amount (1 to 3 ml) of clear, thin serous fluid (Fig. 20.1). This fluid acts as a lubricant and an adhesive agent. Pleural fluid hydrostatically couples the chest wall and lung via the property of surface tension. This hydrostatic coupling

force is analogous to the surface tension force exerted by water placed between two flat glass surfaces. There are several mechanisms for pleural effusion accumulation. Transudative effusions are caused by increased pulmonary interstitial pressure (cardiac failure) or reduced plasma oncotic pressure (renal failure or cirrhosis). Exudative effusions are caused by infection or inflammation involving the pleural space. Malignant pleural effusions are caused by impaired or blocked lymphatic drainage.

The natural tendency of the lungs is to collapse inward. The lung is maintained fully expanded by the outward recoil of the chest wall. Pleural fluid couples the visceral surface of the lung together with the parietal surface lining the chest wall (Fig. 20.2). The normal pleural pressure is between –2 cm H_2O at end expiration and –7 cm H_2O at end inspiration. Excess air or fluid within

Figure 20.1 *Pleural fluid formation is postulated to form from the pressure gradient between the systemic capillary hydrostatic pressure and the pulmonary hydrostatic pressure. The pulmonary lymphatic system is important in humans for absorption of fluid and protein from the pleural space.*

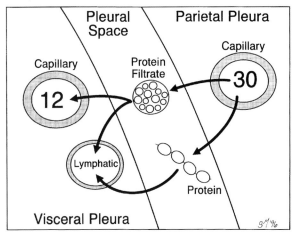

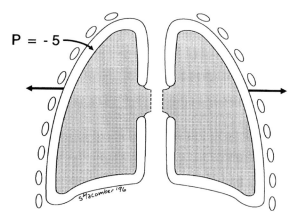

Figure 20.2 *The inward elastic recoil of a lung is counterbalanced by the outward bellow force of the chest wall. This causes a negative pressure within the pleural space. The surface tension of pleural fluid couples the two pleural surfaces together.*

the pleural space disrupts the intrapleural pressure and can impair expansion of the lung. Drainage of air, blood, or fluid from the pleural space requires an airtight system to maintain the negative intrapleural pressure. This is accomplished by a one-wave valve mechanism. A Heimlich flutter valve or a water-seal chamber is the most commonly used antireflux device.

Chest Tube Drainage Systems

The simplest pleural drainage system is the Heimlich valve. A Heimlich valve contains a one-way flutter valve, which opens when there is positive pleural pressure and collapses when there is negative pleural pressure (Fig. 20.3). It is best used for treating pneumothoraces. The advantages of the Heimlich valve are its simplicity, small size, and potential use as an outpatient therapy. The drawbacks are that fluid, blood, or pus can interfere with the function of the flutter valve and the valve can be connected in a reverse direction, which can cause a tension pneumothorax. The thoracic vent is a 13 French urethane catheter with trocar connected to a one-way flutter valve (Fig. 20.4). A signal diaphragm reflects the pressure change in the pleural space and indicates entry of the catheter/trocar into the pleural space. The catheter is then fed over the trocar into the pleural space. Samelson et al. reported successful treatment of 16 simple pneumothoraces using this device.

Suction pleural drainage systems consist of three components for achieving the functions of (1) fluid collection, (2) unidirectional air flow from the pleural space, and (3) suction control. The commercial unitized pleural drainage systems are best understood when they are broken down into these three components and

Figure 20.3 *Heimlich valve. The one-way flutter valve vents air from the pleural space but prevents re-entry. During expiration, the pleural pressure is positive and the air in the pneumothorax will be vented externally. During inspiration, the pleural pressure is negative, which collapses the flutter valve, preventing air reflux.*

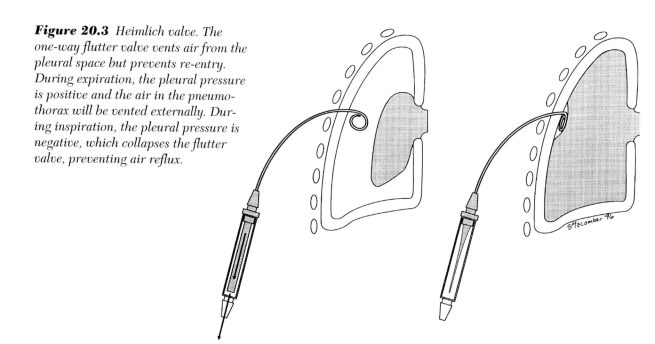

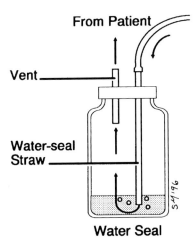

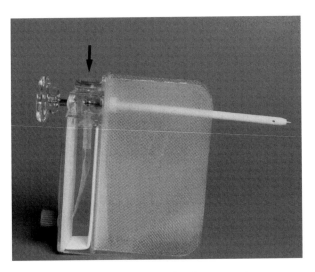

Figure 20.4 *Thoracic vent. This device combines a Heimlich valve with a catheter inserted over a metal trocar. A unique indicator on the top of the vent signals that the pneumothorax has been entered (arrow). Two plastic adhesive wings secure the unit to the patient's chest.*

Figure 20.5 *Diagram of one-bottle pleural drainage system. (Modified from Light RW: Pleural Diseases. 3rd Ed. Williams & Wilkins, Baltimore, 1995, with permission.)*

described based on the bottle systems from which they evolved. A one-bottle collection system consists of a single bottle that is both a collection and a water-seal chamber. The chest tube is connected to a rigid straw inserted into a stopper in a sterile bottle. Enough saline is instilled into the bottle so that the tip of the rigid straw is 2 cm below the surface of the saline solution (Fig. 20.5). This creates a water seal that allows egress of air from the pleural space and prevents reflux of air into the pleural space. This simple system works well for uncomplicated pneumothoraces. The disadvantage of this system occurs when substantial amounts of pleural fluid are draining from the patient's pleural space. The level of the fluid in the bottle rises, which increases the pressure necessary to allow fluid to exit the pleural space.

The two-bottle drainage system addresses the disadvantage of the one-bottle system. The two-bottle system adds a drainage collection bottle before the water-seal bottle (Fig. 20.6). The collection bottle traps the fluid draining from the pleural space and does not allow it to interfere with the level of the fluid in the water-seal bottle. The disadvantage in the two-bottle system is that the air in the fluid collection chamber becomes an extension of the patient's pneumothorax. This creates a dead space of compressible air between

the water-seal chamber and the pneumothorax. This increases the amount of pressure necessary to expel air from the pleural space. The siphon effect that the water seal provides for fluid drainage is lost.

A three-bottle system adds a suction control bottle to the two-bottle system to overcome the dead space effect introduced by the fluid collection bottle (Fig. 20.7). The suction expedites removal of air and

Figure 20.6 *Diagram of two-bottle pleural drainage system. (Modified from Light RW: Pleural Diseases. 3rd Ed. Williams & Wilkins, Baltimore, 1995, with permission.)*

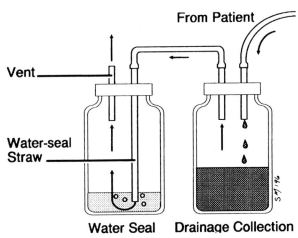

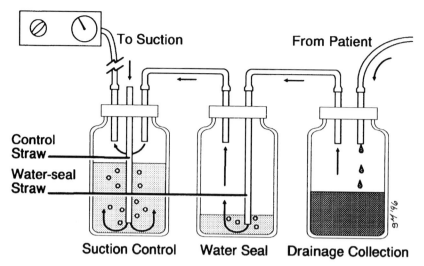

Figure 20.7 *Diagram of three-bottle pleural drainage system. (Modified from Light RW: Pleural Diseases. 3rd Ed. Williams & Wilkins, Baltimore, 1995, with permission.)*

fluid from the pleural space, which facilitates re-expansion of the lung. Ten to 25 cm of water pressure suction is adequate in most cases. The bubbling within the suction control system must be continuous but not vigorous. Vigorous bubbling creates noise and hastens evaporation of the solution. The Emerson three-bottle system can apply suction levels up to 50 cm H_2O. There are several commercially available drainage systems that duplicate the classic three-bottle system in a disposable, compact, unbreakable, and readily transportable apparatus (Fig. 20.8). Examples are Deknatel's Pleur-evac, Argyle's Sentinel Seal, Atrium's Compact 2002, and Davol's Thora-Klex.

Chest Tube Care

The water-seal chamber should be inspected to see whether air bubbles are escaping through the water-seal chamber. This signifies the presence of an air leak within the patient or a false leak from the external pleural drain tubing. If no air bubbles are seen on initial inspection of the water seal, the patient should be asked to cough while observing the water seal for bubbling. Coughing increases the pleural pressure and should demonstrate small air leaks. Leaks in the exter-

nal tubing can be detected by clamping the chest tube at the point where it exits from the chest. This will demonstrate whether the bubbling to the water-seal chamber is from a leak in the drainage system or a leak in the lung. Chest tube blockage was previously treated by milking or stripping the latex connecting tubing. Chest tube stripping is a controversial practice and has fallen out of favor. Obstructed pigtail catheters are opened by guidewire passage, exchanged for new catheters, or flushed open with urokinase.

The water-seal chamber should be inspected with the suction control device turned off. If the chest tube is patent in the pleural space, the level of the fluid should rise in the water-seal chamber on inspiration and fall during expiration. This fluctuation, which mimics changes in pleural pressure, is called "tidaling." Tidaling ceases for two causes. One cause is from kinking or obstruction of the tube. The other cause is when the pneumothorax is evacuated and the lung is re-expanded, tidaling ceases from restored negative pressure and sealing of the pleural around the tube. The fluid within the water-seal chamber rises and responds to the restored negative pressure within the pleural space. A chest radiograph is obtained at this point in time to confirm either the successful pleural drainage or the occlusion of the tube as the cause for the absence of the tidaling.

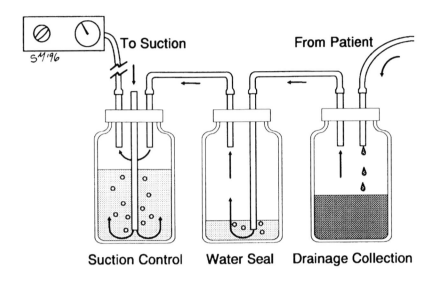

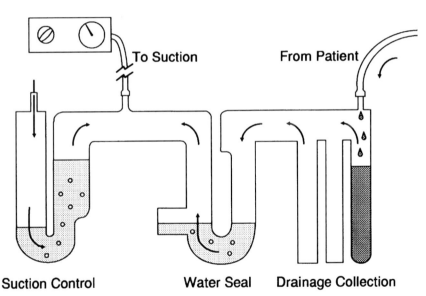

Figure 20.8 *The Pleurovac system is a three-bottle suction drainage system combined into a transportable and compact unit.*

During expiration or coughing, air from the pleural space is expelled. During obstructive inspiration, large subatmospheric pressures up to –80 cm H_2O may be generated so that fluid in the collection chamber may be sucked up into the tubing into the pleural space. To prevent this, the collection chamber should always be placed 100 cm below the chest. Theoretically, if the collection chamber is placed 100 cm below the patient,

suction would not be required. This is because fluid in the drainage catheter forms a hydrostatic column, which generates a subatmospheric pressure up to –100 cm H_2O. However, air pockets produced by dependent loops of connective tubing between the patient and collection chamber can break the continuity of this column, causing a loss of the negative pressure due to the air lock phenomenon.

Air flow within the tubing of a chest drainage system is turbulent. The air flow follows the Fanning equation where flow is proportional to the fifth power of the radius of the drainage tube. A tube with a 6 mm internal diameter allows a maximum flow of 15 L/min of air. A tube with a 12 mm internal diameter allows an air flow rate of 50 to 60 L/min. A 12 French pigtail catheter has an approximate internal diameter of 3 mm. The standard 32 French surgical test tube has an internal diameter of 9 mm. Most air leaks are between 1 and 10 L/min but can be greater than 20 L/min after pulmonary resections. Smaller tubes can be used when the air leak is less than the maximum flow rate as determined by the internal diameter. The consequence of this property is that larger tubes or multiple tubes are required to overcome large air leaks.

Chest Tube Removal

In general, chest tubes for pneumothorax are removed when the lung has expanded and the air leaks stops. A 24- to 48-hour period of water-seal drainage and chest radiographs confirm cessation of the leak. Some advocate a period of clamping a tube before removal. A radiograph is taken to assess for a recurrent pneumothorax. Chest tubes are removed for hemothorax or empyema when the pleural drainage has ceased or is less than 50 ml/day. Chest catheters are removed while the patient performs a Valsalva maneuver. The Valsalva maneuver creates positive pleural pressure and decreases the likelihood of a pneumothorax. The tube is quickly pulled out and the wound covered immediately with an occlusive dressing.

Thoracentesis

Thoracentesis is performed for both diagnostic and therapeutic indications. A diagnostic thoracentesis is designed to determine whether the pleural fluid is transudative, exudative, malignant, or infected. Transudative pleural fluid effusions occur with congestive heart failure, renal failure, and cirrhosis. The fluid contains little protein and few cells. Etiologies of exudative pleural effusions include infections, pulmonary infarcts, neoplasms, pancreatitis, and trauma. Chylous pleural effusions can be due to traumatic rupture of the thoracic duct or rarely to neoplasms.

Laboratory analysis of pleural effusions includes cell count, specific gravity, lactate dehydrogenase (LDH), amylase, pH, Gram stain, glucose, protein, cytology, and culture and sensitivity. Light's criteria are used to differentiate transudative from exudative effusions. The effusion is exudative if the pleural fluid/serum protein ratio is greater than 0.5, the LDH ratio is greater than 0.6, or the pleural fluid LDH is greater than two-thirds the upper normal limit of serum LDH. Elevated pleural fluid amylase indicates a pancreatic related effusion, esophageal perforation, or malignant effusion. Reduced pleural glucose (< 60 mg/dl) indicates a parapneumonic effusion, a tuberculous effusion, a malignant effusion, or a rheumatoid effusion.

The preliminary diagnosis and previous chest radiographs or computed tomography (CT) scans are reviewed to plan the thoracentesis. A diagnostic thoracentesis requires sampling a small volume of fluid for laboratory analysis. Therapeutic thoracentesis is performed for drainage and relief of symptomatic effusions. The thoracentesis can be done for both diagnostic and therapeutic indications. Ultrasound is the first choice for imaging guidance. CT guidance is reserved for loculated effusions not readily visualized by ultrasound or effusions incidentally discovered on CT scan. The patient is examined in the sitting position. The operator should scan the pleural effusion to gain a real-time understanding of the size and variation in the pleural effusion with the patient breathing. Ultrasound is used to mark a posterior or lateral intercostal space that offers the shortest path to the largest collection of pleural fluid. Large pleural effusions can be marked and subsequently drained. Small or loculated effusions are best approached with real-time imaging guidance. A low intercostal approach runs the risk of injury to the spleen or liver. A high intercostal approach increases the chance of lung injury and makes complete evacuation of the pleural effusion more difficult.

The chosen intercostal space is cleansed and generously anesthetized with lidocaine. Both the skin and pleura are anesthetized. The pleura is safely anesthetized by walking the needle over the rib and depositing lidocaine adjacent to the parietal pleura. An 18- to 20-gauge intravenous needle is used for routine diagnostic and simple therapeutic thoracentesis. Commercially available dedicated thoracentesis needles are available that have valves to prevent inadvertent introduction of air into the pleural space. These devices are larger than necessary for diagnostic thoracentesis and are reserved for therapeutic taps. The intravenous needle is connected to a 10 ml syringe. Gentle negative aspiration is applied as the needle is advanced into the pleural fluid collection. Following successful aspiration of fluid, the plastic cannula is advanced into the pleural space. Meticulous care is taken to avoid entry of air into the pleural space. The stopcock and drainage tubing are preassembled before placement of the catheter into the pleural space. This facilitates rapid connection of the external drainage system to the needle. For diagnostic thoracentesis, 50 to 150 ml of fluid are slowly withdrawn and placed into the collecting tubes. A 1 liter evacuation bottle or closed drainage system is used for therapeutic thoracentesis. The evacuation bottle speeds removal of the fluid from the pleural space. It is recommended to aspirate 1 liter of fluid via the vacuum bottle. Larger volumes of fluid that are rapidly removed can result in re-expansion pulmonary edema. Re-expansion pulmonary edema complicates large volume thoracentesis in patients with chronic collapsed lungs or central bronchial obstruction. It is treated by diuresis and supplemental nasal oxygenation. If a large volume thoracentesis is required, placement of a small pigtail catheter and drainage via a Pleurovac device over 1 to 2 hours is recommended. The thoracentesis is stopped if the patient develops symptoms of dyspnea or cough. The needle is removed when the patient performs the Valsalva maneuver. A follow-up chest radiograph documents the amount of fluid removed and evaluates for the presence of a pneumothorax.

Pneumothorax

Image-guided pigtail catheters are used in increasing frequency to treat pneumothoraces. Pigtail catheters are best used to treat small pneumothoraces that are due to intermittent or small air leaks. The goals of treatment are evacuation of the air, re-expansion of the lung, and in secondary cases prevention of recurrence. Indications for image-guided chest catheters include spontaneous pneumothorax, small postoperative persistent air leaks, iatrogenic pneumothorax, and pneumothorax due to underlying lung disease. Image-guided chest catheters can be placed in patients who have small pneumothoraces that cannot be reached by conventional chest tube insertion techniques. The reduced chest wall trauma and smaller size makes these tubes better tolerated by patients.

Either Seldinger or trocar technique can be used to place the chest catheter. Fluoroscopy is used to localize the pneumothorax. The patient can be placed in a semiupright position to collect the air within the apical portion of the hemithorax. The second or third anterior intercostal space is chosen. Local anesthesia is performed by infiltrating lidocaine into the intercostal space and parietal pleura. Regional anesthesia with a bupivacaine intercostal nerve block is easy to perform and well accepted by patients. Bupivacaine is injected underneath the two to three adjacent ribs several inches posterior to the chest catheter insertion site. For Seldinger technique, an 18-gauge needle is passed into the pneumothorax and air is aspirated to confirm needle position. A Superstiff guidewire is placed into the apical pleural space and the tract is dilated. A 12 to 14 French pigtail catheter is advanced over the guidewire into the apex of the hemithorax (Fig. 20.9). The pneumothorax is aspirated and the catheter is connected to a Heimlich valve or Pleurovac. Pleuritic chest pain can be relieved by intrapleural administration of lidocaine. Hospitalized patients are monitored with daily chest radiographs and assessment of the water-seal chamber. When the air leak has stopped, the patient is observed for an additional period of 24 to 48 hours with the pleural drain on water seal. The tube can be removed if no further air leak is seen and the chest radiograph shows re-expansion of the lung and absence of the pneumothorax.

Iatrogenic and spontaneous pneumothoraces are effectively managed with small caliber tubes connected to a Heimlich valve. A reliable patient can be treated as an outpatient with a Heimlich valve. Larger pneumothoraces associated with persistent air leaks or underlying lung disease are best treated by suction drainage. The application of suction helps overcome the leakage of air into the pleural space and allows the pleural surfaces to contact one

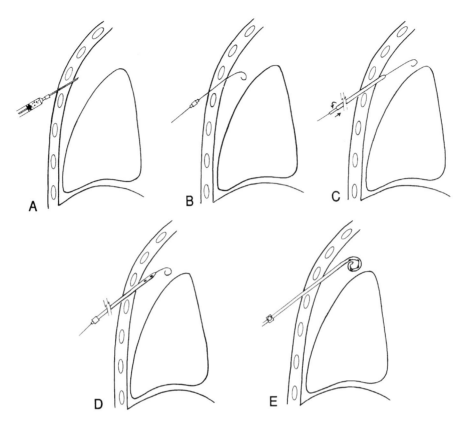

Figure 20.9 *Technique for pigtail catheter drainage of pneumothorax. (**A**) The patient is placed in a semirecumbent position to gravitate the air in the superior and anterior portion of the hemithorax. The second or third anterior intercostal space is anesthetized and punctured with a needle. Aspiration of air confirms the needle position within the pleural cavity. (**B**) A guidewire is inserted and directed into the apex of the hemithorax. (**C**) The intercostal space tract is dilated. (**D**) The pigtail catheter and stiffening cannula are inserted over the guidewire into the apex of the hemithorax. (**E**) The pigtail catheter is formed and positioned within the apex of the hemithorax.*

another. This re-establishes the hydrostatic coupling between the pleural surfaces and promotes closure of air leaks. Most air leaks can be evacuated with 20 to 25 cm H_2O suction generated by the Pleurovac. Larger air leaks can be controlled using the Emerson three-bottle system, which can generate up to 50 cm of suction or by the placement of a larger caliber chest tube. A 12 French pigtail catheter can evacuate 6 L of air/min. This is in comparison to standard surgical chest tubes, which can theoretically evacuate up to 50 to 60 L of air/min but are limited by the resistance of the pleural drainage systems to 30 to 35 L/min.

Chronic air leaks (> 5 days) can be treated using two different strategies. One strategy is long-term drainage with a pigtail catheter attached to a Heimlich valve. The other strategy is to perform a pleurodesis if the pneumothorax can be completely evacuated with the chest catheter in place. The pleurodesis is most successful in patients who have lungs that are re-expandable and have underlying lung disease predisposing to recurrent pneumothoraces. Examples are patients with recurrent spontaneous pneumothoraces or cavitary *Pneumocystis carinii* pneumonia (Fig. 20.10).

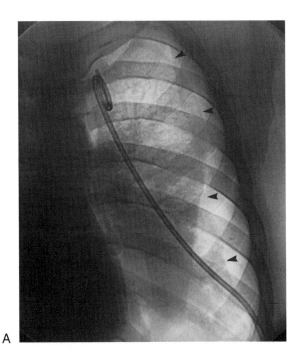

A

Figure 20.10 *Pneumothorax complicating cavitary* Pneumocystis carinii *pneumonia. (A) A 12 French pigtail catheter was inserted between the fourth and fifth left anterior ribs in the midclavicular line. Note the pneumothorax (arrowheads). (B) Lateral chest radiograph showing appropriate position of pneumothorax catheter in apex of hemithorax. (C) The recurrent pneumothorax was treated with talc fluorodesis to prevent recurrence. This resulted in a small accumulation of pleural fluid. There is persistent consolidation and atelectasis in the left lower lobe from the patient's underlying pneumonia.*

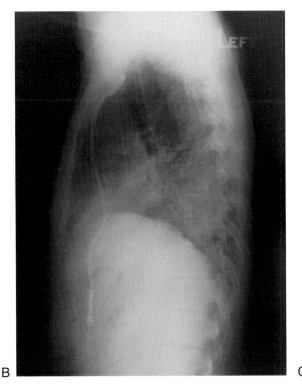

B

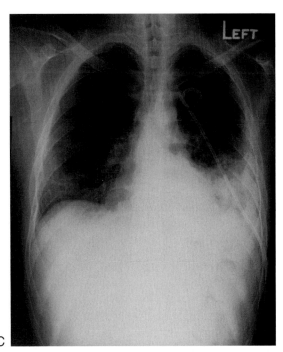

C

Empyema and Infected Hemothorax

Parapneumonic effusions are any effusion associated with a lung infection. The evolution of a parapneumonic effusion into an empyema can be roughly divided into three stages. Stage 1 empyemas are equivalent to parapneumonic effusions. The pH is between 7.2 and 7.4, the glucose is normal, and there is absence of loculation. Antibiotics and thoracentesis are usually adequate for treatment of these exudative effusions. Stage 2 empyemas are fibrinopurulent and characterized by thicker, more turbid fluid. The pH is between 7.0 and 7.2, the glucose is less than 60 mg/dl, and the LDH is elevated. There is loculation due to thin fibrin sheaths forming within the pleural space. This loculation can interfere with chest tube drainage. Stage 3 empyemas are the chronic sequela of infected pleural spaces. They are characterized by thickened pleural peels, entrapment of lung, and restriction of lung motion.

The complex three-dimensional anatomy of the pleural space is best evaluated by cross-sectional imaging. Chest CT scanning gives the best global assessment of the baseline size and distribution of the effusion.

Ultrasound best demonstrates the fibrin septa that loculate stage 2 and 3 empyemas and is useful for directing placement of the catheter (Fig. 20.11). Chest radiographs are useful for following tube position and estimating pleural fluid response to therapy. The catheter should be placed into the most dependent portion of the empyema within the largest cavity. This is usually the posterior costophrenic sulcus. Whenever possible, a lateral approach is used. A catheter placed from a posterior approach can become kinked when the patient lies in the supine position. Imaging guidance can be a combination of ultrasound and fluoroscopy or CT scan. We prefer the combination of fluoroscopy and ultrasound, which provides real-time imaging guidance and fluoroscopic control of guidewire/catheter manipulations. CT scan guidance can be used when the empyema is discovered during diagnostic scanning. Chest CT scan does underestimate the amount of loculation that can be visualized by ultrasound.

An intercostal nerve block is performed to increase the patient's tolerance and comfort level caused by the presence of the drainage catheter. The two to four ribs surrounding the punctured intercostal space are anesthetized. Bupivacaine is injected under the ribs 5 to 10

Figure 20.11 *A transaxillary ultrasound of a left empyema. Note the thick septations and collapsed underlying lung (arrows). The internal septations were not visualized on a CT scan.*

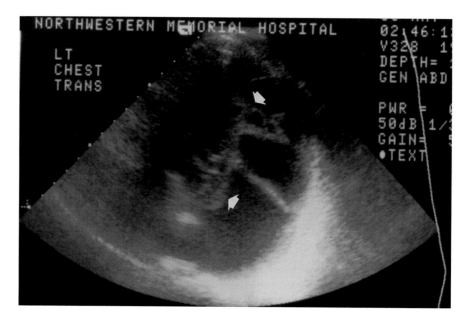

cm proximal to the catheter entry site. A 22- to 25-gauge needle is used to inject 5 ml of bupivacaine under each rib. This significantly lessens the catheter-related pain.

The catheter can be placed using Seldinger or trocar technique. We prefer Seldinger technique and use an 18-gauge needle directed into the effusion/empyema under imaging guidance. A small amount of fluid is aspirated to confirm needle position. A super stiff guidewire is coiled within the pleural space fluid collection. The tract is dilated. Twelve French single lumen pigtail catheters or larger are preferred. Smaller diameter catheters can occlude with debris or become kinked in the intercostal space. The 12 to 14 French single lumen pigtail catheter is advanced over the guide-

wire and positioned in the empyema (Fig. 20.12). The pleural drain is connected to suction drainage. The Pleurovac or similar pleural drainage device has 20 cm H_2O suction continuously applied to the catheter.

The empyema is drained overnight and a chest radiograph is ordered the next day to estimate the amount of remaining fluid. The loculation within empyemas usually prevents complete evacuation by tube drainage alone. This necessitates enzymatic debridement with urokinase, which is performed in the majority of the cases on the first to second day of drainage if the fluid collection is incompletely removed. A mixture of 100 to 150 ml saline and 250,000 units of urokinase is ordered based on the estimated size of the

Figure 20.12 *Technique of pleural fluid drainage. The largest collection of pleural fluid is localized with ultrasound or CT guidance.* **(A)** *The intercostal space is anesthetized and the needle placed over the rib into the pleural fluid.* **(B)** *A wire is coiled within the pleural fluid space.* **(C)** *The intercostal space tract is dilated.* **(D)** *The pigtail catheter with stiffening cannula is inserted over the wire into the fluid collection.* **(E)** *The pigtail catheter is coiled and positioned in the pleural fluid. The fluid is aspirated. Typically the axillary sixth or seventh intercostal space is punctured and the pigtail catheter is directed toward the posterior costophrenic gutter.*

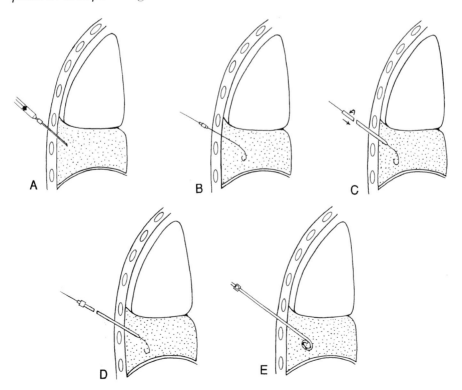

empyema. The reconstituted urokinase is divided into three doses of approximately 83,000 units of urokinase each. Reconstituted urokinase has a shelf life of 24 hours. Two doses are given on the first day, and a third dose is given the morning of the second day. The urokinase dose of 30 to 50 ml is slowly injected into the chest tube. The tube is clamped for 1 hour and then returned to suction drainage. Most empyemas are completely evacuated with three to six doses of urokinase. Infected hemithoraces require six doses. The tube is removed when there is clinical and radiographic evidence of complete drainage of the empyema. Clinical parameters include less than 50 ml of drainage per day, defervescence of fever, and resolution of leukocytosis. Chest radiographs are obtained to evaluate evacuation of the empyema, resolution of the underlying pneumonia, and re-expansion of the involved lung. Because of the complexity of the pleural anatomy, it is frequently necessary to use CT scans to evaluate completeness of empyema resolution (Fig. 20.13).

Figure 20.13 *(A) Right empyema. (B) CT scan 5 days after percutaneous drainage and three doses of urokinase. The effusion has been completely evacuated. The residual pleural thickening will resolve with time. The catheter was inserted through a lateral intercostal approach with the tip positioned in the posterior costophrenic gutter.*

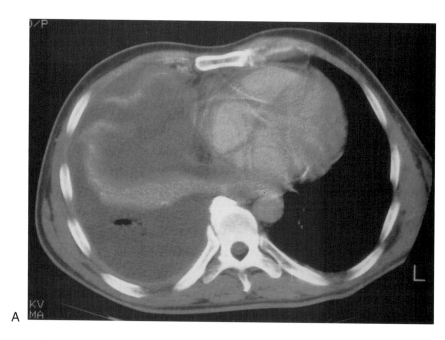

A

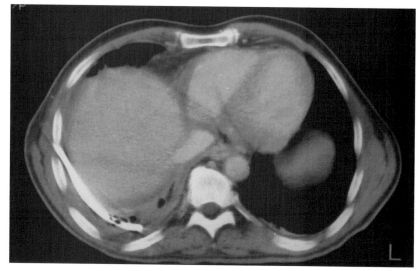

B

Image-guided catheter drainage and intracavitary urokinase can effectively treat empyemas and infected hemothoraces. Fibrinolytic therapy for loculated pleural fluid collections has been used for 45 years. Intracavitary instillation of a lytic agent lyses the fibrin septa and dissolves the fibrinous debris. Most experience has been based on the use of streptokinase, which has a variable success rate and possible allergic or anaphylactic reactions. The cure rates using urokinase are significantly better without the potential side effects of streptokinase. We reviewed the treatment of 37 patients with complicated parapneumonic effusions or frank empyemas. Only 3 of 37 patients were drained completely by catheter drainage alone. Thirty-four of 37 patients required urokinase enzymatic debridement, which resulted in complete radiologic and clinical resolution of the effusions. Six patients with infected hemothoraces responded to six intrapleural instillations of urokinase with clinical and radiographic resolution of the infected hemothorax. There were no associated complications or systemic effects from the intrapleural administration of urokinase. None of the patients required a thoracotomy or decortication surgery.

Malignant Pleural Effusions

The diagnosis of a malignant pleural effusion signals a poor prognosis. Survival times range only to a few months. The treatment of malignant pleural effusion is palliative. The patient's general physical condition, symptoms, and expected survival must be weighed in determining the optimal course of treatment. Debilitated patients with a short expected survival are treated by performing periodic thoracenteses for relief of symptoms. Pleurodesis is reserved for patients with dyspnea who have a longer expected period of survival. Carcinoma of the lung is the most common tumor to result in pleural metastases and malignant pleural effusions. Other malignancies associated with pleural effusions are breast carcinoma, lymphoma, ovarian carcinoma, gastric carcinoma, and malignant mesothelioma. Malignant pleural effusions due to lymphoma, breast cancer, or small cell lung carcinoma can resolve by treatment with systemic chemotherapy. Pleural drainage is performed in these patients to relieve symptoms while undergoing chemotherapy. Pleurodesis is reserved for patients who fail or who are not candidates for systemic chemotherapy.

The indication for chemical pleurodesis is in symptomatic patients with expected survival of greater than 6 to 12 weeks. It is essential to prove that removal of fluid improves the patient's symptoms. Dyspnea is the only symptom likely to be relieved by pleurodesis. Pleurodesis is less likely to be successful but should still be attempted if the pleural fluid glucose is < 60 mg/dl or the pH is < 7.30. Patients who have pleural effusions associated with lymphangitic carcinomatosis, endobronchial obstruction, or chronic atelectasis may not have an improvement in their dyspnea despite complete evacuation of the pleural effusion. It is not helpful to attempt pleural sclerosis if the lung cannot be re-expanded when a main bronchus is obstructed or the lung is entrapped by encasing metastatic disease.

The placement of a pigtail catheter is similar to drainage of empyemas or hemothoraces. An intercostal rib block and local infiltrative anesthesia are used for analgesia. A 12 French pigtail catheter is positioned within the dependent portion of the pleural space in the largest fluid collection via a lateral approach. Serial chest radiographs are obtained to document complete evacuation of the pleural effusion and re-expansion of the underlying lung. The pleural space needs to be drained as completely as possible so that the instilled sclerosing agent is not diluted and the pleural surfaces remain in close contact during the time of the initial inflammatory insult. Malignant effusions are exudative and can become loculated with fibrin septa. Enzymatic debridement with urokinase can expedite complete drainage of malignant effusions. Fibrinolytic therapy expedites complete pleural drainage, reducing the time necessary to perform pleurodesis. If the effusion fails complete drainage after 5 days, intrapleural urokinase is used to complete drainage. In 50 percent of patients refractory to simple drainage, three doses of urokinase administered over 24 hours resulted in complete drainage of the residual effusion, which allowed successful chemical pleurodesis to be performed.

Talc and doxycycline are the available agents for pleurodesis. Talc, the more effective agent, has a 90 to 95 percent success rate. Talc is sterilized by gamma irradiation or autoclave dry heat in aliquots of 4 to 5 g. Doxycycline is readily available but slightly less effective, having a 70 to 80 percent success rate. Sclerotherapy with doxycycline is performed when there is < 100 ml/day of output from the drainage catheter. Talc pleurodesis is effective in patients who have high-output malignant pleural effusions (> 100 ml/day) or small hydropneumothoraces.

Good patient analgesia is important. The pleural space is anesthetized by instilling 20 ml of bupivacaine via the chest tube. The patient is deeply consciously sedated. A talc pleurodesis is performed using 4 to 5 g of talc mixed with 100 ml of normal saline. The talc slurry is instilled into the pleural space with the chest tube clamped for 1 hour. The chest tube is then returned to water suction for 24 hours to promote complete evacuation of the pleural fluid and re-expansion of the underlying lung. A single instillation of talc slurry is effective. Doxycycline pleurodesis is similar. Doxycycline, 500 mg, is mixed in 100 ml of normal saline with 100 mg of lidocaine and instilled into the pleural space for 1 hour. Doxycycline may need to be given two to three times before pleural synthesis is achieved.

Drainage and pleurodesis can be performed on a select group of outpatients. The chest catheter is connected to a Tru-close bag (Uresil; L.P., Skokie, IL) and the patient instructed to record daily output. The reported duration of drainage is similar to conventional suction drainage. Sclerotherapy is performed when the output is less than 100 ml/day.

Lung Biopsy

The indications for lung biopsy are cellular diagnosis of nonoperable lung cancer, diagnosis of recurrent or metastatic tumor, and microbiologic identification of pulmonary infections. Transthoracic lung biopsy can be performed as an outpatient procedure. The radiographs are reviewed to determine the choice of imaging guidance and needle route. Relative contraindications are bleeding disorders, severe pulmonary hypertension, severe pulmonary disease (reduced forced expiratory volume in 1 second [FEV_1]), and vascular lesions. The patient is informed of the small incidence of hemoptysis (5 percent) and the possibility of pneumothorax (20 to 30 percent) requiring a postbiopsy observation period or treatment.

Choice of imaging guidance is based on lesion size and location. Fluoroscopy is preferred for most biopsies because, the real-time imaging guidance shortens the procedure time. Fluoroscopy can be used to sample most peripheral pulmonary nodules seen on chest radiography. CT is used for biopsy of tiny nodules not visible on fluoroscopy, mediastinal masses or lymph nodes, chest wall masses, or pleural based masses (Fig. 20.14). Trans-ster-nal CT-guided biopsy is used to sample anterior mediastinal lymph nodes or masses. CT guidance can be used to place a localization needle adjacent to a tiny pulmonary nodule to help guide subsequent thoracoscopic removal. Ultrasound can be used to guide biopsy of pleural or chest wall masses. Transbronchial biopsy is used for central lesions causing hemoptysis, atelectasis, or postobstructive pneumonitis.

Several biopsy needle systems are available. Fine needle aspirations for cytologic examination use 20- to 22-gauge Westcott or Chiba needles. Coaxial systems have a guiding needle that is placed into the lesion. The stylet is removed and a smaller gauge needle is passed coaxially to obtain cytology aspirations. A core of tissue can be obtained through the guiding needle before its removal. Both systems are successful, and selection is often based on preference of the pathologist interpreting the specimen. We prefer using 22-gauge Westcott needles for most lung biopsies. The Wescott needle passes atraumatically through the lung, and the sample is obtained from a side-cutting port in the needle. The sideport is exposed when the stylet of the needle is removed. Complications are minimized by limiting the length of lung traversed, limiting the number of needle passes, and avoiding bullae and vessels.

The patient is placed in the prone, supine, or oblique positions on the fluoroscopy table depending on the location of the lesion and the approach chosen. The nodule is examined with fluoroscopy from multiple different angles with the patient performing quiet breathing. The intercostal space giving the shortest distance through the lung is chosen. The needle is inserted through the skin into the intercostal space parallel to the fluoroscopy beam. Fluoroscopy is used to direct the needle toward the nodule. The patient is instructed to quietly breathe and avoid coughing or deep breaths. The needle is then passed through the pleural and into the lung to the expected depth of the nodule. Fluoroscopic triangulation is used to determine position of the needle tip relative to the nodule (Fig. 20.15). Fluoroscopy is used to redirect the needle into the lesion or confirm successful needle placement. A 10 ml luerlock syringe is attached to the needle, and suction is applied while gentle up-and-down twisting motions are made until a small drop of blood or fluid just enters the hub of the needle. The suction is released and the needle is removed. The biopsy specimen is processed for cytologic analysis. If an infectious process is suspected, a sample of the specimen is diluted in normal saline for microbiologic analysis. CT-

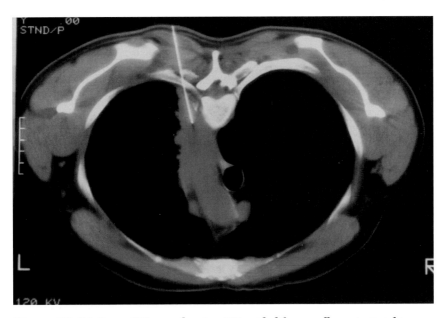

Figure 20.14 *Prone CT scan showing CT-guided fine needle aspiration biopsy of a left posterior mediastinal mass.*

guided biopsy is similar to the techniques used for abdominal mass biopsy. The disadvantage is that the needle is advanced blindly toward the anticipated position of the lesion. A coaxial system is used for transsternal anterior mediastinal biopsy. A 19-gauge needle is carefully pushed or drilled through the sternum toward the lesion. The guiding needle is pushed just through the posterior cortex of the sternum. A 22-gauge is passed through the guiding needle into the target lesion. This allows multiple samples to be taken.

The initial chest film is obtained 30 minutes postbiopsy. Most pneumothoraces (90 percent) are evident on the initial postbiopsy film. A chest radiograph is obtained whenever the patient becomes symptomatic. If no pneumothorax is present and the patient is asymptomatic, a repeat film is obtained at 2 hours postbiopsy. If no pneumothorax is present at 2 hours, the patient is discharged. Treatment of a biopsy-related pneumothorax is dictated by the presence of symptoms, enlarging size, and overall size. Small to moderate size asymptomatic pneumothoraces can be observed and are followed by serial films to assess for any changes in size. If after 3 to 4 hours the pneumothorax is stable or reducing, the patient can be discharged. If the pneumothorax progressively increases in size or is symptomatic, treatment is necessary. Treatment options include

aspiration of the pneumothorax or placement of a chest catheter connected to a Heimlich valve.

Intrathoracic Abscesses

The treatment for lung abscess is a prolonged trial of antibiotic therapy. Drainage is reserved for failures of medical therapy. Percutaneous drainage is an effective alternative or an adjunct to surgical treatment. Chest CT scanning is important to aid in patient selection. Lung abscesses containing fluid adjacent to the chest wall with associated pleural thickening can be approached safely percutaneously. This reduces the likelihood of an empyema or pneumothorax complicating transthoracic drainage. Techniques are similar to drainage of intra-abdominal abscesses. CT guidance offers the accuracy of cross-sectional imaging but lacks the real-time imaging guidance of fluoroscopy, which is helpful for guidewire and catheter manipulations. Either imaging modality can be used. The abscess is approached and punctured where it abuts the chest wall. Catheter size depends on the size of the abscess, ranging from 8 to 14 French single-lumen locking pigtail catheters. Pleurovac drains are used. Duration of drainage is long, ranging from 11 to 18 days.

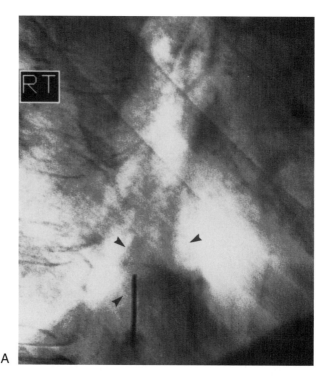

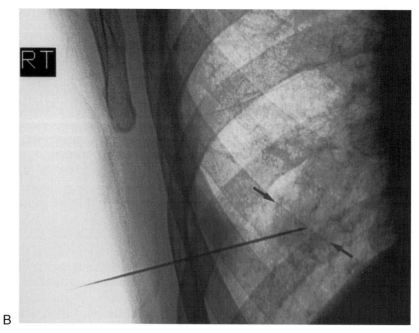

Figure 20.15 *Lung nodule biopsy.* **(A)** *The needle is advanced toward the nodule parallel to the beam of the image intensifier (arrowheads).* **(B)** *Fluoroscopic triangulation documents the needle tip within the nodule (arrows).*

Mediastinal abscesses are a rare but serious infection. Surgical treatment has a high reported morbidity and mortality, often with prolonged hospitalization duration. Etiologies are esophageal leaks, postoperative or post-traumatic in origin. CT scanning is necessary to map out the abscess and choose a percutaneous route into the abscess. The procedure requires careful planning to avoid the mediastinal vascular and airway structures. The pleural space or lung can be crossed to access the abscess as long as no holes on the drainage catheter are placed in the intervening organs to spread the infection or cause a pneumothorax (Fig. 20.16).

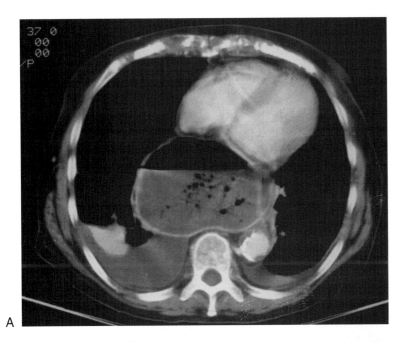

A

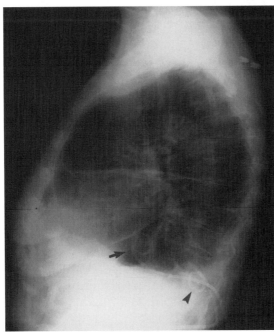

B

Figure 20.16 *Mediastinal abscess drainage. (A) CT scan showing large postoperative mediastinal abscess. The right pleural effusion provided an acoustic window and an extrapulmonary route to drain the abscess. (B) Lateral chest radiograph showing complete resolution of the mediastinal abscess following 3 days of transpleural drainage. The arrow denotes the pigtail within the mediastinal abscess, and the small arrowhead shows right pleural pigtail catheter.*

Tracheobronchial Stents

Tracheobronchial stenosis from both benign and malignant etiologies can be effectively treated with stents. The Wallstent and Gianturco stents can maintain airway caliber following dilatation of the stenosis. The stent interstices allow the epithelium to grow around the stent filaments, incorporating the stent into the wall of the tracheobronchial tree within 3 weeks. Rousseau et al. reported respiratory improvement in 89 percent of 55 patients, with a mean follow-up of 10 months for both malignant and benign stenosis. Complete epithelialization and stent incorporation occur by 6 months. The stents are well tolerated, with little foreign body sensation and few complications.

Indications are nonoperable tracheobronchial stenosis secondary to tumor compression, postoperative strictures, tracheomalacia, and postintubation granulomas. The endoluminal stents are well suited for long strictures (> 6 cm). The lesions are initially evaluated with bronchoscopy to determine the site, etiology, and length of the stricture. CT scanning is used to determine the caliber of the airway and the length of the lesion. Stenosis with active inflammation are treated with other means until the inflammation subsides. Stents are placed with either a combination of bronchoscopy and fluoroscopy for tracheal lesions or fluoroscopy for bronchial lesions. Conscious sedation with or without intubation is necessary for patient comfort. The stricture is outlined by contrast opacification. Strictures are dilated and the stent deployed using routine fluoroscopic techniques. In general, the Wallstent is preferred because of the device's flexibility, durability, and rapid re-epithelialization.

Esophageal Stents

The Celestin plastic endoprosthesis has been widely used to palliate malignant esophageal strictures since 1959. Self-expanding metallic prostheses offer the alternative features of ease of placement with adequate expansile force and low procedural morbidity. The stricture is defined by an esophogram and a stent of appropriate diameter and length chosen. The Wallstent is available in diameters up to 30 mm and lengths of 9 cm. The patient is consciously sedated and the stricture crossed with a stiff guidewire. The stricture is predilated to 12 to 15 mm in diameter. The Wallstent is placed across the stricture and deployed. The stent is dilated if necessary. The patient is placed on a soft diet. An esophogram or endoscopy is used to assess position and expansion of the stent. Once the stent is fully expanded, a regular diet can be resumed.

Percutaneous Balloon Pericardiotomy

Percutaneous balloon pericardiotomy involves the use of percutaneous balloon dilatation to create a pericardial window into the pleural space. Indications are for the treatment of symptomatic pericardial effusions secondary to malignant or benign etiologies. It is becoming the preferred treatment modality for symptomatic malignant pericardial effusions.

Review of the first 50 cases demonstrated success in 46 of 50 patients, with a mean follow-up period of 3.6 months. Two patients required an early operation, and one patient developed bleeding from a pericardial vessel. These were the only major complications. Minor complications included fever and persistent pleural effusion secondary to the drainage of the pericardium into the pleural space.

A pigtail catheter is placed within the pericardial space using ultrasound and fluoroscopic guidance. Seldinger technique is used to place an 8 French pigtail catheter into the pericardial space. The electrocardiogram is monitored carefully. The malignant pleural effusion is gravity drained. A pericardial window is indicated when there is greater than 50 ml/day output after 3 or more days of drainage. The technique starts with a contrast pericardiogram. A small amount of contrast is injected into the pericardial space to outline the parietal pericardium. Two guidewires are placed into the pericardial space. A 15 mm balloon is inflated across the parietal pericardium over the working guidewire, creating a hole into the left pleural space. This hole empties the fluid from the pericardial sac into the left pleural space where it is subsequently reabsorbed (Fig. 20.17). The drainage of contrast through

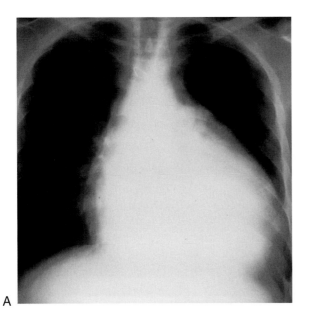

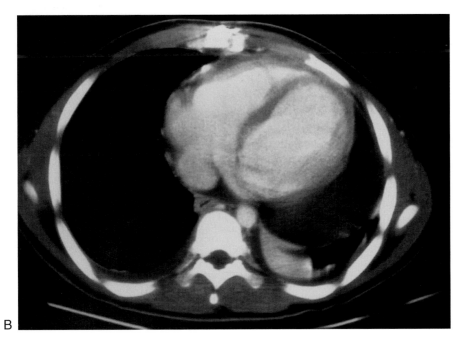

Figure 20.17 *Percutaneous balloon pericar-diotomy.* **(A)** *Chest radiograph showing enlarged cardiac silhouette from pericardial effusion.* **(B)** *CT scan showing large benign pericardial effusion. (Figure continues.)*

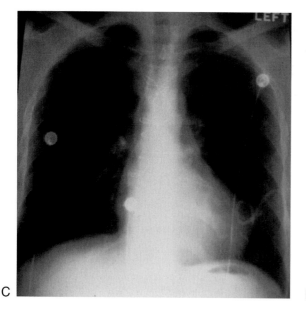

C

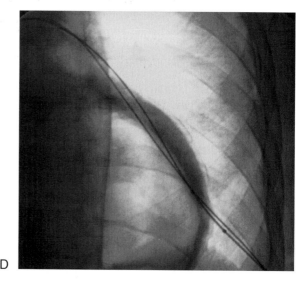

D

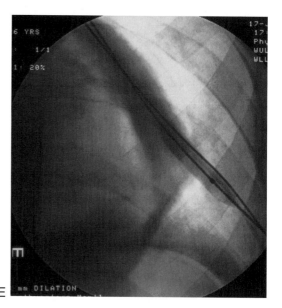

E

Figure 20.17 *(Continued)* *(C) Ultrasound guidance was used to puncture the pericardial effusion from an anterior intercostal approach. The pericardial effusion did not resolve following conservative trial of drainage. (D) A contrast pericardiogram was used to delineate the pericardial space. Two stiff guidewires were placed into the pericardial space. A balloon catheter is positioned across the parietal pericardium over the working guidewire. (E) An 8 mm dilatation of the parietal pericardium is performed to allow internal pleural drainage of the pericardial fluid. The pericardiotomy was subsequently dilated to 15 mm in diameter. The contrast in the pericardial sac is then emptied into the left pleural space.*

the window estimates the effectiveness of the internal drainage. Contrast should readily empty into the left pleural space from the pericardial sac. A second pericardial window can be performed if the fluid within the pericardial space does not adequately drain. If there is good internal drainage, the dilatation apparatus is removed, and the patient is followed-up by serial echocardiography. If the drainage is marginal, the pigtail is left in place and clamped to test the adequacy of the internal window drainage while preserving access.

Suggested Readings

Braun MA, Aronson BA, Nemcek AA Jr, Vogelzang RL: Intracavitary fibrinolysis: effective treatment for empyema and hemothorax. The 79th Scientific Assembly and Annual Meeting of the Radiologic Society of North America. Chicago, November 28–December 3, 1993

Braun MA, Nemcek AA Jr, Vogelzang RL: Drainage and sclerotherapy of malignant pleural effusions with image-guided chest catheters. The 20th Annual Scientific Meeting of the Society of Cardiovascular and Interventional Radiology. Fort Lauderdale, March 25–30, 1995

Cwikiel W: Esophageal stenting. p.134. In Cope C (ed): Current Techniques in Interventional Radiology. 2nd Ed. Current Medicine, Philadelphia, 1995

Ha HK, Kang MW, Park JM et al: Lung abscess: percutaneous catheter therapy. Acta Radiol 34: 362, 1993

Kam AC, O'Brien M, Kam PC: Pleural drainage systems. Anaesthesia 48:154, 1993

Klein JS, Schultz S, Heffner JE: Interventional radiology of the chest; image-guided percutaneous drainage of pleural effusions, lung abscess, and pneumothorax. AJR 164: 581, 1995

Lahorra JM, Haaga JR, Stellato T et al: Safety of intracavitary urokinase with percutaneous abscess drainage. AJR 160: 171, 1993

Lee KS, Im JG, Kim YH et al: Treatment of thoracic multiloculated empyemas with intracavitary urokinase: a prospective study. Radiology 179:771, 1991

Light RW: Pleural Diseases. 3rd Ed. Williams & Wilkins, Baltimore, 1995

Morrison MC, Mueller PR, Lee MJ et al: Sclerotherapy of malignant pleural effusion through sonographically placed small-bore catheters. AJR 158:41, 1992

Moulton JS, Moor PT, Mencini RA: Treatment of loculated pleural effusions with transcatheter intracavitary urokinase. AJR 153: 941, 1989

Patz EF Jr, McAdams HP, Goodman PC et al: Ambulatory sclerotherapy for malignant pleural effusions. Radiology 199:133, 1996

Rousseau H, Dahan M, Lauque D et al: Self-expandable prostheses in the tracheobronchial tree. Radiology 188:199, 1993

Samelson SL, Goldberg EM, Ferguson MK: The thoracic vent: clinical experience with a new device for treating simple pneumothorax. Chest 100: 880, 1991

Tarver RD, Conces DL: Chest intervention: drainage and biopsies. p. 1357. In Castaneda-Zuniga WR (ed): Interventional Radiology. 2nd Ed. Vol. 2. Williams & Wilkins, Baltimore, 1992

van Sonnenberg E, D'Agostino HB, Casola G et al: Lung abscess: CT-guided drainage. Radiology 178:347, 1991

Ziskind AA, Pearce AC, Lemmon CC: Percutaneous balloon pericardiotomy for the treatment of cardiac tamponade and large pericardial effusions: description of technique and report of the first 50 cases. J Am Coll Cardiol 21:1, 1993

Biliary Drainage MICHAEL A. BRAUN
ROBERT L. VOGELZANG

The treatment of obstructive jaundice continues to evolve as advances in surgical, endoscopic, and radiologic techniques provide new options for therapy. Diagnostic percutaneous transhepatic cholangiography has been largely replaced by cross-sectional imaging modalities and endoscopic retrograde cholangiography. It is reserved for cases not amenable to the less invasive techniques and for planning percutaneous treatments. Similarly, the Burhenne technique for removing retained biliary stones has been superseded by endoscopic papillotomy and stone retrieval. However, percutaneous biliary procedures are useful in a wide variety of diagnostic and therapeutic roles (Fig. 21.1).

Percutaneous Transhepatic Cholangiography

Biliary obstruction is initially diagnosed by cross-sectional imaging studies. Percutaneous transhepatic cholangiography is reserved for more accurate mapping of the biliary obstruction and as a prelude to percutaneous drainage. The noninvasive studies are reviewed to plan the approach based on the anticipated level of obstruction. Knowledge of biliary ductal anatomy is important because variation is common. The right lobe of the liver is drained by the posterior and anterior segmental ducts, which form the right main bile duct. The left main bile duct is formed by the medial and lateral segmental ducts. The left main bile duct is longer and slightly larger than the right. Two common variations are the right posterior duct emptying into the main left bile duct and a trifurcation of the main left, right posterior, and right anterior ducts to form the common hepatic duct.

Cholangiography can be performed in many ways. Examples are endoscopic, T-tube, transhepatic, and cholecystic. Optimal projections recommended by LaBerge are the right anterior oblique and left posterior oblique positions, which provide the clearest view of the hilar confluence and use gravity to maximally fill the intrahepatic bile ducts. In patients with obstructive jaundice undergoing cholangiography, we initially perform biliary drainage and delay definitive cholangiography until the obstruction is relieved and the hemobilia resolves. This minimizes septic complications and provides a "cleaner" appearing cholangiogram. The technique of percutaneous cholangiography is similar to biliary drainage and will be described later. Findings of cholangiography are filling defects, leaks, dilatations, narrowings, or obstruction. The shape of a stenosis can predict malignant versus benign etiologies. Malignant strictures are abrupt and shouldered while benign strictures are longer and tapered in appearance. Sclerosing cholangitis predisposes to cholangiocarcinoma, requiring careful review and comparison of sequential cholangiograms. Enlarging strictures and new stenosis associated with dilatation should be biopsied.

Percutaneous biliary biopsy is an adjunct procedure to percutaneous drainage and cholangiography. The stricture can be brushed, scraped, or sampled with an atherectomy device. The brush method is the most simple. The brush catheter is passed across the stricture through the biliary drainage access. The brush is used to scrape the stenosis and then is retracted into the catheter. The catheter and brush are removed, and the brush is cut and submitted in whole to be further processed by pathology. Three specimens are obtained to ensure an adequate specimen. Alternatively, the stricture can be outlined by a cholangiogram and a fine needle aspiration biopsy performed under fluoroscopic guidance.

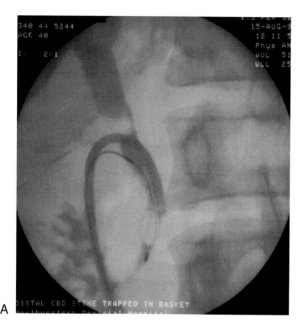

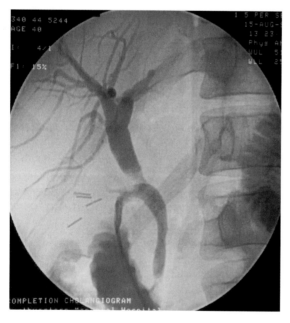

Figure 21.1 *Removal of retained common bile duct stone via a T-tube tract.* **(A)** *A Dormier basket has trapped the stone that was impacted in the distal common bile duct. The stone was then pulled out through the T-tube tract. A safety guidewire preserved access.* **(B)** *Completion cholangiogram showing successful removal of the stone. A balloon sphincteroplasty was performed to dilate the stone-induced stricture.*

Biliary Whitaker

The functional status of a stenosis within the biliary or ureteral tree can be tested by the physiologic variables of flow, volume, and pressure. The Whitaker test was originally described for use in the ureteral system (see Ch. 22). It has subsequently been used within the biliary system. The study is conducted by infusing volumes of saline and contrast into the biliary tree while measuring pressure. Normal biliary pressure is considered < 20 cm H_2O. As the pressure within the biliary tree increases, the sphincter opens and empties the system. This physiologically tests the functional significance of biliary strictures and can help guide future treatment.

The biliary Whitaker test requires a manometer and a means of infusing volumes of dilute contrast into the biliary tree above the stricture or sphincter. The manometer is connected via three-way stopcock to a needle or end-hole catheter placed within the biliary tree above the area of interest. Water is infused into the connecting tubes to eliminate any air bubbles and to zero the manometer. A baseline pressure is measured. This is normally around 5 cm H_2O pressure. Different volumes of 30 percent contrast are infused, and a measurement is obtained after each infusion. The infusion rates are 2 ml/min, 4 ml/min, and 8 ml/min for a duration of 5 minutes each. The procedure is discontinued if the patient becomes symptomatic or if the pressure exceed 30 cm H_2O. The final two infusion rates are 15 ml/min for 3 minutes and 20 ml/min for 2 minutes. The test is considered abnormal if the patient develops symptoms or the pressure exceeds 20 cm H_2O (see box).

Percutaneous Biliary Drainage

Percutaneous biliary drainage is performed for palliative decompression of malignant obstruction, for acute decompression of cholangitis and cholecystitis, and for biliary stone extractions or stricture dilatations. Safe performance of this procedure is vital. Computed tomography (CT) scans and ultrasounds of the liver should be reviewed prior to performance of the procedure. Prophylactic antibiotics are administered before

Biliary Manometry Protocol

Equipment: endhole catheter placed above area of interest, connecting tubing, three-way stopcock, water manometer, injection device

Procedure:
1. Preprocedural antibiotics
2. Zero the saline manometer at the midaxillary line
3. Measure baseline pressure
4. Infuse 30 percent contrast at following rates/durations (rate depends on type and features of injection device)

Rate	Duration
1.9 or 2.0 ml/min	5 minutes
3.8 or 4.0 ml/min	5 minutes
7.6 or 8 ml/min	5 minutes
15 ml/min	3 minutes
20 ml/min	2 minutes

5. Measure pressures at the end of each infusion.
6. Discontinue procedure if:
   a. Patient becomes symptomatic (abdominal pain, chills, nausea)
   b. Biliary pressures exceed 30 cm H_2O

Criteria:
Normal: pressure < 20 cm H_2O at baseline and at all five perfusion rates.
Borderline: minimal elevation (21 to 23 cm H_2O) at maximal infusion rate only; assess cholangiogram, biochemical data carefully; consider clinical trial.
Abnormal: pressure exceeding 20 cm H_2O at any time, or development of symptoms with infusion, with the borderline exception as above.

Note: These criteria as predictors of outcome after therapy for biliary strictures may not apply to patients with sclerosing cholangitis.

performing the procedure to prevent biliary sepsis. The biliary tree is frequently colonized in patients with biliary stones and malignant obstruction. Choice of antibiotics varies among institutions and can be modified by results of culture and sensitivity tests. Intravenous antibiotics are administered 1 hour before the drainage procedure and subsequent catheter manipulations. Pain control is important. An intercostal nerve block using the long-acting agent bupivacaine is effective regional anesthesia. The anesthetic is injected under the rib several centimeters posterior to the anticipated puncture site. One to two ribs above and below the chosen intercostal space are anesthetized. Approxi-

mately 5 ml of bupivacaine are injected under the ribs adjacent to the intercostal nerve. Generous amounts of parenteral fentanyl and midazolam (Versed) are given to provide adequate patient comfort.

There are three routes for percutaneous biliary drainage. Percutaneous cholecystostomy is used if the patient has a gallbladder and the obstruction is distal. The two transhepatic approaches are the right lateral and left subcostal. Our preferred approach to the intrahepatic biliary tree is via a peripheral bile duct in the lateral segment of the left lobe of the liver. The left subcostal approach is less painful and less likely to cause a complication involving the pleural space. A careful choice of the punctured bile duct will facilitate subsequent stages. The entry point should be a peripheral duct. This avoids the major vascular structures and provides an adequate length of central duct for placement of a stent.

There is a choice of either an 18-gauge or 21-gauge needle for bile duct puncture. The 18-gauge needle is easier to see and steer under ultrasound guidance. The 18-gauge needle accepts a 0.035 to 0.038 inch guidewire over which balloon catheters or biliary drains can be placed. The 21-gauge needle systems are used for right lateral fluoroscopic-guided biliary drainage. The 21-gauge needle accepts a 0.018 inch mandrel guidewire. There are several commercially available sets that contain a sheath/dilator/metal cannula system for converting the 0.018 inch wire to a 0.035 to 0.038 inch wire. Examples of these "one-stick" systems are the Accustick (Meditech, Watertown, MA) or the Jeffrey (Cook, Inc., Bloomington, IN). The 21-gauge needle is passed into a bile duct, and placement is confirmed by a small injection of contrast. The 0.018 inch mandrel wire is placed within the biliary tree. The sheath/dilator/metal cannula assembly is passed over the 0.018 inch guidewire into the bile duct. The metal stiffening stylet and the dilator are withdrawn. An 0.038 inch guidewire can be placed through the introducer into the biliary tree alongside the 0.018 inch metal mandrel guidewire. The larger 0.038 inch guidewire is negotiated through the central bile ducts into the duodenum, and the mandrel wire and sheath are removed. An internal/external 8 to 10 French biliary drain is then passed over the 0.038 inch guidewire into the biliary tree (Fig. 21.2).

Percutaneous cholecystostomy is the initial means of providing biliary decompression in patients who have a distal malignant biliary obstruction. A cholecys-

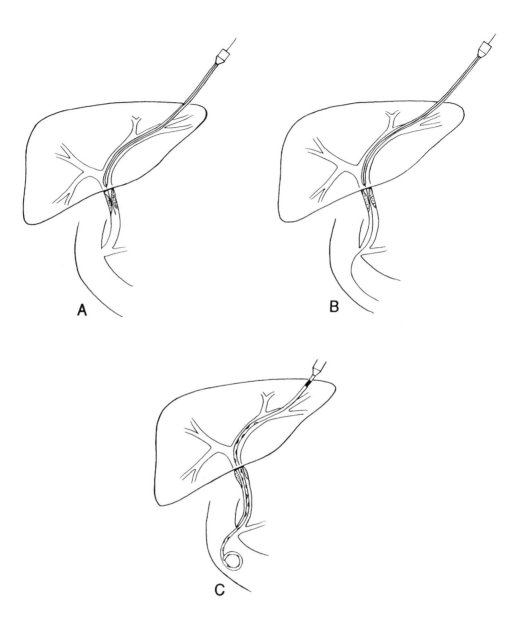

Figure 21.2 *Biliary drainage. (**A**) A steerable catheter and guidewire are used to cross the biliary stricture or obstruction. (**B**) The guidewire is advanced into the duodenum. (**C**) A multisidehole biliary drainage catheter is inserted over a stiff guidewire across the obstruction. The distal tip of the catheter is coiled in the duodenum. Contrast is injected to ensure that all the sideholes are within the biliary tree and relieve the obstruction.*

tocholangiogram can be safely performed after 24 to 72 hours of biliary drainage. This is done carefully under fluoroscopic monitoring to avoid overdistention of the biliary tree and subsequent biliary sepsis. Multiple oblique projections are obtained to optimally visualize the overlapping anatomy. The cholecystocholangiogram is used to direct puncture of a peripheral left bile duct under fluoroscopic guidance. The area near the xyphoid process is sterilely prepped and an 18-gauge needle is directed under fluoroscopic guidance toward an opacified left bile duct. The needle is advanced until it is immediately adjacent to the duct. Triangulation of the C-arm will precisely target the desired duct. A single-wall puncture of the duct facilitates subsequent guidewire passage. A double-wall puncture of the duct tends to direct the guidewire through the bile duct into the liver parenchyma. A Glidewire is used to cannulate the biliary tree and is passed into the duodenum. The tract is dilated and a sheath is placed into the biliary tree. The obstruction or stenosis is dilated with either a dilator or angioplasty balloon. A 10 to 12 French internal/external biliary drain is placed through the biliary tree into the duodenum. A completion cholangiogram is done to assess the position of the catheter drainage holes relative to the obstruction and entry tract.

Transhepatic biliary drainage is required for central biliary obstructions or in patients who have undergone a previous cholecystectomy. When there is intrahepatic biliary dilatation, we prefer an ultrasound-guided puncture of the left bile duct in a subxyphoid approach. Ultrasound is used to target and guide an 18-gauge needle into a left-sided bile duct, usually in the lateral segment of the left lobe. A small contrast injection confirms the intraductal position of the needle. A 0.035 to 0.038 inch guidewire is negotiated into the central biliary tree and preferably into the duodenum. The tract is dilated and a 10 French internal/external biliary catheter positioned across the obstructed ducts to drain both internally into the bowel and externally into a bag (Fig. 21-3). The distal loop of the catheter is formed in the duodenum and secured by the manufacturer's locking system.

The classic route for transhepatic cholangiography and drainage is the right lateral approach. The liver is observed fluoroscopically with the patient in the supine position. The puncture site is in the mid to slightly anterior axillary line. The tenth or lower intercostal space is preferred to minimize pleural complications, but higher (seventh to tenth) intercostal spaces can be used if the

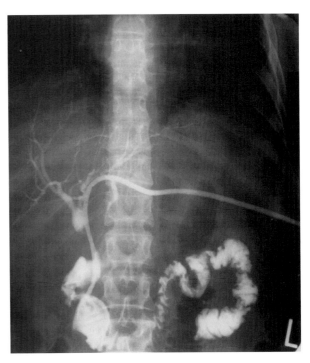

Figure 21.3 *Left biliary internal/external 10 French drain for common hepatic duct malignant obstruction.*

liver is located high under the diaphragm. A 21-gauge 15 cm needle is passed into the liver toward the twelfth vertebral body with the patient performing shallow breathing. Dilute contrast is slowly injected as the needle is withdrawn. Bile ducts are identified by central slow flow of contrast toward the porta hepatis. Hepatic and portal veins are recognized by rapid peripheral flow of contrast. Enough dilute contrast is injected to obtain a spot film to study the punctured duct and the biliary anatomy. The duct is cannulated with the 0.018 inch mandrel guidewire if it is peripheral in location and the entry angle is favorable for further placement of a drain or endoprosthesis. If the duct is unsuitable, then a second 18-gauge needle is directed into a peripheral bile duct visualized with contrast injections into the first needle. Fluoroscopic triangulation guides the duct puncture. A single wall puncture is performed by observing the bile duct wall buckle or tent inward as the needle is advanced. The duct is entered with a slight popping of the needle position. The duct is cannulated with a 0.038 inch guidewire, the tract is dilated, and the biliary catheter positioned across the obstruction.

In cases of a tortuous subcutaneous tract or abrupt angulation of the bile duct puncture site, a stiff 8.3 French Ring (Cook, Inc., Bloomington, IN) catheter can usually be advanced into the biliary tree over a 0.038 inch Superstiff guidewire (Fig. 21.4). Once the tract matures, a softer 10 French biliary catheter can be substituted over a 0.038 inch stiff guidewire. A floppy tip guidewire is used to reverse direction within the biliary tree. The guidewire is buckled in a peripheral duct to reverse direction into the central ducts (Fig. 21.5). An 11 French peel-away sheath can be used to bridge the tract and facilitate passage of the biliary catheter. The internal/external catheter is positioned in the biliary tree and the peel-away sheath removed by pulling the sheath apart and splitting the device as it is pulled out. A contrast injection confirms that the sideholes are within the ducts and adequately drain the obstructed ducts. Sometimes the biliary obstruction cannot be passed on the initial day. An overnight period of external biliary drainage is often enough to clear the hemobilia and relieve the inflammation to allow subsequent crossing of the obstruction. The obstruction is outlined with dilute contrast and probed with an angled-tip catheter and Glidewire combination. The obstruction can usually be successfully crossed with this system.

Secure catheter fixation is necessary to prevent catheter migration or dislodgement. An ostomy stoma wafer center orifice is enlarged to accommodate the catheter. The stoma wafer is threaded over the catheter and is adhered to the skin with skin fixative spray. A piece of cloth tape is looped around the catheter at the exit site to prevent kinking. A 2-0 silk suture is tied around the catheter and tape. The catheter is then attached to the stoma adhesive wafer ring by the 2-0 silk suture. There are several alternative fixation methods. A Molnar disc can be secured to the catheter exit site with the accompanying plastic tie. The Molnar disc can be sutured to the skin or a stoma wafer can be threaded over the catheter and Molnar disc attaching the system to the skin. The disadvantage of Molnar discs are the inability to inspect and clean the catheter exit site. Commercial catheter fixation devices are variants of the previously mentioned techniques. The stoma wafer requires replacement every 2 to 3 weeks. This must be done by home care, nursing, or outpatient visits to the interventional radiology department.

Biliary catheters are initially drained externally to decompress the biliary obstruction and relieve the jaundice. Bilirubin levels should fall at the rate of 1 to 2 mg/dl per day. The patient's symptoms of pruritis should resolve within a few days. The external drainage period for cholangitis is longer compared to noninfected biliary obstruction. The infected biliary

Figure 21.4 *Biliary drainage catheters. The top catheter is an 8.3 French Ring biliary drain. This is a stiff catheter with good pushability but small internal diameter. The middle catheter is a 10 French Meditech biliary drainage catheter. The bottom catheter is a Cook Incorporated biliary drainage catheter.*

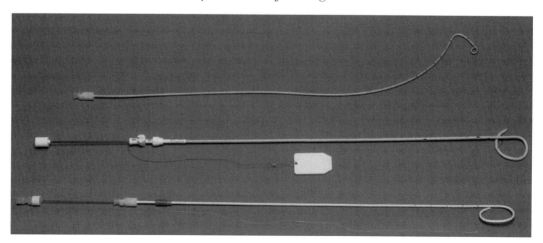

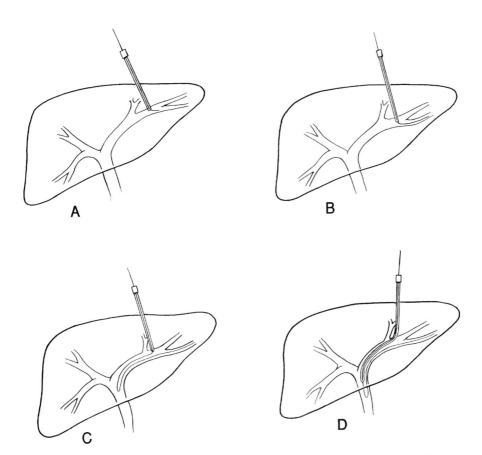

Figure 21.5 *Reversing direction using floppy guidewire. (**A**) The needle is oriented in the biliary tree to direct the wire peripherally rather than centrally. (**B**) A Bentson floppy tip guidewire is inserted through the needle or dilator into the periphery of the bile ducts. (**C**) The floppy guidewire tip buckles back upon itself and extends centrally. (**D**) The catheter is inserted over the guidewire directing it into the central ducts. This reverses the direction of the guidewire safely. It can be used for other applications when direction needs to be reversed.*

tree is externally drained until the fever, leukocytosis, and pain have resolved. Patients with sclerosing cholangitis, cholangiocarcinomas, and benign strictures are treated with long-term internal/external catheters (Fig. 21.6). Internal/external biliary catheters are capped to promote internal drainage in patients treated for prolonged periods of time. This restores the normal enterohepatic circulation of bile salts and prevents electrolyte depletion from external drainage. Biliary catheters become slowly occluded by bile salt encrustation precipitated by bacteria. This necessitates routine exchange every 2 to 4 months. The exchange can be performed on an outpatient basis but requires antibiotic prophylaxis and adequate pain control. The catheter is opened to external drainage and checked if the patient becomes febrile, develops pain, has pericatheter leakage, or if the catheter does not flush. The patient is evaluated on an urgent basis if the catheter migrates or becomes partially withdrawn.

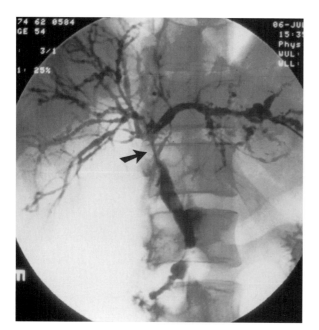

Figure 21.6 *Example of sclerosing cholangitis. Note chain-of-lakes beaded appearance of biliary tree and multiple strictures. There is a long segment stricture involving the common hepatic duct. A left biliary drainage has been performed to treat the patient's obstructive jaundice and low-grade biliary sepsis. Sclerosing cholangitis requires long-term biliary drainage, preferably with external catheters.*

Percutaneous Cholecystostomy

The indications for percutaneous cholecystostomy are cholecystitis, distal common bile duct obstruction, and gallbladder access for stone removal or dissolution. Virtually all patients referred for treatment of cholecystitis are critically ill. This group has a high rate of in-hospital mortality, ranging from 23 to 59 percent, which reflects the severity of coexistent diseases. Percutaneous drainage of the gallbladder is performed empirically in critically ill patients with fevers of unknown origin who are suspected to have acalculous cholecystitis. The response rates are reported to be 15 to 40 percent.

The gallbladder is identified under ultrasound, and a transhepatic route is chosen into the body of the gallbladder. If necessary, a transperitoneal approach to the gallbladder can be used but carries a higher incidence of bile peritonitis. The skin is prepped and draped over the proposed route into the gallbladder. Anesthesia is obtained by local infiltration with lidocaine and a bupivacaine rib block. An 18-gauge standard arterial needle is used to puncture the gallbladder under direct ultrasound guidance (Fig. 21.7). An 0.038 inch movable core J-tipped wire is advanced into the gallbladder. The movable core is partially removed to allow the wire to be coiled several times within the gallbladder. The tract is dilated and an 8 French locking pigtail catheter is placed within the body of the gallbladder (Fig. 21.8). The gallbladder is decompressed by aspirating the excess bile and fluids within it. It is important to send specimens for microbiologic analysis. The catheter is connected to a bag for gravity drainage. The catheter is secured to the skin similar to a transhepatic biliary drain.

Postoperative orders should include careful monitoring of the bile output. Initial gallbladder output should be 200 to 400 ml/day. As the biliary obstruction is

Figure 21.7 *Ultrasound demonstrating transhepatic needle passage into the lumen of the gallbladder. The tip of the needle is seen as a bright specular reflector. Note the thickening of the gallbladder and sludge within the gallbladder lumen, which are ultrasound findings of cholecystitis.*

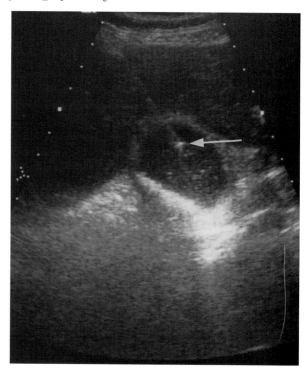

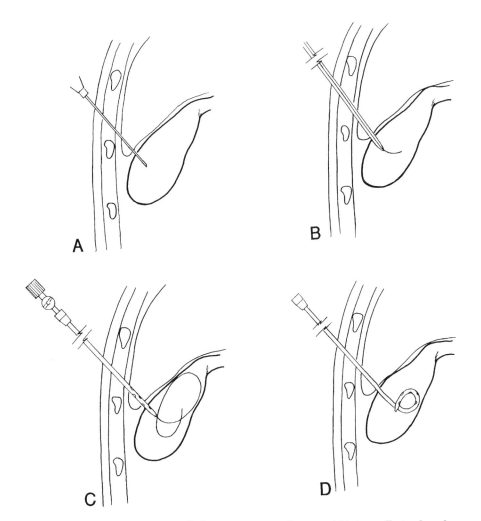

Figure 21.8 *Percutaneous cholecystostomy technique. (**A**) A needle is placed via ultrasound guidance transhepatically into the gallbladder lumen. (**B**) A wire is passed through the needle into the gallbladder. (**C**) A floppy-tipped wire is coiled within the gallbladder lumen to secure the wire position. (**D**) An 8 French pigtail catheter is passed over the wire into the gallbladder lumen. The loop of the pigtail catheter is secured with a suture-locking mechanism.*

decompressed, the output will decrease to 150 ml/day. Provocation of biliary sepsis is avoided by minimizing manipulation of the biliary tree on the first day. Cholangiography is postponed until adequate biliary decompression has occurred. Long-term external biliary drainage can cause dehydration and electrolyte depletion. This is monitored by serum electrolyte analysis.

The cholecystostomy tube can be removed for acalculus disease when the biliary tree is patent, the clinical findings are resolved, and the patient is tolerating a full diet. Normal gallbladder function can be tested by clamping the catheter and administering a fatty meal. Cholecystostomy tubes for biliary diversion for obstruction are removed only after the obstruction has been treated. In calculous disease, the catheter remains in place until the gallbladder or stones are removed. A sinogram of the cholecystostomy tract is performed before the drain is removed. The indwelling drain is removed over a wire coiled within the gallbladder. An 8 French vascular sheath is advanced into the gallbladder. Through the sideport of the vascular sheath, contrast is injected as the sheath is withdrawn along the tract between the gallbladder and the skin. This is done to assess for any potential leakage of bile into the peritoneal cavity once the catheter is removed. If significant extravasation into the peritoneal cavity is noted, the catheter is replaced within the gallbladder, and the tract is allowed to mature for an additional 3 to 5 days.

Biliary Endoprosthesis

Patients with malignant biliary obstruction are best treated by placement of an endoprosthesis. The advantages of an endoprosthesis compared to an external catheter are the elimination of entry site pain and skin irritation and the need for regular catheter care. The absence of an external catheter helps remove the constant reminder to the patient of his or her underlying malignancy. The main disadvantage is the limited life span (6 to 12 months) of the currently available devices; however, this life span approximates the life expectancy of patients with metastatic biliary obstruction.

The two types of endoprostheses are plastic stents and self-expanding metallic stents. Plastic endoprosthesis examples are the Carey-Coons, Ring-Kerlan, and Miller biliary stents. The stents range in size from 12 to 14 French. The larger the stent, the longer it will remain patent. The Carey-Coons stent is L shaped, while the others are straight with malecot or mushroom-type ends. On average, plastic internal biliary stents remain patent for 6 months. The stents eventually occlude either by encrustation from bile salts and bacterial adherence or overgrowth by tumor.

Metallic endoprostheses consist of the self-expanding Wallstent and the Gianturco modified Z-stent. Both stents have at least an 8 mm internal luminal diameter as compared to the 3 mm luminal diameter of the Carey-Coons endoprosthesis. The metallic stents are associated with fewer complications and remain patent slightly longer than plastic stents. Metallic stents are considerably more expensive than plastic stents and are reserved for patients with a life expectancy of greater than 6 months. Patients with Klatskin tumors or complex biliary obstructions at the level of the hilum are best treated with metallic stents. Metallic stents do not become encrusted with bile.

Definitive internal biliary drainage and endoprosthesis placement are best performed at staged intervals. The initial procedure is access into the obstructed biliary tree usually via the left bile ducts. Often, the obstruction cannot be traversed on the same day that access is obtained. An 8 French all-purpose drain is placed within the obstructed ducts and left to external overnight drainage. The temporary external drainage allows for decompression of the contaminated bile ducts, reduces the incidence of sepsis, and allows for clearing of any induced hemobilia. Following external biliary decompression, the malignant obstruction can usually be crossed with a Glidewire directed by a hockey tip-shaped catheter. The catheter is advanced across the obstruction over the Glidewire. The Glidewire is replaced with a stiff 0.038 inch guidewire for subsequent catheter manipulations. A cholangiogram is performed of the biliary tree to determine the position of the obstructing lesion. The malignant stricture is dilated with a balloon catheter or coaxial dilator to facilitate placement of a biliary endoprosthesis. The location and length of the obstruction determine the type of endoprosthesis (Fig. 21.9).

The plastic endoprosthesis is deployed over a 7 French stiffening cannula with an accompanying pushing device. The track is dilated with rigid coaxial dilators and the malignant biliary obstruction dilated with a high pressure angioplasty balloon. The endoprosthesis, stiffening cannula, and pusher are inserted over the guidewire and advanced as a unit into appropriate position. A peel-away sheath with a luminal diameter large enough to accept the endoprosthesis may be necessary to facilitate placement. The stiffening cannula is removed and contrast injected through the pusher to ensure adequate placement. We do not use the subcutaneous button but use the anchor suture to aid in positioning the stent. An external drainage catheter is placed overnight to allow external biliary diversion and preserve access. After 1 or 2 days of external biliary drainage, a cholangiogram is performed to document patency and position of the stent before removing the external access catheter. The external catheter is removed over a guidewire and the tract observed for bleeding.

Metallic endoprostheses combine the advantages of a small tract through the liver and a large lumen once deployed. The Gianturco Z-stent is preferred for benign biliary strictures, and the Wallstent is preferred for malignant disease. The Wallstent is a woven mesh of stainless steel available in a wide variety of diameters (8 to 12 mm). It is resistant to tumor ingrowth

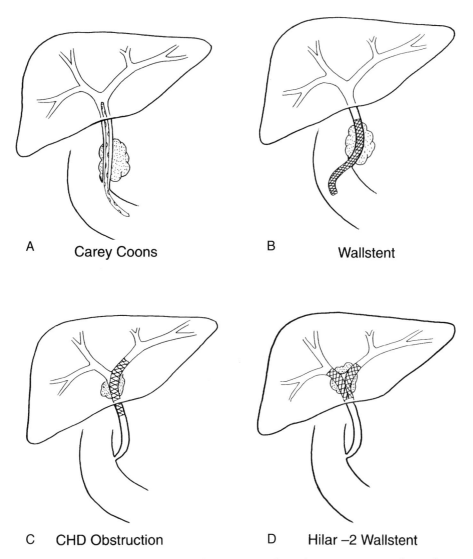

A   Carey Coons

B   Wallstent

C   CHD Obstruction

D   Hilar –2 Wallstent

Figure 21.9 *Biliary endoprostheses. (**A**) L-shaped Carey-Coons endoprothesis placed across distal biliary obstruction. (**B**) Wallstent in distal biliary obstruction extending into duodenum. (**C**) Left-sided Wallstent for common hepatic duct obstruction. (**D**) Bilateral Wallstent for Klatskin tumor of biliary hilum.*

and encrustation. The Wallstent is held contracted around a 7 French introducer catheter by a retractable sheath. The introducer catheter is positioned across the lesion. This is facilitated by radio-opaque marker bands situated adjacent to the ends of the contracted stent. The length of the stent shortens as the stent is expanded. The Wallstent self-expands but can be dilated with angioplasty balloons. The Gianturco Z-stent is formed by a zig-zag cylinder of wires. It is deployed

by collapsing the stent and pushing it through a sheath. Multiple and complex biliary obstructions are best treated with metal stents. Klatskin lesions can be stented by placing both right- and left-sided Wall-stents from a bilateral approach (Fig. 21.10). Alternatively, a left-sided Wallstent can be placed and Gianturco modified Z-stents can be placed within the orifices of right-sided bile ducts from a single left bile duct approach (Fig. 21.11).

Figure 21.10 *(**A**) Cholangiocellular carcinoma caused new obstruction of the right-sided bile ducts and low-grade biliary sepsis. Note the Wallstent in the left-sided bile ducts. (**B**) Cholangiogram through internal/external right biliary catheter. The biliary catheter bridges the obstruction of the right main hepatic duct. (**C**) A Wallstent has been placed across the dilated right hepatic duct obstruction. This has rebuilt the biliary hilum with side-by-side Wallstents.*

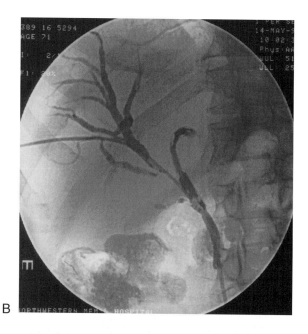

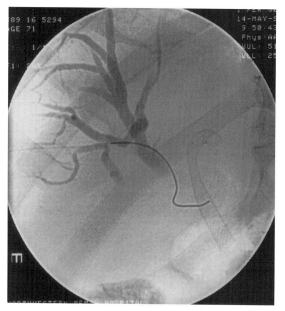

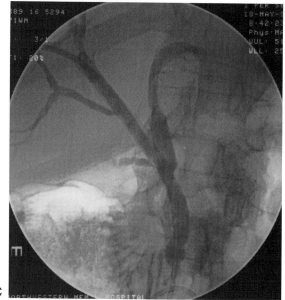

Benign Bile Duct Strictures

The types of benign strictures are postoperative, inflammatory, and traumatic. Postoperative etiologies include cholecystectomy, common bile duct (CBD) exploration, liver transplantation, and biliary enteric anastomosis. Inflammatory etiologies include pancre-

atitis, primary sclerosing cholangitis, biliary stones, infections, and sphincter of Oddi stenosis. Trauma is an uncommon etiology. Left untreated, a stricture can lead to cirrhosis as soon as 2 years.

The management of benign biliary strictures includes surgical revision, endoscopic retrograde cholangiopancreatography (ERCP) dilatation/stenting, and transhepatic dilatation/stenting. Internal/external drains

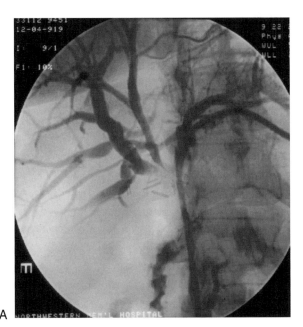 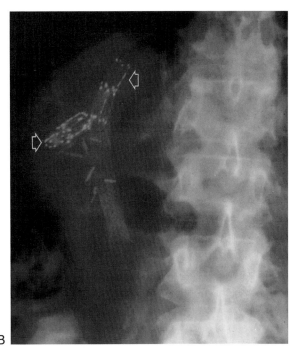

Figure 21.11 **(A)** *Klatskin tumor initially treated with left biliary internal/ external stenting. Note the tapered narrowing of the right posterior and anterior bile ducts.* **(B)** *Gianturco Z-stents were inserted into the dilated stenoses in the origins of the right anterior and posterior bile ducts from the left access (arrows). A Wallstent was then used to bridge the left hepatic duct across the common hepatic duct obstruction into the distal common bile duct.*

are preferred when treating benign strictures due to the limited patency of endoprosthesis (6 to 9 months) compared with the long-term life expectancy of these patients. An exception is the use of Gianturco stents in biliary enteric strictures. The combination of good radial expansion forces and a small amount of metal allows incorporation of the stent into the endothelial lining of the wall with minimal scar reaction. Sclerosing cholangitis is treated by long-term internal/external stenting. Stent exchanges are performed at 3-month intervals. A biliary U-tube facilitates stent exchange by providing control of both ends of the exchange wire. U-tubes are usually created by a surgical biliary enteric anastomosis that is externalized through the skin. A 10 French silicon rubber multisidehole drain tubing is used for U-tubes.

Bile leaks occur infrequently after biliary surgery. Diagnosis is by radionuclide scan, cross-sectional imaging, or ERCP. Bile leaks are treated by drainage of the biloma and diversion of bile. Bile leaks postlaparoscopic cholecystectomy are usually due to incomplete clipping of the cystic duct.

Biliary complications of liver transplantation are obstruction and bile leakage. T-tube cholangiography is performed frequently after liver transplantation due to the variable and nonspecific presentation of biliary problems. The preferred method of biliary reconstruction is an end-to-end anastomosis of the recipient and donor common bile ducts (choledochocholedochostomy) over a T-tube. The T-tube is left in place for 3 months. A liver transplantation T-tube cholangiogram is performed by slow gravity drip infusion of dilute contrast. Biliary manometry is initially performed, and the contrast study is done if the opening pressure is < 20 cm H_2O. Bile leaks occur within the first few weeks post-transplantation. Prolonged drainage and sphincterotomy are common treatments. Biliary strictures are either anastomotic or nonanastomotic. Nonanastomotic strictures are usually multiple and are located within the intrahepatic bile ducts. Proposed etiologies are ischemia, cytomegalovirus infection, rejection, and cold ischemia. These strictures form within 3 months and are treated by dilatation and stenting with modest results. Anastomotic strictures are technical in nature and develop later in the post-transplantation course (3 to 24 months).

Suggested Readings

Adams AN: Metallic biliary endoprostheses. Cardiovasc Interv Radiol 17:127, 1994

Castaneda-Zuniga WR, Irving JD, Herrera MA et al: Biliary tract intervention. p.1053. In Castaneda-Zuniga WR, Tadavarthy SM (eds): Interventional Radiology. Vol. 2. 2nd Ed. Williams & Wilkins, Baltimore, 1992

Gordon RL, Ring EJ, LaBerge JM, Doherty MM: Malignant biliary obstruction: treatment with expandable metallic stents—follow-up of 50 consecutive cases. Radiology 182:697, 1992

LaBerge JM, Venbrux AC (eds): Biliary Interventions. Society Cardiovascular and Interventional Radiology, Fairfax, VA, 1995

Lee MJ, Saini S, Brink JA et al: Treatment of critically ill patients with sepsis of unknown cause: value of percutaneous cholecystostomy. AJR 156:1163, 1991

Lo LD, Vogelzang RL, Braun MA, Nemcek AA Jr: Percutaneous cholecystostomy for the diagnosis and treatment of acute calculus and acalculus cholecystitis. J Vasc Interv Radiol 6:629, 1995

McDonald V, Matalon TAS, Patel SK et al: Biliary strictures in hepatic transplantation. J Vasc Interv Radiol 2:533, 1991

Picus D, Burns MA, Hicks ME et al: Percutaneous management of persistently immature cholecystostomy tracts. J Vasc Interv Radiol 4:97, 1993

Picus D, Hicks ME, Darcy MD et al: Percutaneous cholecystolithotomy: an analysis of results and complications in 58 consecutive patients. Radiology 183:779, 1992

Rossi P, Bezzi M, Salvatori FM et al: Recurrent benign biliary strictures: management with self-expanding metallic stents. Radiology 175:661, 1990

Salomonowitz EK, Antonucci F, Heer M et al: Biliary obstruction: treatment with self-expanding metal prostheses. J Vasc Interv Radiol 3:365, 1992

Stokes KR, Clouse ME: Biliary duct stones: percutaneous transhepatic removal. Cardiovasc Interv Radiol 13:240, 1990

Teplick SK, Harshfield DL, Brandon JC et al: Percutaneous cholecystostomy in critically ill patients. Gastrointest Radiol 16:154, 1991

Trerotola SO, Savader SJ, Lund GB et al: Biliary tract complications following laparoscopic cholecystectomy: imaging and intervention. Radiology 184:195, 1992

van Sonnenberg E, Ferruci JT, Mueller PR et al: Biliary pressure: manometric and perfusion studies at percutaneous transhepatic cholangiography and percutaneous biliary drainage. Radiology 148:41, 1983

Vogelzang RL, Nemcek AA: Percutaneous cholecystostomy: diagnostic and therapeutic efficacy. Radiology 168:29, 1988

Genitourinary Drainage MICHAEL A. BRAUN

Percutaneous Nephrostomy Drainage

The cooperative efforts of radiologists and urologists are required for removal of intrarenal calculi, dilatation of strictures, diversion of urine, and stenting of ureteral leaks. Percutaneous techniques are called on when the retrograde approach fails or is not feasible, as in patients undergoing renal transplantation. The percutaneous access can be used to place ureteral stents or dilated to perform endoscopic stone removal or endopyelotomy. Percutaneous nephrostomy is the preferred treatment for decompression of an infected and obstructed urinary tract. Other indications for percutaneous nephrostomy are the relief of urinary tract obstruction, diversion of urine to heal leaks, urinomas, fistula, and diagnosis and evaluation urinary tract pathology.

The goals of treatment, laboratory studies, and prior radiologic studies are reviewed to plan the procedure. An uncorrectable bleeding diathesis is the only contraindication. Correctable bleeding problems and electrolyte imbalances from renal failure should be addressed before the procedure. Antibiotics should be initiated before attempted percutaneous nephrostomy, especially in patients with stones and infections. Culture-directed antibiotics are preferred. Percutaneous nephrostomy as access for endourologic procedures requires careful planning. The calyx chosen for puncture must provide optimal access for the subsequent procedure. Radiographic studies are reviewed to plan the approach into the collecting system and to choose the imaging guidance method. The position of any intervening organs (spleen or colon) are noted. Anesthesia is by semiconscious sedation and local infiltrative analgesia.

The patient is placed in the prone position. The posterolateral approach aligns the needle passage parallel to the vasculature of the kidney, minimizing bleeding complications. A subcostal approach is preferred, especially when subsequent dilatation for endoscopic surgery is planned. The ideal approach is end on into the middle of a posterior calyx of the middle or renal lower pole (Fig. 22.1). Puncture of the renal infundibula or pelvis is avoided because there is a higher risk of vascular injury. All nephrostomy catheters should traverse the renal parenchyma before entering the collecting system. The parenchyma provides a secure seal around the catheter.

Imaging guidance is by ultrasound, fluoroscopy, or, rarely, computed tomography (CT) scan. Ultrasound is preferred in obstructed and dilated collecting systems and can be used in the majority of the cases. Ultrasound guidance allows continuous monitoring and guiding of the needle tip relative to the targeted calyx. Visualization by ultrasound avoids adjacent and possibly overlapping organs. Ultrasound technique is limited in obese individuals and in precise puncturing of the middle of a calyx for stone removal. Fluoroscopy can be used in conjunction with intravenous contrast injection, blind landmark puncture, or puncture onto a renal calculus.

The collecting system can be punctured with a 21-gauge or an 18-gauge trocar stylet needle. The 18-gauge needle is readily directable and better visualized under ultrasound using standard biopsy guidance technique. Another advantage is that 18-gauge needles accept 0.038 inch stiff or torquable guidewires. The 21-gauge systems are used when performing fluoroscopic guidance. The collecting system can be targeted by a stone in a calyx or intravenous contrast material injection. Traditional double-stick technique is 21- to 22-gauge puncture of the renal pelvis identified by urine return or small contrast injections (Fig. 22.2). A contrast pyelogram directs second needle puncture of the desired posterior calyx. Air can be injected to aid in identification of the anterior or posterior position of the calyces. The 21-gauge needle accepts a 0.018 inch

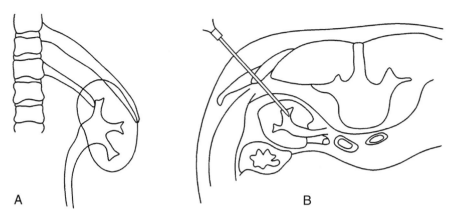

A   B

Figure 22.1 *(**A**) Prone view of relationship between ribs and renal collecting system. A subcostal approach is preferred and is usually feasible into the middle and lower pole calyces. (**B**) Transverse view showing optimum plane for accessing the posterior calyx of the middle or inferior pole collecting system.*

Figure 22.2 *(**A**) Two-needle fluoroscopic nephrostomy technique. Initial needle placed into renal pelvis to opacify collecting system. (**B**) An 18-gauge needle is directed into desired calyx via opacification with a 21-gauge pyelogram needle. (**C**) Ultrasound guidance using biopsy guide technique. (**D**) Renal calculus used as fluoroscopic landmark to guide calyceal puncture. (**E**) The tract into the kidney is dilated over a guidewire placed within the collecting system. (**F**) An 8 to 10 French nephrostomy catheter is coiled within the renal pelvis. (Modified from Elyaderani MK, Kandzari SJ, Castaneda WR, Lange PH: Invasive Uroradiology: A Manual of Diagnostic and Therapeutic Techniques. DC Heath, Lexington, MA, 1984, with permission.)*

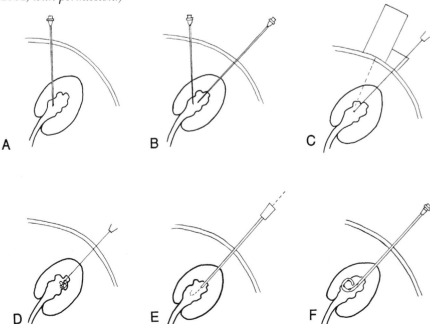

A   B   C

D   E   F

mandrel guidewire, which is advanced into the renal pelvis or ureter. A metal cannula/dilator/sheath system is passed over the mandrel wire into the collecting system. Several commercially available products are based on this system designed by Cope. The stiff metal cannula does not make bends and is intended to prevent buckling in the tract. The metal cannula and dilator are removed, leaving the sheath and 0.018 inch wire in place. A return of urine reassures position in the collecting system. The 0.018 inch wire can be replaced with a 0.038 inch stiff wire, or the new 0.038 inch wire can be placed alongside the 0.018 inch mandrel wire in the Accustick system (Meditech, Watertown, MA). The 0.038 inch guidewire is coiled in the collecting system or advanced down the ureter. The tract is dilated up to 10 French in size.

A 10 French self-retaining Cope loop-type nephrostomy catheter is recommended. The self-retaining pigtail catheter is straightened out on the metal cannula. The catheter and cannula are advanced over the wire through the access tract into the renal parenchyma. The metal cannula cannot make a bend and is meant to bridge the subcutaneous tract. The catheter is fed off the cannula over the wire into the renal pelvis. The self-retaining loop is formed in the renal pelvis by pulling the retaining suture and secured by the catheter's locking mechanism. If the catheter buckles in the tract, a peel-away sheath can be used to bridge the access tract. Rarely, the guidewire will pass into the subendothelial plane. The course of the guidewire will parallel the collecting system, but the guidewire will not advance freely or coil within the pelvis. A contrast injection will demonstrate persistent staining of fascial planes or lymphatic filling. Before termination of the procedure, a gentle injection of contrast material through the nephrostomy tube is performed to confirm satisfactory position and function of the tube. An antegrade pyelogram with multiple different views is performed in patients who are going to undergo endourologic procedures to fully map out the punctured calyx and collecting system.

The nephrostomy tube is secured to the patient's skin. Several methods are available similar to attaching biliary and abscess catheters. We prefer placing a piece of tape around the catheter, which is attached to a stoma pad ring with 2-0 silk suture. Alternatively, the catheter can be sutured to the skin or have a Molnar disc attached. The Molnar disc prevents internal migration and can be further secured with a stoma pad or skin sutures. The Molnar disc does hamper skin care of the exit site. Stoma pads require renewal every 2 to 3 weeks. Samples of urine are sent for laboratory analysis. The nephrostomy catheter is connected to a drainage bag, which should allow gravity decompression of the urinary tree. Hematuria is routine for up to 72 hours after nephrostomy tube placement. A postobstructive diuresis can be anticipated following relief of the obstruction. The urine output is carefully monitored every hour and the fluid volume replaced orally or intravenously. The nephrostomy tube is removed over a guidewire under fluoroscopic control whenever a ureteral stent is present to prevent dislodgement of the ureteral stent. The self-retaining loop is freed by cutting the catheter hub off before attempting removal. Occluded nephrostomy tubes that require exchange infrequently cannot be removed over a guidewire. In these cases, a 2-0 or stronger suture is attached to the cut external end of the catheter. A peel-away sheath one size larger than the catheter is slid over the occluded nephrostomy and suture. When the sheath is in the collecting system, the occluded nephrostomy can be removed by pulling on the suture and replaced.

Ureteral Perfusion Test

The ureteral perfusion test or Whitaker test is a method to determine the functional significance of a stricture or anastomosis. The test differentiates between the upper and lower urinary tract. The test is performed through a percutaneous nephrostomy or skinny needle placed into the collecting system. Simultaneous pressures are measured in the bladder and renal pelvis using water manometers (Fig. 22.3). A baseline pressure measurement is made in the resting state with the bladder empty. This is normally less than 10 cm H_2O and is abnormal when greater than 25 cm H_2O. The collecting system is challenged with a volume of dilute contrast and pressures recorded simultaneously in the bladder and renal pelvis. The volume is infused at 5 to 10 ml/min for 10 minutes. Dilute contrast allows visualization of any strictures and monitors for distention of the collecting system. In dilated systems, a larger volume at 20 ml/min may be necessary to challenge the system. The test is repeated with a full bladder. A gradient between the renal pelvis and bladder of 15 cm H_2O or less is normal at a flow rate of 10 ml/min for 10 minutes. A gradient of 20 cm H_2O or greater is abnormal while gradients between 15 and 20 cm are equivocal. Pressures > 30 cm H_2O are best avoided to prevent overdistention of the collecting system.

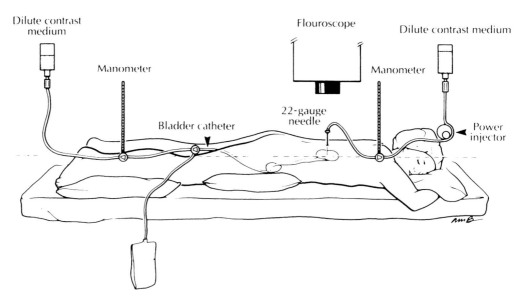

Figure 22.3 *Schematic diagram of the ureteral perfusion test. (From Dyer R: Handbook of Basic Vascular and Interventional Radiology. Churchill Livingstone, New York, 1993, with permission.)*

Ureteral Stenting

Ureteral stents are placed for the maintenance of ureteral patency in patients with stones, strictures, and obstructions. In addition, stents are placed as mechanical aids to enhance healing in patients with ureteral fistulas or perforations and following ureteral dilatations. Ureteral stents can be inserted from a percutaneous antegrade, perurethral retrograde, or transconduit retrograde approach. Percutaneous stent insertion is performed when retrograde insertion fails or is not feasible (e.g. renal transplantation). Ureteral stent placement provides the benefits of urine drainage and diversion without the inconvenience of a bag or catheter.

Percutaneous nephrostomy is initially performed, and the tract is allowed to mature and hematuria resolve before placement of a ureteral stent. An antegrade nephrostogram is helpful in planning ureteral placement. This helps direct subsequent canalization of a partially obstructed or tortuous ureter. A Glidewire and steerable catheter are used to cross the obstructed ureter. The catheter is advanced over the guidewire into the bladder. The Glidewire is removed and the ureters length measured using the double bend tech-

nique. The wire's tip is positioned just within the bladder, and the wire is bent 90 degrees to mark this point. The wire is withdrawn into the renal pelvis and bent at this point. The wire is removed and the distance between the two bends measured. A 22 or 24 cm long ureteral stent is almost always adequate in most cases. Shorter length stents are available for transplant ureters. A super stiff guidewire is placed through the catheter into the bladder. The obstruction or stricture may need dilatation before stent placement. This can be accomplished with a 5 to 8 mm angioplasty balloon.

Ureteral stents come in 8 and 10 French calibers. A 10 French size is preferred since it will require less frequent exchange. For conventional antegrade stent placement, the ureteral stent is mounted on its stiffening cannula and assembled together with a pushing device. A suture at the proximal end of the pigtails aids in the subsequent positioning of the proximal pigtail within the collecting system. The stent is passed over the super stiff guidewire so that at least 10 cm of the distal end of the stent is within the bladder. The wire and stiffening cannula are slowly withdrawn, allowing the distal pigtail to form. The proximal pigtail of the ureteral stent is positioned in the renal calyx using the suture material or pusher device. Special care must be maintained when removing the wire from the proximal end of the ureteral stent. Access to the collecting system must be preserved to allow placement of a temporary percutaneous nephrostomy. A percutaneous nephrostomy is left within the proximal collecting system to aid in temporary urinary diversion (Fig. 22.4). An antegrade pyelogram is performed before subsequent withdrawal of the percutaneous nephrostomy. This will reveal the patency and position of the ureteral stent before removing percutaneous access.

Long-term care of patients with ureteral stents is assumed by the urology service. These stents are periodically exchanged every 6 months or removed via cystoscopy. Alternatively, the bladder can be catheterized with a Foley catheter and a snare used to capture the ureteral stent within the bladder and remove it per the urethra. The wire is passed up the indwelling stent into the kidney's collecting system over which a new stent is deployed. This is readily performed in female patients but is not always feasible in male patients because of the longer length of the urethra. A second alternative is placement of a nephroureteral stent, which can be changed percutaneously when stent occlusion occurs. Nephroureteral stents are used in patients in whom retrograde stent exchange would be difficult due to bladder disease. The disadvantage of these stents is that there is an external component that requires catheter care and reminds the patient of the underlying disease process.

In patients with bowel conduits, a guidewire is passed into the ureter either through an antegrade access or through the conduit. The stent is passed in a retrograde manner with a pigtail end positioned in the renal pelvis and the other end exiting the stoma into the ostomy bag. A 7 French pigtail catheter with additional holes punched into the ureteral portion of the catheter or a retrograde ureteral stent can be used.

Renal Calculus

Percutaneous removal of symptomatic renal and rarely ureteral calculi are cooperative efforts performed by both the interventional radiologist and the urologist. The development of extracorporeal shockwave lithotripsy (ESWL) has dramatically changed the indications for and the applications of percutaneous nephrolithot-omy. Almost all ureteral stones and most renal stones can be treated with ESWL. Percutaneous stone removal methods are now reserved for patients who are not ESWL candidates or have a staghorn calculus or stone larger than 3.0 cm.

The approach for placement of a percutaneous nephrostomy for removal of calculus is similar to placement of a nephrostomy for other indications. However, the tract will subsequently be dilated to 30 French to accept the endoscope. Endourologists prefer a tract that courses under the rib cage rather than through the intercostal space. Placement of the nephrostomy through the middle of the calyx is necessary. Careful planning is necessary to choose the nephrostomy access through a calyx, which facilitates the subsequent stone extraction. Access may be required through several calyces to remove large or multiple stones within the collecting system.

Large stone burdens hamper the passing of wires through the collecting system and into the ureter. For this reason, Glidewires and Glide catheters are frequently necessary. A 7 French pigtail is used to provide a nephroureteral stent for subsequent tract dilatation and stone removal in the operating room. The nephroureteral stent facilitates subsequent guidewire manipulation within the urology suite. Tract dilatation can be by sequential passage of dilators or balloon dilatation. A 30 French sheath is passed over the inflated balloon to bridge the tract. The sheath vents the irrigation fluid and prevents a hydrothorax during an intercostal approach. Stone removal is by irrigation, basketing, grasping, and contact lithotripsy. A large Mallecot drain is left in the collecting system after the procedure.

Urinoma

A urinoma is an encapsulated collection of chronically extravasated urine. Usually these are located in the perirenal space, frequently following renal transplantation. Urinomas are best drained under ultrasound guidance. Frequent contrast sinograms are required to determine any communication with the collecting system. This may not be seen initially and becomes evident only after the inflammation subsides. Urinomas that are caused by ureteral obstructions or anastomotic

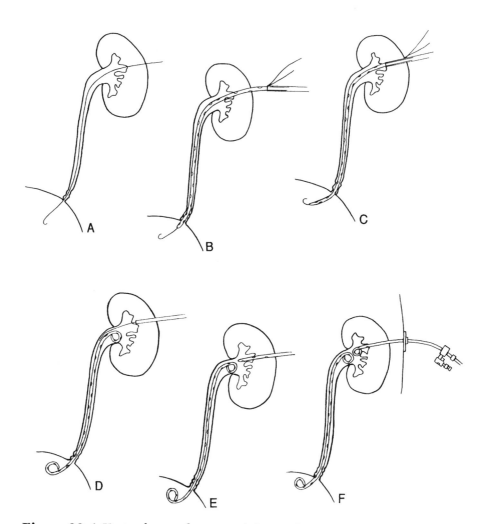

Figure 22.4 *Ureteral stent placement. (A) A guidewire is advanced through the nephrostomy tract across the distal ureteral obstruction into the bladder. (B) The ureteral stent mounted on a stiffening cannula with a pusher is advanced over the wire across the dilated ureteral obstruction. (C) The ureteral stent is placed 10 cm into the bladder. The wire is withdrawn, allowing the distal pigtail to form within the bladder. (D) The pushing device or suture is used to optimally position the proximal pigtail within the renal pelvis. Careful attention is paid to preserving access into the collecting system when removing the wire from the proximal end of the ureteral stent. (E) A new nephrostomy is advanced over the wire into the collecting system. (F) The nephrostomy catheter is coiled within the renal pelvis adjacent to the proximal ureteral stent pigtail. (Modified from Elyaderani MK, Kandzari SJ, Castaneda WR, Lange PH: Invasive Uroradiology: A Manual of Diagnostic and Therapeutic Techniques. DC Heath, Lexington, MA, 1984, with permission.)*

strictures frequently require stenting of the collecting system (Fig. 22.5). Obstructing calculi need to be removed and the ureteral strictures dilated. Ureters obstructed by malignancy require placement of a stent.

Ureteral Stricture

The age, etiology, location, and length of ureteral strictures influence the treatment. Overall, 50 percent of strictures respond to the first dilatation attempt. The low morbidity of balloon dilatation makes it a suitable alternative to surgery. Fresh strictures and traumatic strictures respond best to transluminal dilatation. Long-standing strictures and long-segment strictures respond poorly and are best treated by stenting. Malignant strictures are best treated by stenting or diversion. Four to 6

Figure 22.5 *Left pelvic renal transplant nephro-ureteral stent. The donor kidney had a duplicated collecting system joined at the renal pelvis. A urinoma formed secondary to a ureteral leak at the junction between the upper and lower pole collecting systems. The ureteral leak healed by urinary diversion through nephroureteral stents and urinoma drainage.*

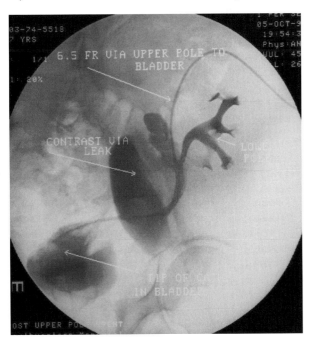

mm balloons are favored for strictures of the ureter and 6 to 10 mm balloons for ureteral pelvic junction strictures. The stricture is dilated until the waist disappears. This may require repeat inflations for several minutes per inflation. Following dilatation, a nephroureteral stent is placed for 6 to 8 weeks. The efficacy of the dilatation is assessed with nephrostograms and Whitaker tests before catheter removal.

Fallopian Tube Recanalization

Occlusion of the fallopian tubes is the most common cause of female infertility (30 to 40 percent). Etiologies of tubal obstruction are fibrosis, salpingitis isthmica nodosa, endometriosis, inflammation, intramural polyps, iatrogenic, and congenital. Selective salpingography is best at differentiating spasm and transient plugs from intrinsic lesions. The probing of the proximal fallopian tube with a small guidewire is effective in dislodging debris or breaking up fine adhesions that cause tubal occlusion and result in infertility. Patients with obstructed tubes in the proximal isthmus portions of the tube (within 3 cm of the uterine cavity) are candidates for this procedure.

Fallopian tube recanalization can be performed using fluoroscopic guidance with injection of contrast, ultrasound guidance, or by hysteroscopy. The procedure is performed during the follicular phase of the patient's menstrual cycle, which is at least 2 days after bleeding has stopped. The patient receives doxycycline, 100 mg orally, twice a day for 5 days before the procedure. A vacuum cup device, cervical balloon, or an acorn device are used to provide access into the uterine cavity. The Thurmond-Rösch Hysterocath is a typical device. A coaxial catheter system is used to engage the tubal ostium. A 9 French Teflon sheath and a 5.5 French angled-tip catheter are advanced over a 0.035 inch J guidewire. The 9 French sheath is placed in the lower third of the uterus to stabilize the system. The 5.5 French catheter is advanced through the 9 French sheath into the uterine cornu. Through the 5.5 French catheter, a Glidewire is advanced into the tube (Fig. 22.6). If the proximal tubal obstruction persists, a 0.014 inch guidewire with a platinum tip and a 3 French Teflon catheter are advanced together through the 5.5 French catheter. When the guidewire passes the obstruction, the catheter is advanced coaxially over the guidewire. Con-

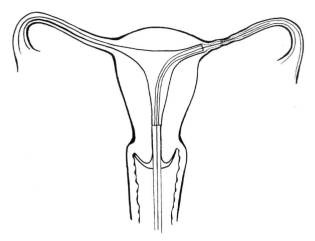

Figure 22.6 *Fallopian tube recanalization. The ostium of the left fallopian tube has been selectively catheterized. A guidewire is passed through the diseased segment of the proximal fallopian tube recanalizing the lumen.*

trast is injected through the catheter to demonstrate satisfactory recanalization and spillage into the peritoneal cavity. If the other side is blocked, the procedure is repeated in an attempt to open both tubes.

Tubal microsurgery; in vitro fertilization; and hysteroscopic, laparoscopic, and fluoroscopic procedures offer treatment options for obstructed proximal fallopian tubes. Hysterosalpingography and selective salpingography remain important diagnostic tools in the evaluation of tubal disease. The place of fluoroscopically guided fallopian tube recanalization has not yet achieved widespread acceptance within the gynecology community. The evaluation of the pregnancy rates following this treatment is difficult because of the multiplicity of causes for infertility. Technical success rates are reported to be as high as 90 percent. After successful recanalization, approximately one-third of the women conceived within 1 year, which compares favorably with but is slightly less than conception after hysteroscopic-guided recanalization. In patients who do not conceive, approximately 50 percent of the tubes reocclude within 6 months.

Suggested Readings

Banner MP: Interventional radiology in the kidney. p.35. In Mueller PR, vanSonnenberg E, Becker GJ (eds): Syllabus: A Categorical Course in Diagnostic Radiology Interventional Radiology. RSNA Publications, Oak Brook, IL, 1991

Banner MP, Amendola MA, Pollack HM: Anastomosed ureters: fluoroscopically guided transconduit retrograde catheterization. Radiology 170:45, 1989

Castaneda-Zuniga WR, Tadavarthy SM, Hunter DW et al: Interventional uroradiology. p. 777. In Castaneda-Zuniga WR, Tadavarthy SM (eds): Interventional Radiology. Vol. 2. 2nd Ed. Williams & Wilkins, Baltimore, 1992

Confino E, Risquez F: Transcervical Procedures on the Fallopian Tubes. Ex Libris, Caracas, 1994

Dyer R: Handbook of Basic Vascular and Interventional Radiology. Churchill Livingstone, New York, 1993

Elyaderani MK, Kandzari SJ, Castaneda WR, Lange PH: Invasive Uroradiology: A Manual of Diagnostic and Therapeutic Techniques. DC Heath, Lexington, MA, 1984

Lang EK: Interventional radiology of the lower urinary tract. p.49. In Mueller PR, van Sonnenberg E, Becker GJ (eds): Syllabus: A Categorical Course in Diagnostic Radiology Interventional Radiology. RSNA Publications, Oak Brook, IL, 1991

Lang EK, Glorioso LW: Antegrade transluminal dilatation of benign ureteral strictures: long-term results. AJR 150:131, 1988

Machan LS: Gynecologic interventional radiology. J Vasc Interv Radiol Suppl 7:S273, 1996

Matalon TAS, Thompson MJ, Patel SK et al: Percutaneous treatment of urine leaks in renal transplantation patients. Radiology 174:1049, 1990

Newhouse JH, Pfister RC, Hendren WH, Yoder IC: Whitaker test after pyeloplasty: establishment of normal ureteral perfusion pressures. AJR 137:223, 1981

Thurmond AS, Uchida BT, Rösch J: Device for hysterosalpingography and fallopian tube canalization. Radiology 176:283, 1990

Whitaker RH: An evaluation of 170 diagnostic pressure flow studies of the upper urinary tract. J Urol 121:602, 1979

Yedlicka JW, Aizpuru R, Hunter DW et al: Retrograde placement of internal double-J ureteral stents. AJR 156:1007, 1991

Index

Page numbers followed by *f* indicate figures; those followed by *t* indicate tables.